2-99

D1473724

UNDERSTANDING MOTOR DEVELOPMENT: INFANTS, CHILDREN, ADOLESCENTS

2nd EDITION

David L. Gallahue
Indiana University

Benchmark Press, Inc.
Indianapolis, Indiana

Library of Congress Cataloging in Publication Data:

GALLAHUE, DAVID L., 1943-

UNDERSTANDING MOTOR DEVELOPMENT: INFANTS, CHILDREN,
ADOLESCENTS
2nd Edition

Cover Design: Gary Schmitt

Art: Craig Gosling

Copy Editor: Lynne Voorhies

Manufactured By: Edwards Brothers
Ann Arbor, Michigan

Library of Congress Catalog Card number: 87-70628

ISBN: 0-936157-22-4

Printed in the United States of America
10 9 8 7

DEDICATED TO:

My Children, David Lee and Jennifer;
and my wife, Ellie.

"You Are the Sunshine of My Life."

CONTENTS

SECTION THREE: CHILDHOOD

SECTION FIVE: PROGRAMMING

Foreword

The second edition of *Understanding Motor Development* has accomplished what editors and readers expect but rarely receive from such a revision—it has made an outstanding book even better. Author David Gallahue has avoided the common temptation of delaying a revision until much of the information is dated. Rather, he has kept pace with the rapidly developing research in such areas as self-concept, movement competence, physical fitness, and curricula for young children and has included this new information in a timely second edition.

The current market in the area of motor skill acquisition during infancy, childhood, and adolescence offers the reader five or six books that I regard as accurate, comprehensive, and pertinent. I chose to endorse *Understanding Motor Development* because of author Gallahue's outstanding ability to bridge the gap between the theory and practice of movement skill acquisition in infancy and childhood. His ability to translate oft-times sterile research studies into practical applications for care-givers of infants, teachers in early childhood programs, physical educators, and those who teach infants and children with physical, mental, and perceptual handicaps is unequaled in any of the contemporary texts. David Gallahue's interpretation of research reflects his broad background as a researcher, teacher, and supervisor of teachers. The selection of content, as reflected by the extensive bibliography, focuses on the theme of *theory into practice*. The naive reader has been spared an introduction to countless references that purport to study movement skill acquisition, but in reality, do not lead to a better understanding of motor development.

A pervasive theme in each of the 22 chapters is the importance of movement to the intellectual, social, physical, and emotional development of infants and children. This book counteracts the impression held by many educators that movement skill development is a natural, continuous, and unalterable process. It identifies the variables that influence motor development and underscores the ages and stages when their effects are likely to be most profound. The reader is reminded, through numerous practical applications, of the important interaction between maturation, opportunities for practice, and experience that must take place if learners are to achieve their potential for motor prowess.

The organization of *Understanding Motor Development* will enhance the reader's ability to digest and retain its content. Section One provides the background of motor development that is essential in an introductory text. The following sections on infancy, childhood and adolescence apply the principles of Section One to the dynamic learner. Section Five translates the concepts of movement skill development into curricula and underscores the problems that currently impede our attempts to provide appropriate movement experiences for individuals from infancy through adolescence. New features that are certain to aid the reader include a list of competencies that serve as *advanced organizers*, and three categories of information, termed *Chapter Concepts, Terms to Remember*, and *Critical Readings*, that provide a summary for each chapter.

The ultimate utility of information contained in a book is the degree to which it empowers the reader to absorb and understand current concepts for the further acquisition of information. *Understanding Motor Development* enables teachers and care-givers to enter a new relationship with infants, children, and adolescents because they will now be able to observe and interpret movement from an elevated level of comprehension. The emerging emphasis in education to incorporate movement in the total educational experience of children, especially during the early childhood years, reinforces the emphasis that David Gallahue has placed on translating research into practice. The new generation of readers who assimilate the information in this second edition will be on their way to a new appreciation for the role that movement has in human well-being.

Vern Seefeldt
Michigan State University

Preface To The Second Edition

Understanding Motor Development is designed for undergraduate and graduate students taking a first course in growth and motor development. It is written in an easy-to-understand and easy-to-use manner in order for it to be of significant value to educators from a variety of disciplines including physical education, special education, early childhood education, elementary and secondary education. The text attempts to provide a descriptive profile of the individual from birth through the adolescent period with each chapter beginning with a list of Chapter Competencies. These competencies are taken directly from the *Physical Education NCATE Guidelines* (AAHPERD, 1987) for an introductory course in motor development. Chapter Competencies are followed by an introduction to the specific topic and an up-to-date researched-based discussion. The Summary and Chapter Concepts found at the end of each chapter provide the reader with a condensed overview and delineation of the major points discussed. A list of Terms To Remember is also presented for the student who desires a quick self-test on important terms used in the chapter. Furthermore, each chapter contains a wealth of tables, figures, and line drawings designed to provide the reader with a clearer understanding of the process of motor development.

Development is a process that begins at conception and continues throughout life. However, because of the still-limited knowledge base about adult development and aging, I have chosen to limit the discussion of motor development to infancy, childhood, and adolescence. Also, I have chosen to include the primary cognitive and affective factors that impact on one's motor development during these periods.

The text is divided into five sections. Section One provides background information on the study of motor development. Chapter 1, Understanding Motor Development: An Overview, examines the history, methods of study, research problems, and terminology used in the study of motor development. Chapter 2 provides a discussion of models of child development. Particular attention is given to the theoretical models of Jean Piaget, Eric Erikson, and Robert Havinghurst and their implications for motor development. In Chapter 3, Motor Development: A Theoretical Model, a systematic approach to the study of motor development is presented. The phases and stages of this lifespan model serve as the theoretical and organizational framework for the remainder of the text. Chapter 4 focuses on a variety of biological, environmental, and physical factors that affect motor development.

Section Two deals with the topic of Infancy. Chapter 5 is devoted to a wide variety of parental factors that may affect later motor development. Prenatal and infant growth is the topic of Chapter 6. Chapter 7 examines the reflexive movements and rhythmical stereotypies of the young infant with particular attention given to their integration into the expanding movement repertoire of the young child. Chapter 8 is devoted to the rudimentary movement phase of infancy. The major locomotor, manipulative and stability tasks of this period are discussed and summarized. An extensive discussion of infant perception in Chapter 9 concludes the section on infancy, and relates perception to the motor behavior of the infant.

Section Three deals with the period of Childhood. Chapter 10 provides the reader with a general overview of cognitive, affective and psychomotor characteristics during both early and later childhood. This sets the stage for the three chapters that follow. Chapter 11 examines the fundamental movement abilities of childhood. A three-stage approach (initial, elementary, mature) is utilized with mechanically correct line drawings depicting each stage. Physical Abilities of Children is the topic of Chapter 12. A review of the latest information on children's health-related fitness and motor fitness is presented along with information on fitness training for children. Perception and perceptual-motor development during childhood is the theme of Chapter 13. Important new information on both of these topics is reviewed and synthesized. Chapter 14 concludes the section on childhood with a discussion of self-concept development during childhood. The latest information on self-esteem is reviewed with a view toward movement as an important facilitator of a positive self-concept.

Section Four is devoted to Adolescence. Chapter 15 examines the topics of adolescence growth, puberty, and reproductive maturity. Chapter 16 Specialized Movement Abilities, centers on the topics of youth sport participation, fostering improvement, and the developmental sequence of specialized skills. This is followed by a discussion of the changing nature of health-related and performance-related fitness abilities during adolescence in Chapter 17. Chapter 18 concludes the section on adolescence with a discussion of the socialization process during adolescence, with particular attention given to the role of physical activity in this process.

Section Five synthesizes information from the proceeding sections and deals with the topic of Programming. Chapter 19 examines children's play, toys, and play spaces. Chapter 20 focuses on the education of children, with particular attention given to the motor development dilemma, educational programs for young children, and the interaction between learning to move and learning through movement. Chapter 21, Developmental Physical Education: A Curricular Model, may be the most important to the field professional. This chapter presents a developmental approach to the physical education program during the preschool, elementary and secondary school years. Numerous diagrams are used to synthesize the concepts presented in this chapter. Chapter 21 forms the basis for a companion text to this book: *Developmental Physical Education For Today's Elementary School Children* (Macmillian, 1987), which puts the concepts and principles dealt with here to practical use through the implementation of developmentally appropriate movement programs. Finally, Chapter 22 takes a critical look at selected motor development assessment instruments with a view to their strengths and weaknesses, and utility in a variety of settings.

As with all authors there are numerous people to thank for their many contributions both direct and indirect. With this second edition of *Understanding Motor Development* I would especially like to acknowledge the following:

> My Professional Colleagues: for their diligence, and persistence in the pursuit and acquisition of knowledge.
>
> My Graduate Students: for their enthusiasm, inquisitive minds, and dedication to personal as well as professional excellence.
>
> My Publisher and Editor: for their confidence in my abilities.
>
> My Typists: for their patience and tolerance.
>
> My Family: for their support, acceptance, and love.
>
> My God: for His constant presence and the knowledge that in Him all things are possible.

David L. Gallahue

SECTION I
BACKGROUND

**THE
HOURGLASS:**

*A Life Span Model
of
Motor Development*

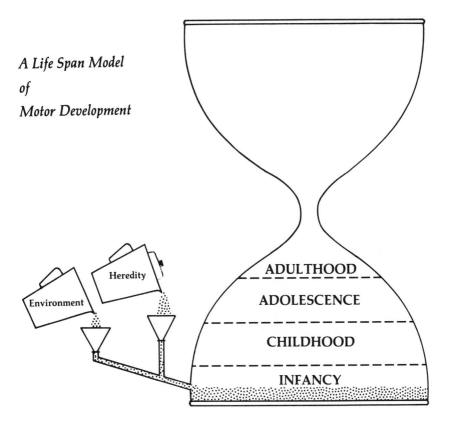

1

Understanding Motor Development: An Overview

CHAPTER COMPETENCIES

Upon Completion of This Chapter You Should Be Able To:

* *Describe the research of several historical and contemporary scholars in motor development.*

* *Compare and contrast motor development with other study in human movement (motor learning, exercise physiology, biomechanics).*

* *Demonstrate knowledge of the various forms of ananysis that are used in the study of motor development.*

* *Discuss advantages and shortcomings of the major methodologies associated with the study of change.*

* *Identify key methods of assessing biological maturity.*

* *Define terms unique to physical growth and biological maturation.*

● *Describe common problems associated with the study of motor development.*

● *List the chronological age classifications of human development across the lifespan.*

The study of human growth and development has been of keen interest to scholars and educators for many years. Knowledge of the processes of development lies at the very core of education, whether it be in the classroom, in the gymnasium, or on the playing field. Without a

*PLEASE NOTE: The competencies marked by an asterisk at the beginning of each chapter are from "Guidelines and Standards for Undergraduate Motor Development contained in the 1987 *Physical Education NCATE Guidelines* sponsored by the National Association for Sport and Physical Education, Reston, VA: AAHPERD. Competencies marked by a dot are covered in addition to the NCATE guidelines.

sound knowledge of the developmental aspects of human behavior, one can only guess at the appropriate educational techniques and intervention procedures to use in skill development. Considerable research has been conducted and a number of texts have been written on the processes of development. Although a fair amount of research has been conducted on the developmental aspects of movement behavior, it is of considerably less scope and magnitude than the amount conducted on the cognitive and affective processes of development.

Developmental psychologists tend to be slightly interested in motor development, and only frequently as a visual indicator of cognitive functioning. Likewise the social psychologist often is interested in affective development, but only fleeting attention is given to movement and its influences on the social and emotional development of the individual. Since the primary thrust of research and study has come from the many branches of psychology, it is only natural that motor development has been viewed in terms of its potential influences on other areas of behavior and as a convenient and readily observable means of studying behavior, instead of a phenomenon worthy of study for its own sake.

The study of motor development as a specialized field is relatively new, not gaining impetus until the 1960s. Motor development cuts across the fields of exercise physiology, biomechanics, motor behavior, and motor control, as well as the fields of developmental psychology and sociology. The early and continuous work of individuals such as Helen Eckert, Anna Espenschade, Ruth Glassow, Lolas Halverson, and G. Lawrence Rarick did much to kindle interest in the study of motor development by physical education scholars. The quest for understanding progressed at a slow but steady pace into the 1960s. Then, the pace began to escalate as physical educators and psychologists shifted their focus away from achievement-oriented norms back to the study of underlying developmental processes. During the 1970s an ever-expanding body of research led by a new generation of scholars heightened interest in the study of motor development. An unprecedented amount of significant research has been conducted in the 1980s, with developmentalists from a variety of fields interfacing with motor development scholars. The study of motor development has taken its place as a legitimate area of study and research within the fields of physical education and psychology.

Unfortunately, the process of human development is often studied from a compartmentalized standpoint, which has led to a rather unbalanced view of growth and development. Development has been studied in terms of domains (cognitive, affective, psychomotor), age-related behaviors (infancy, childhood, adolescence, adulthood, middle age, old age), and from a biological or an environmental bias (Figure 1.1). It is crucial that those interested in the study of motor development not compound the errors of compartmentalization. The study of motor development

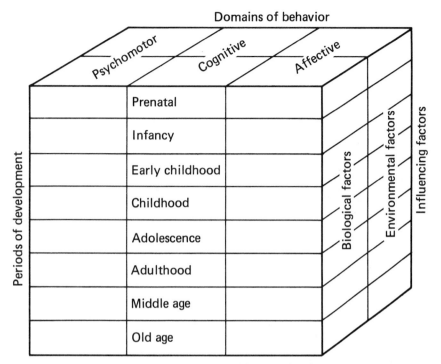

Figure 1.1. The compartmentalized view of human development

must be viewed from the perspective of the totality of humankind. It must encompass both the biological and environmental aspects of cognitive and affective behavior that impact on motor development, and it must look across various age periods of development. If it is to be of any real value to the practitioner, the study of motor development must not focus only on the skilled performer in a controlled environment, but it must instead analyze and document what individuals of all ages can do under normal and augmented circumstances. Figure 1.2 provides a schematic representation of the interrelated nature of the study of motor development.

The information contained in this book is not the "last word" on the process of physical growth and motor development, but it is the "latest word." Research and study in this area are still in their infancy in comparison to other areas of developmental study. Our knowledge base is constantly expanding.

STUDY OF THE DEVELOPMENTAL PROCESS

Development is a continuous process that begins at conception and ceases only at death. Development encompasses all aspects of human be-

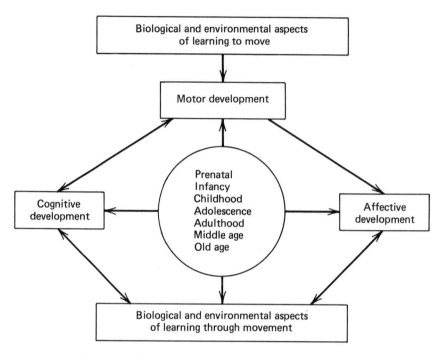

Figure 1.2. The interrelated nature of the study of motor development

havior, and as a result may only be artificially separated into domains, categories, or age periods. The growing acceptance of the concept of "life-span" development is important. Just as study of the skilled athlete during adolescence and adulthood is important, so is the study of movement during infancy, childhood, and later life. There is much to be gained by learning about motor development at all ages and by viewing it as a continuous process.

Motor development is highly specific. The once accepted notion of general motor ability has been disproved. Superior ability in one area does not guarantee similar ability in others. The outmoded concept that one either possesses or does not possess ability in movement activities has been replaced by the concept that each person has specific capabilities within each of the many performance areas.

Various factors involving movement abilities and physical abilities interact in complex ways with cognitive and affective abilities. Each of these abilities is in turn affected by a wide variety of biologically and environmentally related factors.

The process of development, and more specifically the process of motor development, should constantly remind us of the individuality of the learner. Each individual has his or her own unique timetable for the development and acquisition of movement abilities. Although our "biological clock" is rather specific when it comes to the sequence of acquisition of abilities, the rate and extent of development are individually determined. Typical age periods of development are just that: typical, and no more. Age periods represent approximate time ranges during which certain behaviors may be observed. Over-reliance on these time periods would negate the concepts of continuity, specificity, and the individuality of the developmental process.

The study of growth and motor development dates back only to the 1930s. Since then a number of methods of study have evolved, and a variety of problems have influenced both the quantity and quality of available information. The following sections briefly review the history, methods of study, and problems encountered in the study of motor development.

History

The first serious attempts at the study of motor development in children were made in the 1930s by Bayley (1935), Gesell and Thompson (1934), McGraw (1935), Shirley (1931), and others. Since their early pioneering efforts, their names have become legend in motor development research. The surge of interest their research brought about was motivated by interest in the relationship of the processes of maturation and learning to cognitive development. In their separate but remarkably similar studies, the early researchers chronicled the well-known sequences of motor development during infancy. Their naturalistic observations of children provided a great deal of information about the sequential nature of the progression of normal development from the acquisition of early rudimentary movements to mature patterns of behavior. Although the rate at which children acquired selected movement abilities varied somewhat, the investigations revealed that the sequence of acquisition was universal and invariant.

The studies of Gesell and Thompson (1929) and McGraw (1935) are classics in the use of the co-twin control method of studying development. Their research provided considerable insight into the influence of augmented and restricted practice on the acquisition of various movement abilities, and raised numerous questions concerning early practice and the acquisition of various movement abilities. The study of throwing behavior by Monica Wild (1938) marked the beginning of the study of developmental movement patterns in children. Unfortunately, after her study, which was outstanding in terms of depth and completeness, little interest was shown in the study of the various aspects of motor development for several decades. With the exceptions of the unpublished doctoral dissertation of Dorothy Deach (1951) and the continuing research of Espenschade, Rarick, and Glassow, little significant research was conducted until the early 1960s.

Since 1960 there has been a steadily growing knowledge base in the study of motor development. The work of Halverson and several of her graduate students at the University of Wisconsin on the acquisition of fundamental movement abilities did much to revive interest in children's research because of its emphasis on identifying the mechanisms behind the acquisition of skill instead of on the final skill itself. *Fundamental Motor Patterns* (1983) by Ralph Wickstrom, and the excellent research conducted by Vern Seefeldt (1972) and his associates at Michigan State University on fundamental movement did much to set the stage for the research and study now being conducted. Now, due in part to the youth sport phenomenon, and to the formation of the Motor Development Academy within the American Alliance for Health, Physical Education, Recreation, and Dance (AAHPERD), significant research is being conducted throughout North America and much of the rest of the world on the topic of motor development from infancy through adulthood.

Methods

There are two basic ways in which motor development is studied: the *longitudinal study*, and the *cross-sectional study*. Because motor development research involves the study of changes that occur in motor behavior over time, the longitudinal method of study is ideal in many ways. Longitudinal data collection attempts to explain behavior changes over time and involves charting various aspects of the individual's growth and/or motor performance for several years. The longitudinal approach allows one to observe changes over time on selected variables and, although time-consuming, permits the study of motor development as a function of maturity rather than age. The Medford Boys Growth Study conducted by H. Harrison Clarke (1971) from 1956 to 1968 is one of the most complete longitudinal studies of growth ever carried out. The motor development study begun in 1966 by Vern Seefeldt at Michigan State University and carried on today by John Haubenstricker and Crystal Branta (1987) has collected extensive anthropometric data and film footage on children performing selected fundamental movement skill. Both are fine examples of longitudinal studies of growth and motor development.

It easily can be seen that the longitudinal method of data collection is very time-consuming. The drop-out rate because of children moving, illness, or disability is often great. Therefore, large numbers of children need to be tested in hopes of still having a representative sample at the end of the five- to 10-year study period. Problems in methodology and design are also likely to creep into the longitudinal study. The reliability and objectivity of changing testers over the course of the study period may cause problems in data interpretation. The potential learning effects over time from repeated performances on the measured items has also been shown to be a difficult variable to deal with (Beumen et al., 1980). Because of these difficulties, many researchers have opted for the cross-sectional approach to studying motor development.

The cross-sectional method of study permits the researcher to collect data on different groups of people at varying age levels at the same point in time. Although this method yields only average changes in groups over time and not individual changes, the basic assumption is that random selection of subjects will provide a representative sample of the population for each age group tested. Cross-sectional studies can describe only typical behaviors at the specific ages studied. The vast majority of research on motor development uses a cross-sectional approach; it is a simpler and more direct technique. Also, it should be noted data collected from longitudinal studies, in general, do seem to substantiate the results of cross-sectional data collection studies even though the learning effects of repeated performances are still present (Wickstrom, 1983).

In recent years, development psychologists and motor development researchers have begun to look more closely at the application of both cross-sectional and longitudinal research designs. This sequential method of studying development, or *mixed-longitudinal method*, as it is often termed, combines the best aspects of the cross-sectional and longitudinal methods in that it covers all of the possible data points necessary for both describing and explaining developmental change (Schaie and Baltes, 1975).

Both longitudinal and cross-sectional methods of study may be applied in a variety of research formats. Table 1.1 provides a brief overview of these formats for studying development. An investigation may take the form of an experimental study, the most powerful method because of the rigid controls required, or it may be cross-cultural, involving naturalistic observation, surveys, interviews, case history reports, or a combination of these techniques.

Over the years there has been a shift in the study of motor development from process to product, and back to process again. The early researchers emphasized the importance of *process-oriented research*, that is, form and function. H. M. Halverson (Halverson et al., 1931; Halverson, 1937), Shirley (1931), and Wild (1938) all focused on the sequential acquisition of movement patterns. Their suggestions for studying the process of motor skill development went largely unheeded until the 1960s when interest in such study was again revived; since then, it has been a focus of motor skill development research. The use of cinematography, electro-goniometry, and electromyographic techniques in conjunction with

Table 1.1 Primary Methods of Studying Motor Development

Longitudinal study: The same subjects are studied over a 5- to 10-year period	Cross-sectional study: Different subjects representing a variety of ages are studied at the same point in time

Experimental method: Random assignment of subjects to treatment conditions. Rigid control of influencing variables

Cross-cultural: May or may not be experimental design. Comparison of various factors across different cultures

Naturalistic observation: Nonobtrusive observation of behavior in the natural environment

Survey: Group or personal interviews on a series of selected topics to reveal attitudes, opinions

Case history: Report on individual subjects providing a variety of detailed background information

computer analysis has enhanced our knowledge of the process of movement.

Product-oriented research, or research on the performance capabilities of individuals has been conducted for many years. This type of research is typically concerned with the outcome of the individual's performance. The distance a ball travels, the velocity with which it can be kicked, or how far one can jump are examples of movement performance scores. Strength, endurance, power, balance, and flexibility as measured by a particular battery of tests are examples of performance scores.

The relationship between process and product, or form ratings and performance scores, is an interesting and largely unresearched area. Wickstrom (1983, p. 6) has indicated, however, that: "There is a positive but not direct causal relationship between form and performance. Mature form enhances performance, but good performance is not totally dependent upon mature form." The factors that influence performance, such as strength, speed of movement, agility, coordination, and reaction time have an impact on performance abilities but may not influence form to any significant degree.

Problems

Data collection, whether it be product or process oriented, can be difficult when investigating infants and children. In fact, one of the chief causes of the lag in the motor development research information on infants and children has been problems associated with data collection. Infants and preschoolers tend to be difficult subjects unless procedures are adopted that take into account their natural independent natures. The two primary problems associated with good data collection are inhibited or exaggerated performance, and inconsistency in performance. Special precautions must be taken to eliminate, as far as possible, the potential bias of the data caused by these factors.

In an attempt to put the child at ease, time-consuming orientation periods, and modified data collection procedures that simulate a more naturalistic setting are frequently employed. This still will not ensure consistency in performance. For example, when asked to "throw the ball overhand as far as you can," the young child may throw first with the right hand and then just as casually begin throwing with the left. Some throws may be overhand, others sidearm or underhand, even after precise instructions as to the particular type of throw desired. Some throws may go several yards, other only a few feet. Some throws may closely approximate a mature pattern of action; others may look like a shot-put attempt or grenade-tossing exercise. As a result, the experimenter is required to exercise considerable patience and to work with the child until he or she has demonstrated what the experimenter judges to be a maximum or representative effort using the most characteristic pattern of movement. The potential problems this may cause are serious. Learning and fatigue factors may contaminate the data, as may errors in experimenter judgment.

Another problem that plagues the developmental researcher is *inter-rater reliability.* It is crucial, for example, that observational assessment be systematically analyzed and that observers be carefully trained in how to observe and in what to look for. The most serious problem facing the researcher involves the reliability and validity of the measuring instrument itself. A variety of motor development assessment devices are available. Some have been meticulously designed, while others represent a combination of measures for which there is only a vague notion as to their reliability with much less known about their validity.

However, the benefits to be gained from motor development research far outweigh the problems and pitfalls. As information gradually accumulates and is replicated, we are gaining a more accurate picture of the processes involved in motor development. Research efforts that use longitudinal and cross-sectional approaches, that focus on form and performance, and that recognize the need for patient, unbiased data collection are making significant contributions to our understanding of motor development.

AGE CLASSIFICATIONS OF DEVELOPMENT

It is interesting to note that the classification of developmental levels may be done in a variety of ways. Without a doubt the most popular, but often the least accurate method, is classification by chronological age.

Chronological age, one's age in month's and/or years, is probably the most popular technique because of its universal usage and that it represents a constant for all. By knowing one's birthdate we can easily calculate age in years, months, and days. Table 1.2 provides a conventional chronological classification of age from conception through old age. As you review this table, keep in mind that although development is age related it is not age dependent. Chronological age provides only a rough estimate of one's developmental level which may be more accurately determined through other means.

The *biological age* of an individual provides a record of his or her rate of progress toward maturity. It is a variable age that corresponds only roughly to chronological age, and may be determined by measures of: (1) morophological age, (2) skeletal age, (3) dental age, or (4) sexual age.

Morophological age is a comparison of one's attained size (height & weight) to normative standards. Normative size has been determined by Wetzel (1948) and others through exhaustive charting of heights and weights of thousands of individuals. The Wetzel Grid (1948) was used for many years by most pediatricians as the primary means of determining the morophological age of their patients. Although not used as frequently today due to secular changes in height and weight, the Wetzel Grid was at one time the most popular method of determining morophological age.

Skeletal age provides a record of the biological age of the developing skeleton. Skeletal age can be very accurately determined by x-ray of the carpel bones of the hand and wrist (Greulich and Pyle, 1959; Tanner and Whitehouse, 1975). It is, however, an infrequently used measure of biological age outside the laboratory because of cost, inconvenience, and the accumulative effects of radiation.

Dental age is another accurate, but also infrequently used, means of determining biological age. The sequence of tooth development from first appearance of the cups to root closure provides a measure of calcification age. Eruption age also may be determined by charting the progressive emergence of the teeth.

Sexual age is a fourth method of determining biological age. Sexual maturation is determined by the variable attainment of primary and secondary sexual characteristics. The Tanner pubic hair scale (Tanner, 1962) provides an accurate and easy to determine means for assessing sexual maturity. Figures 15.3-15.6 (pages 387-393) provide a description of the Tanner scales. It should be noted that although this method is an easy and quite accurate predictor of biological maturity, it is still infrequently used because of social and cultural factors. In fact, to date, only New York State requires an estimate of sexual maturity in its preparation sports physical examination (Caine and Broeknoff, 1987).

Table 1.2 Conventional Chronological Classifications of Age

PERIOD	APPROXIMATE AGE RANGE
I PRENATAL LIFE	(CONCEPTION TO BIRTH)
A. Period of the Zygote	Conception-1 week
B. Embryonic Period	2 weeks-8 weeks
C. Fetal Period	8 weeks-Birth
II INFANCY	(BIRTH TO 24 MONTHS)
A. Neonatal Period	Birth-1 month
B. Early Infancy	1-12 months
C. Later Infancy	12-24 months
III CHILDHOOD	(2 YEARS TO 10 YEARS)
A. Toddler Period	24-36 months
B. Early Childhood	3-5 years
C. Middle/Later Childhood	6-10 years
IV ADOLESCENCE	(10-20 YEARS)
A. Prepubescence	10-12 years (F)
	11-13 years (M)
B. Post Pubescence	12-20 years (F)
	14-20 years (M)
V YOUNG ADULTHOOD	(20-40 YEARS)
A. Novice Period	20-30 years
B. Settling Period	30-40 years
VI MIDDLE ADULTHOOD	(40-60 YEARS)
A. Mid Life Transition	40-45 years
B. Middle Age	45-60 years
VII OLDER ADULTHOOD	(60+ YEARS)
A. Young Old	60-70
B. Middle Old	70-80
C. Frail Old	80+

A variety of other methods of age classification exist. They include measures of: (1) emotional age, (2) mental age, (3) self-concept age, and (4) perceptual age. *Emotional age* is a measure of one's socialization and ability to function within a particular social/cultural setting. *Mental age* refers to one's mental potential as a function of both learning and intelligence. *Self-concept age* is a measure of one's perception of self and often fluctuates within one's lifetime. *Perceptual age* is an assessment of the rate and extent of one's perceptual development.

All measures of maturity are variable; they are related to chronological age, but are not dependent upon it. Therefore, care must be taken by all those dealing with people, whether they are infants, children, adolescents, or adults not to subscribe to a chronological classification of age because of its ease and convenience.

TERMINOLOGY USED IN MOTOR DEVELOPMENT

A working knowledge of the terms commonly used in any area of study is an important first step in understanding that field. Whether it is medicine or law, special education or economics, there is jargon typical to each field of study. Motor development is no exception. Over the years a variety of terms have come into common usage. These terms are presented in this section. As with the jargon in most areas of study, agreement on the meaning of each term is not universal. We must strive for greater consistency of meaning. Words have meaning, and ideally their meanings should be universal. It is with this concept in mind that the following terms are presented.

Growth and Development

The terms "growth" and "development" are often used interchangeably, but there is a difference in emphasis implied by each. In its purest sense, *physical growth* refers to an increase in the size of the body or its parts as the child progresses toward maturity. In other words, physical growth is an increase in the structure of the body brought about by the multiplication or enlargement of cells. The term "growth," however, is often used to refer to the totality of physical change. As a result, it becomes more inclusive and takes on the same meaning as development.

Development, in its purest sense, refers to changes in the individual's level of functioning. Keoph and Sugden (1985, p. 6) define development as "adaptive change toward competence." Although development is most frequently viewed as an emerging and broadening of one's ability to function on a higher level, we must recognize that the concept of development is much broader, and that it is in fact a lifelong process. The study of development is concerned with what occurs and how it occurs in the human organism in its journey from conception through maturity to death. Development is a continuous process of change that encompasses all of the interrelated dimensions of our existence, and care must be taken not to consider these dimensions as autonomous, or limited to the growing years of childhood.

The interwoven elements of maturation and experience play a key role in the developmental process. *Maturation* refers to qualitative changes that enable one to progress to higher levels of functioning. Maturation, when viewed from a biological perspective, is primarily innate; it is genetically determined and resistant to external or environmental influences. Maturation is characterized by a fixed order of progression in which the pace may vary but the sequence of appearance of characteristics generally does not. For example, the progression and approximate ages at which an infant learns to sit, stand, and walk are highly influenced by maturation. The sequence of appearance of these abilities is fixed and resistant to change with only the rate of appearance being altered by the environmental influences of learning and experience.

Experience refers to factors within the environment that may alter or modify the appearance of various developmental characteristics through the process of learning. The experiences that children are exposed to may have an effect on the rate of onset of certain patterns of behavior.

The developmental aspects of both maturation and experience are interwoven. Determining the separate contribution of each of these processes is impossible. In fact, a heated debate in the literature over the relative importance of the two has raged for well over a century. As a result, the term *adaptation* is often used to refer to the complex interplay between forces within the individual and the environment. Figure 1.3 illustrates how the factors of growth, maturation, experience, and adap-

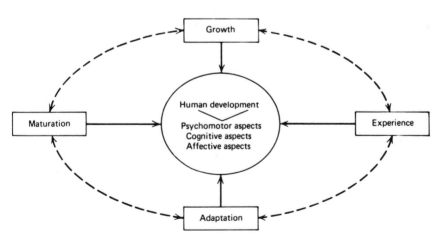

Figure 1.3. The interrelated components of human development

tation are all directly related to the developing individual and to one another.

Domains of Behavior

The classification of human responses into *domains of behavior* was first popularized by Bloom and his associates (1956) and Krathwohl et al. (1964) in their pioneering attempt to establish a taxonomy of educational objectives. Their separation of behavior into cognitive (intellectual behavior), affective (social-emotional behavior), and motor (motor behavior) domains has, unfortunately, caused many to deal with each domain as an independent entity of human development and learning. We must not lose sight of the interrelated nature of development and the three domains of human behavior even though we may tend to separate them for the sake of convenience in our discussion and study of human development.

Motor development is the process of change in motor behavior brought about by interaction between heredity and the environment. Movement may result from cognitively mediated processes in higher brain centers (motor cortex), from reflexive activity in lower brain centers, or from the central nervous system. Motor development is a lifelong process. It encompasses all physical change and the acquisition, stabilization, or diminution of motor skills. Motor development may be categorized into the development of physical abilities and the development of movement abilities. *Physical abilities*, or motor performance abilities, as they are sometimes called, are the terms used to lump the various components of health-related fitness (muscular strength, muscular endurance, aerobic endurance, flexibility, and body composition) and performance-related abilities (speed of movement, agility, coordination, balance, and power) together. Physical abilities are associated with the capacity to perform motor tasks. *Movement abilities* is a comprehensive term used to group together the three *categories of movement* (locomotion, manipulation, and stability). Thus, one may be interested in an aspect of motor development as it relates to understanding physical abilities and as it applies to the performance of a variety of movement abilities across age, gender, or social class.

Cognitive development, as applied to the study of movement behavior, involves the functional relationship between mind and body. The reciprocal interaction of mind and body has been dealt with from as far back as the philosophical musings of Socrates and Plato to the developmental theorists of the twentieth century. Jean Piaget (1952), known for his theory of cognitive development, is an example of a modern theorist who recognized the important role of movement, particularly during the early years of life. Piaget's work has done much to spread the notions of perceptual-motor development and the development of academic concept readiness through the medium of movement.

The term *perceptual-motor* has come into use in recent years to signify the important influence that sensory cues and the perceptual process have on motor activity. In its broadest sense, a perceptual-motor act is any voluntary movement that relies on sensory data to process information used in the performance of that act. All voluntary movement may be viewed as perceptual-motor in nature. Movements that are subcortically controlled (reflexes) are the only forms of movement of the skeletal muscles that do not require some element of perception.

Affective development, as related to the study of human movement, involves feelings and emotions as applied to self and others through movement. Movement confidence, perceived competence, self-esteem, peer relations, and play are areas of interest to students of motor development. *Self-esteem* may be thought of as one's personal feelings of self-worth, or worthlessness. It is influenced by a variety of factors, two of which are movement confidence and perceived physical competence (Weiss, 1987; Harter, 1981).

Peer relations refers to the level of social interaction evidenced by an individual. Play behavior has been shown to have a developmental base that manifests itself in changing peer relations and more sophisticated levels of functioning (Ellis, 1973; Coakley, 1987).

These definitions of the psychomotor, cognitive, and affective domains as they influence, and are influenced by, developmental processes permit us to clarify a variety of terms that contain the word "motor" or "movement." What follows is not an exercise in semantics. It is important that we impose similar meanings on words because subtle differences in words often make gigantic differences in the thought or concept being presented.

Motor Development

The term *motor,* when used alone, refers to the underlying biological and mechanical factors that influence movement. The term, however, is rarely used alone, but serves as a suffix or prefix to such terms as: "psychomotor," "perceptual-motor," "sensorimotor," "motor learning," "motor control," and, of course, "motor development." The terms psychomotor, perceptual-motor, and sensorimotor have gained popularity with psychologists and educators. Physical educators, however, have tended to limit use of the prefixes of these words to discussions that focus specifically on that aspect of the motor process. The term "motor" is used as a prefix to describe specific areas of study. The following is a brief description of several of these terms as they are commonly used.

Learning is defined as a relatively permanent change in behavior resulting from experience and training interacting with biological processes. Learning is shaped by the individual's state of development, and is a function of practice (Piaget, 1964). Learning is a phenomena in which experience is prerequisite, whereas development is a process that *may* occur relatively independent of experience. *Motor learning* is that aspect of learning in which movement plays a major part. *Motor behavior* is a generic term defined here as motor learning that embodies learning and performance factors and maturational processes associated with movement performance. Motor behavior research is concerned with the study of motor learning, motor control, and motor development.

Motor control is that aspect of motor learning that deals with the study of isolated tasks under specific conditions. Study in this area concentrates on the underlying processes involved in the performances of a movement act that are consistent from trial to trial.

Motor development is that aspect of motor behavior that is primarily concerned with the study of changes in movement throughout the entire life span. Rarick (1981, p. 163) defines motor development as a "specialized field of inquiry concerned with studying the origins and development of motor behavior in humans." Study of the underlying biological and environmental processes of motor development is typically viewed in stages (infancy, childhood, adolescence, adulthood, old age) that reflect the particular interest of the investigator.

The terms *motor pattern, fundamental motor pattern, motor skill*, and *perceptual-motor skill* all refer to the *underlying* sensory, integrative, and decision-making processes that precede the performance of an observable movement. Perception and cognition are important variables because they influence underlying motor processes. Underlying motor processes are involved in the performance of *all* voluntary movement.

Movement Forms

The term *movement* refers to an actual observable change in position of any part of the body. Movement is the culminating act of the underlying motor processes. The word movement is often linked with others to broaden or clarify its meaning, but in general it refers to the overt act of moving. The following is a brief description of some movement terms as they are commonly used.

A *movement pattern* as defined by Wickstrom (1983, p. 5) is "a combination of movements organized according to a particular time-space sequence." A movement pattern is an organized series of related movements. More specifically, a movement pattern represents the performance of an isolated movement that in and of itself is too restricted to be classified as a fundamental movement pattern. For example, the sidearm, underarm, or overarm patterns of movement alone do not constitute the fundamental movements of throwing or striking, but merely represent an organized series of movement. A *fundamental movement pattern*, therefore, refers to the observable performance of basic locomotor, manipulative, and stabilizing movements. Fundamental movement patterns involve the combination of movement patterns of two or more body segments. Running, jumping, striking, throwing, twisting, and turning are examples of fundamental movement patterns.

Although the terms movement pattern and movement skill are often used interchangeably a *movement skill* is viewed here as a fundamental movement pattern performed with greater accuracy, precision, and control. In a movement skill, accuracy is stressed; therefore, extraneous movement is limited. In a fundamental movement pattern, movement is stressed but accuracy is limited.

A *sport skill* is the combination of fundamental movement patterns or movement skills applied to the performance of a sport related activity. Therefore, the fundamental movement patterns of twisting the body and striking may be developed to a high degree of precision and applied in their horizontal form to batting in the sport of baseball, or in their vertical form to playing golf or serving a tennis ball. The performance of a sport skill requires making increasingly precise alterations in the basic patterns of movement as higher levels of skill are achieved.

Movement education is a term that has been defined in a variety of ways, all of which seem somewhat restrictive and shortsighted. It has been defined as a method, as a process, and as an aspect of the physical education program generally limited to children. Logsdon et al. (1985, p. 12) take a more global view of movement and define it as follows: "Movement education is a lifelong process of change. This process of motor development and learning has its beginning in the womb and proceeds through a never-ending series of changes until death." For the purpose of our discussion we will view movement education as the lifelong process of changes in movement behavior brought about by opportunities for practice, encouragement, and instruction. Input from qualified instructors, positive motivation, and reinforcement, as well as appropriate facilities and equipment, facilitate the process of movement education. However, it is not entirely restricted to these conditions nor to specific age ranges.

Gross and Fine Movements

Movement, whether it takes the form of a movement pattern or a movement skill, may be classified in a variety of ways. There is not a clear delineation between the terms *gross* and *fine*, but movements are often classified as one or the other. A *gross motor movement* involves movement of the large muscles of the body. Most sport skills are classified as gross motor movements, with the exception perhaps of target shooting, archery, and a few others. *Fine motor movements* involve limited movements of parts of the body in the performance of precise movements. The manipulative movements of sewing, writing, and typing are generally thought of as fine motor movements.

Discrete, Serial, and Continuous Movements

On the basis of its temporal aspects, movement also may be classified as discrete, serial, or continuous. A *discrete movement* has a very definite beginning and ending. Throwing, jumping, kicking, and striking a ball are examples of discrete movements. *Serial movements* involve the performance of a single, discrete movement several times in rapid succession. Rhythmical hopping, basketball dribbling, and a soccer or volleyball volley are typical serial tasks. *Continuous movements* are movements that are repeated for a specified period of time. Running, swimming, and cycling are common continuous movements.

Open and Closed Movements

Fundamental movement patterns and movement skills are often referred to as open tasks, or closed tasks (Poulton, 1957). An *open movement task* is performed in an environment where the conditions are constantly changing. These changing conditions require the individual to make adjustments or modifications in the actual pattern of movement to suit the demands of the situation. Plasticity, or flexibility, in movement is required in the performance of an open skill. Most dual and group activities involve open skills that depend on external and internal feedback for their successful execution. For example, the child taking part in a typical game of tag, requiring running and dodging in varying directions, is never using the exact same patterns of movement during the game. The child is required to adapt to the demands of the activity through a variety of similar but different movements. Performance of an open movement task differs markedly from performance of a closed movement task.

Closed movement tasks may be thought of as movements that "require a constancy of movement pattern and are performed under an unchanging environment" (Sage, 1984, p. 19). A closed movement skill, or fundamental movement pattern, demands rigidity of performance; it depends on kinesthetic, rather than visual and auditory, feedback from the execution of the task. The child who is performing a headstand, throwing at a target, or doing a vertical jump is performing a closed movement task.

You are cautioned not to be arbitrary in the classification of movement as either gross or fine; discrete, serial, or continuous; and open or closed. The vast majority of movement involves some elements of each.

Distinct separation and classification of movements is not always possible, nor is it always desirable. We are dynamic, moving beings, constantly being acted upon and interacting with many subtle environmental factors. The arbitrary classification of movement should serve only to focus attention on the specific aspect of movement under consideration. Table 1.3 provides a schematic representation and brief description of terms commonly used in the study of learning and development. You will find it useful to carefully review these terms, paying particular attention to how they interrelated. The terms motor and movement, pattern and skill, which are commonly used interchangeably, have particularly subtle differences.

Table 1.3 The Interrelated Nature of Terms Commonly Used in Motor Development

Motor behavior: Study of change in motor learning, motor control, and motor development brought about by the interaction of learning and biological processes

Motor control: Underlying changes in the performance of isolated tasks	*Motor performance*: Underlying learning and biological processes involved in motor learning

Motor development: Progressive change in motor behavior brought about by the interaction of both maturation and experience throughout the life cycle

Motor: Underlying factors affecting movement	*Movement*: The observable act of moving
Motor pattern: Common underlying biological and mechanical processes	*Movement pattern*: An organized series of related movements (e.g., a side-arm pattern)
Fundamental motor pattern: Common underlying process of basic movements	*Fundamental movement pattern*: An organized series of basic movements (e.g., striking)
Motor skill: Common underlying process of control in movement	*Movement skill*: Form, accuracy, and control in performance of a movement (e.g., striking an oncoming object or splitting wood)

Sport skill: The combination of a fundamental movement pattern with form, accuracy, and control in the performance of a sport-related activity (e.g., batting in baseball or softball)

Movement education: The lifelong process of change in movement behavior brought about by the environmental factors of opportunities for practice, encouragement and instruction (e.g., change in striking abilities over time)

SUMMARY

A cursory review of most growth and development texts and many physical education texts will reveal statements such as: "Children, youth, and adults need plenty of daily vigorous physical activity in order to develop their movement and fitness abilities." Although physical activity is an important part of one's day, this statement needs to be qualified and broadened if it is to have real meaning. We may, and generally can, find time during the course of the day to pursue vigorous physical activity. Often, however, we fail to take advantage of this time due to (1) lack of opportunities, (2) lack of encouragement, and (3) lack of qualified instruction.

The daily routines of millions have been programmed from the minute they wake up until the moment they go to sleep. Demands are constantly placed on our time; little time is left for regular participation in vigorous physical activity, unless we consciously program such activity into our daily schedule. The best way to ensure that all school age youth have the opportunity to take part in regular vigorous physical activity is through the scheduling of quality *daily* physical education at all grade levels. For adults it is a somewhat different matter. Analysis of one's daily routine and a reordering of priorities is essential if vigorous movement is to play a significant role.

For too many years it has been assumed that through maturation and lifestyle alone individuals will *automatically* develop their movement and fitness abilities. This is false. Children, youth, and adults need adequate opportunity for practice, encouragement, and instruction in a variety of daily, vigorous activities in order to develop their unique movement and physical abilities to their optimum level.

CHAPTER CONCEPTS

1.1 Interest in the study of motor development began in the 1930s, but waned until the 1960s.

1.2 The study of motor development has, until recently, been overshadowed by study of the cognitive and affective processes of development.

1.3 There has been a rapidly expanding knowledge base in motor development over the past 30 years, and it is now viewed by many as a cornerstone of the physical education profession.

1.4 Motor development research involves the use of a variety of techniques that use both longitudinal and cross-sectional research techniques.

1.5 Data collection in controlled experiments is often very difficult with young children.

1.6 Although chronological age is the most commonly used means of age classification, it is frequently the least accurate.

1.7 Motor development is age related but not age dependent.

1.8 The terminology used in motor development must be understood in order to grasp essential concepts.

1.9 There is often overlap in the terms used to describe movement; yet many subtle differences are implied.

1.10 Motor development is an important aspect of one's total development, a process which begins at conception and does not end until death.

TERMS TO REMEMBER

Longitudinal Study
Cross-Sectional Study
Mixed-Longitudinal Study
Process-Oriented Research
Product-Oriented Research
Interrater Reliability
Chronological Age
Biological Age
Morphological age
Skeletal Age
Dental Age
Sexual Age
Emotional Age
Mental Age
Self-Concept Age
Perceptual Age
Physical Growth
Development
Maturation
Experience
Adaptation
Domains of Behavior
Motor Development
Physical Abilities
Movement Abilities

Categories of Movement
Cognitive Development
Perceptual-Motor
Affective Development
Self-esteem
Peer Relations
Motor
Learning
Motor Learning
Motor Behavior
Motor Control
Movement
Movement Pattern
Fundamental Movement Pattern
Movement Skill
Sport Skill
Movement Education
Gross Motor Movement
Fine Motor Movement
Discrete Movement
Seriel Movement
Continuous Movement
Open Movement Task
Closed Movement Task

CRITICAL READINGS

Gallahue, D. L. (1989) "Motor Developmentalists—All?" *Motor Development Academy Newsletter*, 10, 1.
Haubenstricker, J. and Seefeldt, V. (1986). "Acquisition of Motor Skills During Childhood." In Seefeldt, V. (ed.). *Physical Activity and Well-Being*. Reston, VA: AAHPERD, (p. 42-46).
Keogh, J. and Sugden, D. (1985). *Movement Skill Development*. New York: Macmillian, (Chapter 1).
Lockhart, A. (1964). "What's in a Name?" *Quest*, 2, 9-13.
Magill, R. A. (1989) *Motor Learning,—Concepts and Applications*. Dubuque, IA: Wm. C. Brown, (Chapter 1).
Rarick, G. L. (1981). "The Emergence of the Study of Human Motor Development" In Brooks, G. A. (ed.) *Perspectives on the Academic Discipline of Physical Education*, Champaign, IL: Human Kinetics, (Chapter 10).
Sage, G. H. (1984). *Motor Learning and Control: A Neuropsychological Approach*. Dubuque, IA: Wm. C. Brown, (Chapter 2).
Seefeldt, V. (1989) This Is Motor Development. *Motor Development Academy Newsletter*, 10, 1.
Wickstrom, R. L. (1983). *Fundamental Motor Patterns*. Philadelphia: Lea and Febiger, (Chapter 1).

2

Models of Human Development

CHAPTER COMPETENCIES

Upon Completion of This Chapter You Should Be Able To:

* *Compare and contrast maturational, environmental and interactionist views of causation in motor development.*

* *Discuss changes in cognitive processing across the life span.*

* *Describe variations in cognitive processing mechanisms within an age group.*

• *Demonstrate familiarity with a variety of theoretical models of human development.*

• *Classify theories of development into various conceptual viewpoints.*

• *Analyze changes in psychosocial development across the life span.*

• *Identify the major developmental tasks across the life span.*

During the past half century several developmental theorists have closely studied the phenomena of human development. Sigmund Freud, Erik Erikson, Arnold Gesell, Robert Havighurst, and Jean Piaget, among others, have made valuable contributions to our knowledge of development. Each has constructed theoretical models of development that depict the many phases and stages passed through on the journey from childhood to maturity. Each of the models has several similarities but reflects its originator's philosophical learnings and particular interests in the study of development. This chapter will take a brief look at the models of growth and development proposed by these theorists. In order to provide a basis for a more detailed study of development, we also will examine characteristic ways in which theorists view the phenomena of development and examine three of the most popular theories of development, namely those of Erikson, Piaget, and Havighurst.

THEORETICAL MODELS OF HUMAN DEVELOPMENT

Freud's *psychoanalytic theory* of human behavior (1927) may be viewed, in part, as a model of development even though his work centered around personality and abnormal functioning in adults. His famous psychosexual stages of development reflected various zones of the body with which the individual seeks gratification of the id (the unconscious source of motives, desires, passions, and pleasure-seeking) at certain general age periods. The ego mediates between the pleasure-seeking behavior of the id and the superego (common sense, reason, and conscience). Freud's oral, anal, phallic, latency, and genital stages of personality development represent the terms applied to the pleasure-seeking zones of the body that come into play at different age periods. Each stage relies heavily on physical sensations and motor activity.

Psychoanalytic theory has received its share of criticism, primarily due to the inability to scientifically objectify, quantify, and validate its concepts. It has, however, stimulated considerable research and study and served as the basis for the notable works of Erik Erikson.

Erikson a student of Freud's, focused on the influence of society, rather than of sex, on development. His *psychosocial theory* (1963) describes eight stages of the human life cycle and puts them on a continuum, emphasizing factors in the environment, not heredity, as facilitators of change. Erikson's view of human development acknowledges that factors within the individual's experiential background have a primary role in development. His view of the importance of motor development is more implicit than explicit, but he clearly points out the importance of success-oriented movement experiences as a means of reconciling the developmental crises through which each individual passes.

Gesell's (1945) *maturational theory* of growth and development also emphasizes the physical and motor components of human behavior. Gesell documented and described general age periods for the acquisition of a wide variety of rudimentary movement abilities and viewed these maturationally-based tasks as important indicators of social and emotional growth. Gesell also described various ages when children are in "nodal" periods or when they are "out of focus" with their environment. A nodal stage is a maturational period during which the child exhibits a high degree of mastery over situations in the immediate environment, is balanced in behavior, and is generally pleasant to be with. On the opposite end when a child is out of focus he or she exhibits a low degree of mastery over situations in the immediate environment, is behaviorally unbalanced or troubled, and is generally unpleasant to be with. Maturational theory is not widely accepted today, but it played a significant role in the evolution of child development as an area of study.

A fourth developmental model, that of Robert Havighurst (1952), views development as an interplay between biological, social, and cultural forces by means of which children are continually enhancing their abilities to function effectively in society. Havighurst's *environmental theory* viewed development as a series of tasks that must be achieved within a certain time frame to ensure the proper developmental progression of the individual. According to Havighurst's model, there are teachable moments when the body is ready and when society requires successful completion of a task. As with the other models discussed, the tasks described by Havighurst rely heavily on movement, play, and physical activity for their development, particularly during infancy and childhood.

A currently popular developmental theory among educators is that of Jean Piaget (1969). Piaget's *cognitive development theory* places primary emphasis on the acquisition of cognitive thought processes. He gained insight into the development of cognitive structures through careful observation of infants and children. The genius in Piaget's work lies in his uncanny ability to detect subtle clues in children's behavior that give us indications of their cognitive functioning. Piaget viewed these subtle indicators as milestones in the hierarchy of cognitive development. Movement is emphasized as a primary agent in the acquisition of increased cognitive functioning, particularly during infancy and the preschool years. Piaget identified the developmental periods as sensorimotor (birth to 2 years), preoperational (2 to 7 years), concrete operations (7 to 11 years), and formal operations (12 years and over). Piaget did not concern himself with development beyond age 15 because he believed that highly sophisticated intellectual capabilities were developed by this time.

All theorists look at the phenomena of development from somewhat different points of view. Close inspection, however, reveals remarkable congruence on many aspects. Each theorist emphasizes movement, motor development, and play as important facilitators of enhanced functioning. Also, each tends to be more descriptive of human behavior than explanatory. They each differ, however, in the particular aspect of development emphasized. The multidimensional facets of development require a comprehensive model to explain behavior. In this regard, all of the theories have shortcomings, and care must be taken not to subscribe to one to the exclusion of the others. We must be aware of the interrelatedness of human behavior and dispel the notion that the psychomotor, cognitive, and affective domains of human behavior are independent of

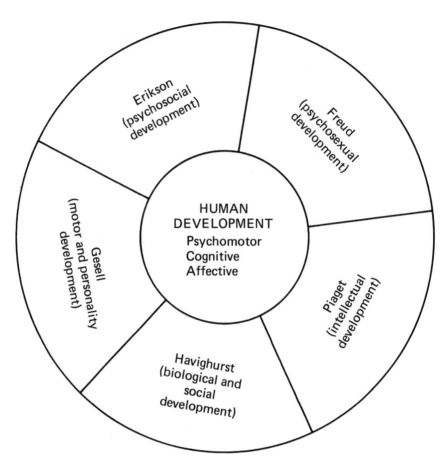

Figure 2.1. The interrelationship of theoretical models of human development

one another. Figure 2.1 illustrates the interrelatedness of each of the developmental models discussed and the particular area of interest of each theorist.

CONCEPTUAL VIEWPOINTS OF DEVELOPMENT

Close inspection of the five models of development as well as study of others reveals a distinct tendency for each to group around one of three similar but independent conceptual frameworks. These frameworks are classified here as (1) phase-stage, (2) developmental task, or (3) developmental milestone, concepts of human development.

Phase-Stage Theory

The *phase-stage approach* to developmental theory is the oldest of the conceptual viewpoints, and is sometimes referred to as "classical theory" or simply as "developmental theory" (Lerner, 1986). All classical developmental theorists (i.e., stage theorists), whether studying cognitive, moral, personality, or motor development, contend that there are universal age periods that are characterized by certain types of behavior. These behaviors occur in phases or stages, last for arbitrary lengths of time, and are invariant. In other words, stages are sequential and cannot be skipped or reordered. Furthermore, stage theory focuses on broad-based changes rather than narrow or isolated behaviors. Each phase (i.e., typical behavior) generally covers a period of one year or more and may be accompanied by one or more other stages. Some theorists sub-divide particular phases into smaller stages. Others prefer to view the phase as typical of one period of time. Most theorists who propose a phase-stage scheme have divided childhood, or even the entire life cycle, into 10 or fewer periods. The phase-stage concept is probably the most popular among parents and educators and is often reflected in our thinking and speech when we say, "she is just going through a stage" or "I will be happy when he is out of that phase." Freud, Erikson, and Gesell each viewed child development as a stage-related process. Stages have been proposed for several fundamental movement tasks (Wild, 1938; Seefeldt et al. 1972; Wickstrom, 1977; McClenaghan and Gallahue, 1978a). Robertson (1977), however, questioned the viability of a rigid stage theory of motor development and has suggested a more flexible stage model based on the components of a movement rather than on the total body configuration. It must be remembered that any phase-stage theory describes only general (i.e., groups, or normative) developmental characteristic for a generic human being that are postulated to be common to all people. It gives us a view of the big picture but must not be too closely adhered to lest we fail to see the details.

Developmental Task Theory

A second conceptual viewpoint of development is the *developmental task approach*. A developmental task is an important accomplishment individuals must achieve by a certain time if they are to function effectively and meet the demands placed on them by society. Proponents of developmental task theory view the accomplishment of particular tasks within a certain time span as prerequisite to smooth progression to higher levels of functioning. This concept of development differs from the age-stage view in that it is predictive of later success or failure based on the individual's performance at an earlier stage and does not merely attempt to describe typical behavior at a particular age. Havighurst's view of development uses the developmental task concept to describe and predict behavior from infancy through adolescence. Also, the hemispherical dominance theory and threatment techniques for individuals with learning as proposed by Delacato (1966) follow a developmental task approach.

Developmental Milestone Theory

The *developmental milestone approach* is the third and final conceptual framework from which development is viewed. Developmental milestones are similar to developmental tasks except for their emphasis. Instead of referring to accomplishments that are necessary for the individual's environmental adaptation, this approach refers to strategic indicators of how far development has progressed. The accomplishment of a developmental milestone may or may not, in itself, be as crucial to adjustment in the world as it is with a developmental task. Milestones are merely convenient guidelines by which the rate and extent of development can be gauged. As with stage theory, they are more descriptive than predictive, but unlike stage theories, they view development as a continual unfolding and intertwining of developmental processes, not as a neat transition from one stage to another.

Recognition of the fact that most models of human development tend to fall under one of these three concepts enables us to view the phenomena of growth and development more objectively. Each concept has merit and operates to a certain degree throughout the developmental process. The years of infancy and early childhood do, in fact, require the achievement of certain important tasks such as learning to walk, talk, and take solid foods by a certain age in order for normal functioning to be established. These years also encompass a variety of stages that children pass through at more or less the same age in addition to a variety of milestones that are achieved as subtle indicators of how far development has progressed throughout life.

THREE LEADING THEORIES OF DEVELOPMENT

In this section summaries of three theories, each representing a different conceptual point of view, are presented. The age-stage theory of Erik Erikson, the developmental milestone theory of Jean Piaget, and the developmental task theory of Robert Havighurst have been selected because of their thoroughness, popularity, and important implications for motor development.

Erik Erikson

The psychosocial theory of Erik Erikson (1963) adheres to the phase-stage approach to studying human development. It is an experience-based theory widely acclaimed by educators and psychologists. The following overview of Erikson's theory is presented in outline form for clarity and ease of understanding. Note the numerous implications for movement throughout the theory, particularly during the first four stages.

A. ACQUIRING A SENSE OF BASIC TRUST VERSUS MISTRUST (infancy).
   1. For the neonate, trust requires a feeling of physical comfort and a minimum of fear or uncertainty.
   2. A sense of basic trust helps the individual to accept new experiences willingly.
   3. Bodily experiences provide the basis for a psychological state of trust.
   4. The infant learns to trust "mother," oneself, and the environment through mother's perception of his or her needs and demands. Mutual trust and a willingness to face situations together are established between mother and child.

B. ACQUIRING A SENSE OF AUTONOMY VERSUS DOUBT AND SHAME (toddler).
   1. Continued dependency creates a sense of doubt about capacity.
   2. Children are bombarded by conflicting pulls of asserting themselves and denying themselves the right and capacity to make this assertion.
   3. Children need guidance and support lest they find themselves at a loss and become forced to turn against themselves with shame and doubt.
   4. Children explore and accomplish new feats.
   5. Proper development of the ego, which spells healthy growth, permits awareness of self as an autonomous unit.
   6. Children experience frustration as a reality of life (a natural part of life, not a total threat).
   7. Play allows children to develop autonomy within their own boundaries.
   8. Autonomy is developed in children through the realization that they and the environment can be controlled. Children develop concepts of forward, backward, upward, downward, and so on.
   9. Children violate mutual trust to establish autonomy in distinct areas.

C. ACQUIRING A SENSE OF INITIATIVE VERSUS GUILT (play age).
   1. Avid curiosity, feelings of guilt, and anxiety develop. The conscience is established.
   2. Specific tasks are mastered. Children assume responsibility for themselves and their world. They realize that life has purpose.
   3. Children initiate behavior, the implications of which go beyond themselves. This includes feelings of discomfort and guilt through the frustration of the autonomy of others. Their guilt and desire to curtail all initiative conflict with the pull toward continuing their searching initiative.
   4. Children discover that in their greater mobility they are not unlike the adults in their environment. Their use of language has improved, permitting them to expand their fields of activity and imagination.
   5. Children incorporate into their conscience what the parents really are as people and not merely what the parents try to teach them.
   6. Awareness of sex differences develops. Children find pleasurable accomplishment in manipulating meaningful toys.
   7. Most guilt and failure quickly become compensated for by a sense of accomplishment. The future absolves the past.
D. ACQUIRING A SENSE OF INDUSTRY VERSUS INFERIORITY (school age).
   1. This stage is marked by development of the skills necessary for life in general and preparation for marriage and family life.
   2. Children need to find a place among their peers instead of among adults.
   3. Children need to work on mastering social skills. They need to become competent and self-striving, and to obtain a sense of accomplishment for having done well. They ward off failure at any price.
   4. Activities tend to reflect competition.
   5. Boys and girls play separately. Play begins to lose importance at the end of this phase.
   6. Beginning with puberty, involvement in play merges into semiplayful and, eventually, real involvement in work.
   7. Children recognize that they must eventually break with accustomed family life.
   8. Dependence on parents as children's major influence shifts to dependence on social institutions.
E. ACQUIRING A SENSE OF IDENTITY VERSUS ROLE CONFUSION (puberty-adolescence).
   1. During this stage there is rapid body growth and sexual maturation. Masculine or feminine identity develops. Feelings of accep-

tance or rejection by peers are important. Conflict arises when peers say one thing and society says another.
2. Identity is essential for making adult decisions (vocation and marriage partner).
3. Youths will select as significant adults people who mean the most to them.
4. The individual slowly moves into society as an interdependent member.
5. A sense of identity assures the individual a definite place within his or her own corner of society.

F. ACQUIRING A SENSE OF INTIMACY VERSUS ISOLATION (young adult—late teens, early twenties).
1. The individual accepts himself or herself and goes on to accept others by fusing his or her personality with them.
2. Childhood and youth are at an end. The individual settles down to the task of full participation in the community and begins to enjoy life with adult liberties and responsibilities.
3. The individual shows readiness and ability to share mutual trust and to regulate cycles of work, procreation, and creation.

G. ACQUIRING A SENSE OF GENERATIVITY VERSUS SELF-ABSORPTION (adulthood).
1. The individual shows interest in the next generation rather than being caught up with his or her own problems (i.e., wants to advance the coming generation).
2. Generativity refers to the course one establishes and pursues with one's mate in society in order to assure for the next generation the hope, virtues, and wisdom he or she has accumulated. It also includes parental responsibility for society's efforts and interests in child care, education, the arts and sciences, and traditions.

H. ACQUIRING A SENSE OF INTEGRITY VERSUS DESPAIR (mature adult and old age).
1. The individual accomplishes the fullest sense of trust as the assured reliance on another's integrity.
2. A different love of one's parents is established. Integrity provides a successful solution to an opposing sense of despair.
3. Fulfillment of this stage involves a sense of wisdom and a philosophy of life which often extends beyond the life cycle of the individual and which is directly related to the future of new developmental cycles.

Jean Piaget

The developmental milestone theory of Jean Piaget (1952, 1954, 1957, and 1969) is currently among the most popular of the theories postulated by experts in the field of child development because of clarity, insight into, and understanding of the development of cognitive abilities. Cognitive development, according to Piaget, occurs through the process of *adaptation*. Adaptation involves one's making adjustments to environmental conditions and intellectualizing those adjustments through the complimentary processes of assimilation and accommodation. A summary of Piaget's theory presented in outline form follows. Note the numerous implications for movement throughout the phases of development, particularly during the sensorimotor phase.

A. SENSORIMOTOR PHASE (birth to 2 years): The major developmental tasks are coordination of the infant's actions or movement activities and perceptions into a tenuous whole.
   1. *Use of reflexes* (birth to 1 month): There is a continuation of prenatal reflexes. They are spontaneous repetitions caused by internal and external stimulation. Rhythm is established through practice, and habits are formed that later emerge as voluntary movements.
   2. *Primary circular reactions* (1 to 3 months).
      a. Reflexive movement is gradually replaced by voluntary movements.
      b. Neurological maturity must be reached before sensations can be understood.
      c. What previously had been automatic behavior is repeated voluntarily.
      d. More than one sensory modality can be used at a time.
      e. Accidentally acquired responses become new sensorimotor habits.
      f. Primary circular reactions refer to the *assimilation* (i.e., interpreting new information based on present interpretations) of a previous experience and the recognition of the stimulus that triggers the reaction.
      g. New or past experiences have no meaning unless they become part of the primary circular reaction pattern.
   3. *Secondary circular reactions* (3 to 9 months).
      a. The infant tries to make events last and tries to make events occur.
      b. The focus of the infant is on retention, not repetition.
      c. The infant tries to create a state of permanency.
      d. Primary circular reactions are repeated and prolonged by secondary reactions.
      e. Two or more sensorimotor experiences as related to one expe-

riential sequence or schema. (*Schema* is Piaget's term for a pattern of physical or motor action.)

   f. Vision is the prime coordinator, but other sensory modalities are also used.

   g. Imitation, play, and emotion begin to appear at this stage.

4. *Application of the secondary schemata to new situations* (8 to 12 months).

   a. This is characterized by the child's ability to distinguish means from ends (i.e., producing the same result more than one way).

   b. Children use previous behavioral achievements primarily as the basis for adding new achievements to their expanding repertoire.

   c. There is increased experimentation; ends and means are differentiated by experimenting.

   d. *Accommodation* (i.e., adaptation that the child must make to the environment when new and incongruent information is added to his or her repertoire) is a result of experimentation.

   e. The infant can experience action by observation.

5. *Tertiary circular reactions* (12 to 18 months).

   a. Discovery of new means through active experimentation.

   b. Curiosity and novelty-seeking behavior are developing.

   c. Reasoning comes into play and is developed.

   d. Failure to remember is failure to understand.

   e. The infant develops spatial relationships upon discovering objects as objects.

   f. Imitation develops.

   g. Play is very important because it repeats the action phase.

6. *Invention of new means through mental combinations* (12 to 24 months).

   a. There is a shift from sensorimotor experiences to an increased reflection about these experiences. This is the steppingstone to the next phase, which is an advanced level of intellectual behavior.

   b. Children discern themselves as one object among many. They perceive and use objects for their own intrinsic qualities.

   c. Children begin to relate the objects to new actions without actually perceiving all of the actions.

   d. Sensorimotor patterns are slowly replaced by semi-mental functionings.

   e. Imitation copies the action itself or the symbol of the action.

   f. Parallel play appears.

   g. Identification, as a mental process, becomes evident at the end of this phase. It depends on the level of intellectual development of the child.

h. This period is characterized by the creation of means and not merely the discovery of means (i.e., insight begins).

B. PREOPERATIONAL PHASE (2 to 7 years).
  1. This is a period of transition from self-satisfying behaviors to rudimetary socialized behaviors.
  2. Continuous investigation of one's world develops.
  3. The child knows the world only as he or she sees it.
  4. The child is egocentric rather than autistic, as in the sensorimotor phase.
  5. Assimilation is the paramount task of the child.
  6. Play occupies most of the waking hours. Emphasis on "how" and "why" becomes a primary tool for adaptation.
  7. Imaginary play is important.
  8. Language begins to repeat and replace sensorimotor activity.
  9. Events are judged by outward appearance regardless of their objective logic.
  10. Either the qualitative or quantitative aspects of an event are experienced, but not both simultaneously. The child cannot merge concepts of objects, space, and causality into interrelationships with a concept of time.
  11. There is widening social interest in the world about the child.
  12. Egocentricity is reduced and social participation increases.
  13. The first real beginning of cognition occurs.
  14. Speech replaces movement to express thinking.
  15. The child can think of only one idea at a time.
  16. The child tries to adjust new experiences to previous patterns of thinking.
  17. The child becomes aware of relationships.
  18. Conservation of quantity (i.e., object permanence), such as permanence and continuity, must be mastered before a concept of numbers can be developed.
  19. Play enacts the rules and values of elders.
  20. Parallel play continues.
C. CONCRETE OPERATIONS PHASE (7 to 11 years).
  1. The child becomes aware of alternative solutions.
  2. The child acquires *reversibility* (i.e., the capacity to relate an event or thought to a total system of interrelated parts in order to consider the event or thought from beginning to end or from end to beginning).
  3. Operational thought develops mental capacity to order and relate experience to an organized whole.

4. The concrete operational thought level presupposes that mental experimentation still depends on perception.
5. The child examines parts to gain knowledge of the whole.
6. The child establishes systems of classifications of organizing parts into a hierarchical system.
7. Perceptions are more accurate.
8. The child applies interpretation of perceptions of the environment knowingly.
9. Play is used for understanding the physical and social world.
10. Play loses its assimilative characteristics and becomes a balanced, subordinate process of cognitive thought.
11. Curiosity finds expression in intellectual experimentation instead of in active play.
12. The child becomes interested in rules and regulations.

D. FORMAL OPERATIONS PHASE (12 to 15 years).
1. Childhood ends and youth begins.
2. The individual enters the world of ideas.
3. There is a systematic approach to problems.
4. There is logical deduction by implication.
5. The individual thinks beyond the present (e.g., vertically).
6. The individual can dream and does not need reality.
7. Deduction by hypothesis and judgment by implication enable reasoning beyond cause and effect.

Robert Havighurst

The theory of Robert Havighurst (1952, 1953, 1972; Havighurst and Levine, 1979) is based on the concept that successful achievement of developmental tasks leads to happiness and success with later tasks, whereas failure leads to unhappiness, social disapproval, and difficulty with later tasks. It is interesting to note his disagreement with any theory that proposes an innate basis of growth and development. He believes that living is learning and growing is learning (Havighurst, 1972). Development, then, according to Havighurst, is the process of learning one's way through life. Havighurst views successful development as mastering a series of tasks. At each level of development the child encounters new social demands. These demands, or tasks, arise out of three sources. First, tasks arise from physical maturation. Such things as learning to walk and talk and to get along with one's age-mates are maturation-based tasks. Second, tasks arise out of the cultural pressures of society, such as learning how to read and learning to be a responsible citizen. The third source is oneself. Tasks arise out of the maturing personality and the individual's values and unique aspirations.

Havighurst's theory has implications for all age levels. His theory is of particular importance to educators because it emphasizes that when the body is "ripe," when society requires, and when the self is ready to achieve a certain task, the teachable moment (readiness period) has arrived. We can, therefore, better time our teaching efforts by identifying the tasks that are suitable for a particular level of development, being fully aware that one's level of readiness is influenced by biological, cultural, and self factors all interacting with one another.

Havighurst has suggested six major periods of development: infancy and early childhood (birth through 5 years), middle childhood (6 through 12 years), adolescence (13 through 18 years), early adulthood (19 through 29 years), middle adulthood (30 through 60 years), and later maturity (61 years and up). A summary of Havighurst's developmental tasks in outline form follows. The reader is cautioned to be flexible in the interpretation of these tasks with respect to age. Ages are only convenient approximations and should not be viewed as rigid time frames. Significant deviation beyond these age boundaries, however, would, according to Havighurst, represent failure in a developmental task, resulting in unhappiness and great difficulty with succeeding tasks.

A. INFANCY AND EARLY CHILDHOOD (birth to 5 years).
   1. Learning to walk.
   2. Learning to take solid foods.
   3. Learning to talk.
   4. Learning to control the elimination of bodily wastes.
   5. Learning sex differences and sexual modesty.
   6. Acquiring concepts and language to describe social and physical reality.
   7. Readiness for reading.
   8. Learning to distinguish right from wrong and developing a conscience.
B. MIDDLE CHILDHOOD (6 to 12 years).
   1. Learning physical skills necessary for ordinary games.
   2. Building a wholesome attitude toward oneself.
   3. Learning to get along with age-mates.
   4. Learning an appropriate sex role.
   5. Developing fundamental skills in reading, writing, and calculating.
   6. Developing concepts necessary for everyday living.
   7. Developing a conscience, morality, and a scale of values.
   8. Achieving personal independence.
   9. Developing acceptable attitudes toward society.

C. ADOLESCENCE (13 to 18 years).
1. Achieving mature relations with both sexes.
2. Achieving a masculine or feminine social role.
3. Accepting one's physique.
4. Achieving emotional independence of adults.
5. Preparing for marriage and family life.
6. Preparing for an economic career.
7. Acquiring values and an ethical system to guide behavior.
8. Desiring and achieving socially responsible behavior.
D. EARLY ADULTHOOD (19 to 29 years).
1. Selecting a mate.
2. Learning to live with a partner.
3. Starting a family.
4. Rearing children.
5. Managing a home.
6. Starting an occupation.
7. Assuming civic responsibility.
E. MIDDLE ADULTHOOD (30 to 60 years).
1. Helping teenage children to become happy and responsible adults.
2. Achieving adult social and civic responsibility.
3. Satisfactory career achievement.
4. Developing adult leisure-time activities.
5. Relating to one's spouse as a person.
6. Accepting the physiological changes of middle age.
7. Adjusting to aging parents.
E. LATER MATURITY (60 years and up).
1. Adjusting to decreasing strength and health.
2. Adjusting to retirement and reduced income.
3. Adjusting to death of spouse.
4. Establishing relations with one's own age group.
5. Meeting social and civic obligations.
6. Establishing satisfactory living quarters.

SUMMARY

The process of development is commonly viewed as hierarchical. That is, the individual proceeds from general to specific and from simple to complex in gaining mastery and control over his or her environment. Erik Erikson's age-stage theory, Jean Piaget's developmental milestone theory, and Robert Havighurst's developmental task theory make it obvious that the human organism throughout all aspects of its development is moving from comparatively simple forms of existence to more complex and sophisticated levels of development. These levels of development have been expressed primarily in terms of the cognitive and affective behaviors of the individual, with only indirect attention given to motor development.

Although the theoretical formulations of Erikson, Piaget, and Havighurst are of value, none adequately addresses motor development. It is, therefore, appropriate that a theoretical model of motor development be put forth in order to describe and explain this important aspect of development. The following chapter is dedicated to this end.

CHAPTER CONCEPTS

2.1 There are numerous theories of development, each of which reflects the originator's interests and biases.

2.2 Theories of development are molar in nature. That is, they attempt to explain all aspects of behavior and, by necessity, break down at some point.

2.3 No one theory of development is complete or totally accurate. Each offers us a better but still incomplete understanding of the individual and should generate testable hypotheses.

2.4 Most theories of development do not deal with movement as an integral part of the model but view movement in terms of how it impacts on cognitive and affective development.

2.5 Developmental theory may be subdivided into distinct conceptual viewpoints.

2.6 Erikson's theory focuses on the affective development of the individual throughout life and has numerous implications for movement.

2.7 Piaget's theory focuses on the cognitive development of the individual from birth to about age 15. The sensorimotor phase has particular implications for the child's motor development.

2.8 Robert Havighurst focuses on crucial tasks throughout life that impact on later development in the cognitive, affective, and psychomotor domains.

2.9 Close examination of developmental theories provides us with a clearer understanding of the intricate physical and mental processes involved in development and help us construct theoretical models for the process of motor development.

TERMS TO REMEMBER

Psychoanalytic Theory
Psychosocial Theory
Maturational Theory
Environmental Theory
Cognitive Development Theory
Phase-Stage Approach
Developmental Task Approach

Developmental Milestone Approach
Trust
Autonomy
Initiative
Industry
Identity
Intimacy

Generativity

Integrity

Sensorimotor Phase Reflexes

Primary Circular Reactions

Secondary Circular Reactions

Assimilation

Schema

Accommodation

Tertiary Circular Reactions

Invention of New Means

Preoperational Phase

Concrete Operations Phase

Reversibility

Formal Operations Phase

CRITICAL READINGS

Erikson, E. (1963). *Childhood and Society*. New York: Norton.

Havighurst, R. (1972). *Developmental Tasks and Education*. New York: David McKay.

Lerner, R. M. (1986). *Concepts and Theories of Human Development*. New York: Random House. (Chapter 7).

Maier, H. W. (1978). *Three Theories of Child Development*, New York: Harper & Row, (Chapters 2-3).

Payne, V. G. and Isaacs, L. D. (1987). *Human Motor Development a Lifespan Approach*. Mountain View, CA: Mayfied, (Chapter 2).

3

Motor Development:
A Theoretical Model

CHAPTER COMPETENCIES

Upon Completion of This Chapter You Should Be Able To:

* *Define life span motor development.*
* *View an individual's motor behavior as "more" or "less" advanced on a developmental continuum rather than as "good" or "bad."*
* *Demonstrate an understanding of neural, physiological, perceptual, and cognitive changes across the life span.*
* *Distinguish between inductive and deductive theory formulation.*
* *Describe the Phases of Motor Development.*
* *List and describe the stages within the Phases of Motor Development.*

A major function of theory is to integrate existing facts, to organize them so they are meaningful. Theories of development take existing facts about the human organism and provide a developmental model congruent with these facts. Theory formulation, therefore, serves as a basis for fact testing, and vice versa. Facts are important but alone do not constitute a science. The development of a science depends on the advancement of theory as well as on the accumulation of facts. In the study of human behavior, especially in the areas of cognitive and affective development, theory formulation has gained increased importance over the past several years. Theory has played a critical dual role in both of these areas; namely, it has served and continues to serve as an integrator of existing facts and as a basis for the derivation of new facts.

Unfortunately, the recent surge of interest in motor development has been concerned primarily with describing and cataloging data, with little interest in developmental models leading to a theoretical explanation of behavior. This research has been necessary and very important to our knowledge base, but at present only a limited number of comprehensive developmental models exist, and there is no comprehensive theory of motor development. Researchers and scholars have focused on the performance of specific movement tasks at specific developmental levels. This research has produced both process oriented information (i.e., biomechanical and observational assessment along various levels) and product-oriented information (i.e., normative data on the physical and movement abilities of specific age groups). At this point in our knowledge of human motor development, a comprehensive model leading to a theory of motor development should be put forth in an effort to explain motor development and generate new facts about this aspect of behavior.

The first function of a theory of motor development should be to integrate the existing facts encompassed by the area of study. The second function should be to generate new facts. One might argue that the facts could be interpreted from different theoretical perspectives. This is entirely possible and, in fact, desirable. Different viewpoints generate theoretical arguments and debates sparking research that sheds new light on different theoretical interpretations. Even if theoretical differences do not exist, research should be undertaken to determine whether the hypotheses derived from the theory can be experimentally supported.

Theory should undergird all research and science, and the study of motor development is no exception. Developmental theory must be both *descriptive* and *explanatory*; the developmentalist is interested in what people are like at particular age periods (description), and what makes these changes occur (explanation). Without a theoretical base of operation, research in motor development often yields little more than isolated facts. Without an existing body of knowledge (facts), we cannot formulate theory, but without the formulation and constant testing of theory, we cannot hope for a higher level of understanding and awareness of the phenomenon that we call motor development.

A theory is a group of statements, concepts, or principles that integrate existing facts and lead to the generation of new facts. The model of The Phases of Motor Development presented in this chapter is not based solely on the accumulation of facts. Such a model would result from using an inductive method of theory formulation. That is, in the *inductive method* the researcher first starts with a set of facts and then tires to find a conceptual framework within which to organize and explain them. The *deductive method* of theory formulation, as used here, is based on inference and has three qualifications: (1) The theory should integrate existing facts and account for existing empirical evidence that affects the content of the

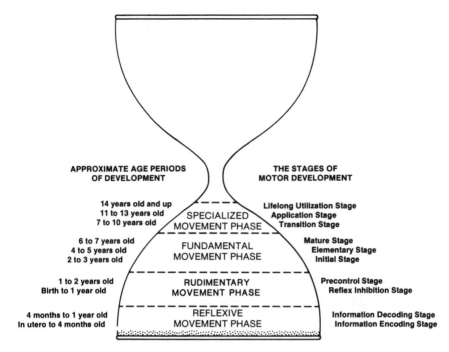

Figure 3.1. The Phases of Motor Development

ing and sucking reflexes are thought by some to be primitive survival mechanisms. Without them, the newborn would be unable to obtain nourishment.

Postural reflexes are the second form of involuntary movement. They are remarkably similar in appearance to later voluntary behaviors but are entirely involuntary. According to Wyke (1975), these reflexes seem to serve as a "neuromotor testing time" for locomotor, manipulative, and stability mechanisms that will be used later with conscious control. The primary stepping reflex and the crawling reflex, for example, closely resemble later voluntary walking and crawling behaviors. The palmar grasping reflex is closely related to later voluntary grasping and releasing behaviors. The labyrinthine righting reflex and the propping reflexes are related to later balancing abilities. The reflexive phase of motor development may be divided into two overlapping stages.

Information Encoding Stage. The information encoding (gathering) stage of the reflexive movement phase is characterized by observable involuntary movement activity during the fetal period until about the fourth month of infancy. During this stage lower brain centers are more developed than the motor cortex and are essentially in command of fetal and neonatal movement. These brain centers are capable of causing involuntary reactions to a variety of stimuli of varying intensity and duration. During this stage reflexes serve as the primary means by which the infant is able to gather information, to seek nourishment, and to seek protection through movement.

Information Decoding Stage. The information decoding (processing) stage of the reflex phase begins around the fourth month. During this time there is a gradual inhibition of many reflexes as higher brain centers continue to develop. Lower brain centers gradually relinquish control over skeletal movements and are replaced by voluntary movement activity mediated by the motor area of the cerebral cortex. The decoding stage replaces sensorimotor activity with perceptual-motor behavior. That is, the infant's development of voluntary control of skeletal movements involves processing sensory stimuli with stored information, not merely reacting to stimuli.

Chapter 7 focuses on primitive and postural reflexes as they relate to the information encoding and decoding stages. Special attention is given to the relationship between the reflex phase of development and voluntary movement.

Rudimentary Movement Phase

The first forms of voluntary movement are rudimentary movements. They are seen in the infant from birth to about age 2. Rudimentary movements are maturationally determined and are characterized by a highly predictable sequence in their appearance. This sequence is resistant to change under normal conditions. The rate at which these abilities appear will vary from child to child and is dependent on both biological and environmental factors. The rudimentary movement abilities of the infant represent the basic forms of voluntary movement that are required for survival. They involve stability movements such as gaining control of the head, neck, and trunk muscles; the manipulative tasks of reach, grasp, and release; and the locomotor movements of creeping, crawling, and walking. The rudimentary movement phase of development may be subdivided into two stages that represent progressively higher orders of movement control.

Reflex Inhibition Stage. The reflex inhibition stage of the rudimentary movement ability phase may be thought of as beginning at birth. At birth, reflexes dominate the infant's movement repertoire. From then on, however, the infant's movements are increasingly influenced by the developing cortex. Development of the cortex causes several reflexes to be inhibited and gradually to disappear. The primitive and postural reflexes are replaced by voluntary movement behavior. At the reflex inhibition level, voluntary movement is poorly differentiated and integrated. That is, the neuromotor apparatus of the infant is still at a rudimentary stage of development. Movements, though purposeful, appear uncontrolled and unrefined. If the infant wishes to make contact with an object, there will be global activity of the entire hand, wrist, arm, shoulder, and even trunk. In other words, the process of moving the hand into contact with the object, although voluntary, lacks control.

Precontrol Stage. Around one year of age, children begin to bring greater precision and control to their movements. The process of differentiating between sensory and motor systems and integrating perceptual and motor information into a more meaningful and congruent whole takes place. The rapid development of higher cognitive processes and motor processes causes rapid gains in rudimentary movement abilities during this stage. Given the short time they have in which to develop these abilities, children learn to gain and maintain their equilibrium, to manipulate objects, and to locomote throughout the environment with an amazing degree of proficiency and control. The maturational process may explain the rapidity and extent of development of movement control during this phase, but the growth of motor proficiency is no less amazing.

Chapter 8 provides a detailed explanation of the development of rudimentary movement abilities. Particular attention is paid to the interrelationship between the stages within this phase and the stages within the reflexive phase of development. Attention is also focused on the critical function that the rudimentary movement phase serves in preparing the child for the development of fundamental movement abilities.

Fundamental Movement Phase

The fundamental movement abilities of early childhood are an outgrowth of the rudimentary movement phase of infancy. This phase of motor development represents a time in which young children are actively involved in exploring and experimenting with the movement capabilities of their bodies. It is a time for discovering how to perform a variety of locomotor, stability, and manipulative movements, first in isolation and then in combination with one another. Children who are developing fundamental patterns of movement are learning how to respond with adaptability and versatility to a variety of stimuli. They are gaining increased control in the performance of discrete, serial, and continuous movements as evidenced by increased fluidity and control in movement. Fundamental movement patterns are basic observable patterns of behavior. Locomotor activities such as running and jumping, manipulative activities such as throwing and catching, and stability activities such as the beam walk and stick balance are examples of fundamental movement abilities that should be developed during the early childhood years.

A major misconception about the developmental concept of the fundamental movement ability phase is the notion that these abilities are maturationally determined and are little influenced by environmental factors. Some child development experts (not in the motor development area) have written repeatedly about the "natural" unfolding of the child's movement or play skills and about the idea that merely by growing older (maturation), these abilities will develop. Maturation does, in fact, play a role in the development of fundamental movement abilities. It should not, however, be viewed as the only influencing factor. The factors of opportunities for practice, encouragement, and instruction all play important roles in the degree to which fundamental movement abilities develop.

Several investigators and assessment instrument developers have attempted to subdivide fundamental movements into a series of identifiable sequential stages. For the purpose of our model we will view the entire fundamental movement phase as having three separate but often overlapping stages, namely the initial, elementary, and mature stages. These stages are dealt with briefly here and in greater detail in Chapter 11.

Initial Stage. The initial stage of the fundamental movement ability phase represents the child's first goal-oriented attempts at performing a fundamental movement pattern. Movement itself is characterized by missing or improperly sequenced parts, markedly restricted or exaggerated use of the body, and poor rhythmical flow and coordination. In other words, spatial and temporal integration of movement are poor during this stage. Typically, the locomotor, manipulative, and stability movements of the 2-year-old are at the initial level. Some children may be beyond this level in the performance of some patterns of movement, but most are at the initial stage.

Elementary Stage. The elementary stage involves greater control and better rhythmical coordination of fundamental movements. The temporal and spatial elements of movement are better coordinated, but patterns of movement at this stage are still generally restricted or exaggerated, although better coordinated. Children of normal intelligence and physical functioning tend to advance to the elementary stage primarily through the process of maturation. (McClenaghan and Gallahue, 1978a). Observation of the typical 3- or 4-year-old child reveals a variety of abilities at the elementary stage. Many individuals fail to develop beyond the elementary stage in many patterns of movement and remain at this stage throughout life.

Mature Stage. The mature stage within the fundamental movement phase is characterized by mechanically-efficient, coordinated, and controlled performances. The majority of available data on the acquisition of fundamental movement skills suggest that children have the development "potential" to be at the mature stage by age 5 or 6 in most fundamental skills. Manipulative skills which require tracking and intercepting a moving object (catching, striking, volleying), however, mature somewhat later because of the sophisticated visual-motor sequence. Even a casual glance at the movements of children and adults reveals that a great many have not developed their fundamental movement abilities to the mature level. Although some children may reach this stage primarily through maturation and with a minimum of environmental influences, the vast majority require ample opportunities for practice, encouragement to learn, and instruction. Failure to include these factors in the lives of individuals makes it virtually impossible for them to achieve the mature stage within this phase and will inhibit complete development in the next phase.

Specialized Movement Phase

The specialized or sport related[1] phase of motor development is an outgrowth of the fundamental movement phase. During this phase, movement, instead of continuing to be closely identified with learning to move for the sake of movement, now becomes a tool that may be applied to a variety of specialized movement activities. It is a period when fundamental locomotor, manipulation, and stability skills are progressively refined, combined, and elaborated upon in order to be used in increasingly demanding activities. The fundamental movements of hopping and jumping, for example, are now applied to rope-jumping activities, to performing folk dance activities, and to performing the triple jump (hop-step-jump) in track.

The onset and extent of skill development within the specialized phase depends on a variety of cognitive, affective, and psychomotor factors. Reaction time and movement speed, cordination, body type, height and weight, customs, peer pressure, and emotional makeup are but a few of the factors. The specialized movement phase may be subdivided into several stages depending on the sophistication of the observer. A three-stage approach is advocated here, and recommended for those who must rely on naked eye observation as their primary means of assessment.

Transitional Stage. Somewhere around the seventh or eighth year of life, children commonly enter a transitional,[2] or general movement,

---

[1] The term sport is used in its broadest sense. It should not be construed to apply solely to competitive sports but also encompasses rhythmical and recreational activities and games of a gross motor nature.
[2] Vern Seefeldt, Michigan State University, is credited with popularization of this term.

skill stage. During the transitional movement stage the individual begins to combine and apply fundamental movement skills to the performance of sport-related skills. Walking on a rope bridge, jumping rope, and playing kickball are examples of common transitional skills. Transitional movements contain the same elements as fundamental movements but great accuracy and control of movement are now evident. The fundamental movement abilities that were developed and refined for their own sake during the previous stage are now applied in play, game, and sport situations. Transitional sport skills are simply an application of fundamental movements in somewhat more complex and specific forms.

The transitional stage is an exciting time for the parent and the teacher as well as for the child. During this stage children are actively involved in discovering and combining numerous movement patterns and skills and are often elated by their rapidly expanding abilities. The goal of the concerned parent and teacher during this stage should be to help the child develop and expand his or her abilities in a wide variety of sport-related activities. Care must be taken not to cause the child to specialize or restrict his or her activity involvement. A narrow focus on skills during this stage is likely to have undesirable effects on the last two stages of the sport related phase.

Application Stage. From about age 11 to age 13 (the middle school years) interesting changes take place in the skill development of the individual. During the previous stage the limited cognitive abilities, affective abilities, and experiences of the child, coupled with a natural eagerness to be active, cause the normal focus (without adult interference) on movement to be broad and generalized to all activity. During the application stage, increased cognitive sophistication and a broadened experience base enable the individual to make numerous learning and participation decisions based on a variety of factors. For example, the five feet, ten-inch-tall 12-year-old who likes team activities and applying strategy to games, who has reasonably good coordination and agility, and who lives in Indiana may, based on specific physical, cognitive, and cultural factors, choose to specialize in the development of basketball playing abilities. A similar child who does not really enjoy team efforts may choose to specialize in improving his or her abilities in a variety of track and field activities. In other words, the individual begins to make conscious decisions based on a variety of likes and dislikes, strengths and weaknesses, opportunities and restrictions, to narrow his or her activity base. The child begins to seek or avoid participation in specific activities. Increased emphasis should now be placed on form, skill, and accuracy of performance. This is a time for more complex skills to be refined and used in the performance of advanced lead-up activities and in the chosen sport itself.

Lifelong Utilization Stage. The lifelong utilization stage of the specialized phase of motor development begins around the fourteenth year of life and continues through adulthood. The lifelong utilization stage represents the pinnacle of the development process and is characterized by the individual's desire to participate in a limited number of movement activities over a period of years. The interests, abilities, and choices made during the previous stage are carried over to this stage and further refined. Factors such as available time and money, equipment, and facilities for participation affect this stage. The level of activity participation will depend on the individual's talents, opportunities, physical condition, and motivation. One's lifetime performance level may range anywhere from the professional levels and the Olympics, to intercollegiate and interscholastic competition, to participation in organized or unorganized, competitive or cooperative, recreational sports.

In essence, the lifelong utilization stage represents a culmination of all preceding phases and stages. It should, however, be viewed as a continuation of a lifetime process. One of the primary goals of education is to develop individuals to a point where they become happy, healthy, contributing members of society. We must not lose sight of this lofty but worthy goal. We must view the hierarchical development of movement abilities as stepping stones to the specialized movement skill level. We must cease in viewing children as miniature adults who can be programmed to perform at this stage in such potentially high-pressure, physiologically and psychologically questionable activities as Little League Baseball and Pee Wee Football. We must view children as developmentally immature individuals, and structure meaningful movement experiences appropriate for their particular developmental level. Only when we recognize that the progressive development of movement abilities in a developmentally appropriate sequence is imperative to the balanced motor development of children will we begin making significant contributions to the total development of the individual. Specialized skill development can and should play a role in our lives, but it is unfair to require children to specialize in one or two skill areas at the expense of developing their abilities in and appreciation for many other areas.

THE HOURGLASS: A LIFE SPAN PROCESS

The age ranges for each phase of motor development should be viewed as general boundaries only. Children will often be functioning at different phases depending on their experiential background and genetic makeup. For example, it is entirely possible for a 10-year-old to function at the specialized movement phase at the lifelong utilization stage in stability activities involving gymnastic movements but only at the elementary stage of the fundamental movement phase in manipulative or locomotor activities such as throwing, catching, or running. Although we should continue to encourage this precocious behavior in gymnastics, we should also be concerned that the child catches up to his or her age-mates in the other areas and develops an acceptable level of proficiency in this stage as well. Rigid adherence to age classifications is unwise and in direct conflict with the principle of individual differences. Development is a life-long process and so too should be the development of movement skills that have utility throughout life.

It is important that we gather facts about the process of motor development. In fact, throughout this text we will discuss study after study, but if I fail to provide you with a theoretical framework and a conceptual grasp of the process of motor development, I will have accomplished little more than providing you with isolated facts that tell you little about their implications for successful developmental teaching. I would, therefore, like to propose a theoretical model for the process of motor development and work through this model with you. This model as presented is not a comprehensive theory of motor development. It is an outline and is intended to serve as a springboard for the development of a more comprehensive model.

In order to present this model in a meaningful fashion, picture yourself as an hourglass (Figure 3.2). Into your hourglass we need to place the stuff of life: "sand." Sand gets into your hourglass from two different containers. One is your hereditary container, the other your environmental container. When we look at the heredity container, we see that there is a lid on its top. In other words, at conception our genetic makeup is determined and the amount of sand in that container is fixed. In the second container, however,—our environmental container—we don't have a lid. This signifies that sand may continually be added to this container and to your hourglass. For example, we could take your environmental container, reach down into the "sand pile" (i.e., the environment) and get more sand to put into your hourglass.

The two buckets of sand signify that the process of development is influenced by our environment as well as by our unique individual heredity. The relative contributions of each has been a volatile topic of debate for years. Arguing the relative importance of each is a meaningless exercise because sand is actually funneled from both containers into your hourglass through a single tube. In the final analysis, it does not matter if your hourglass is filled with hereditary sand or environmental sand. What is important is that somehow sand gets into your hourglass and that this stuff of life is the product of both heredity and the environment.

Now, what do we know about motor development during the early phases of life? When we look at the reflexive and rudimentary phases of

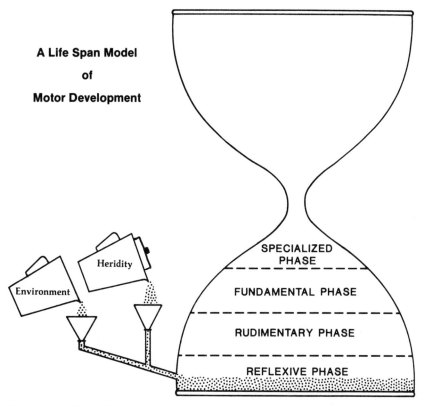

THE HOURGLASS:

A Life Span Model

of

Motor Development

Heridity

Environment

SPECIALIZED PHASE

FUNDAMENTAL PHASE

RUDIMENTARY PHASE

REFLEXIVE PHASE

Figure 3.2. Filling the hourglass with "sand" (ie the stuff of life)

motor development, we know that sand pours into the hourglass primarily, but not exclusively, from the hereditary container. In other words, the sequential progression of motor development during the first few years of life is quite rigid and resistant to change except under environmental extremes. Therefore, we know that in the first two phases of motor development the sequence of development is highly predictable. For example, children all over the world learn how to sit before they stand, how to stand before they walk, and how to walk before they run. What we do see, however, is considerable variability in terms of the rate at which the very young acquire their rudimentary movement abilities. This is something that researchers and program developers have become increasingly interested in over the past few years. We have seen a rapid rise in the number of infant stimulation programs and infant-toddler movement programs. Some make elaborate claims about the worth of these programs and their ultimate importance to the child. Unfortunately, we have little hard evidence at this juncture to either support or refute these claims. What we do know, however, is that children the world over will develop their rudimentary movement abilities in the same sequence. The rate may differ somewhat if a child receives additional stimulation, but the amount, type, and duration of this extra stimulation is still open to speculation.

The fundamental movement phase is that point in time where boys and girls are beginning to develop a host of basic movement abilities. Such things as running, hopping, jumping, throwing, catching, kicking, and trapping are generally considered to be fundamental movements. Unfortunately, many professional early childhood and elementary educators have the notion that children somehow "automatically" learn how to perform these fundamental movements. Many naively think that children at this phase of development will, through the process of maturation, develop mature fundamental movement abilities. This simply is not so for the vast majority of children. Most children must have some combination of those three important environmental conditions of opportunities for practice, encouragement and instruction. These three conditions are crucial to helping them through each of the stages within the fundamental movement phase.

In the specialized skill phase, successful performance of the mechanics of sport skills is dependent upon mature fundamental movements. Once beyond the transitional stage we progress to the final stages which involve the application of specialized movements skills to the sport activities of one's culture for a lifetime of recreational and competitive sport experiences.

Hopefully, you have the abilities, knowledge, and interest to be involved in vigorous physical activity of some form for your lifetime, because at some point our hourglass turns over (Figure 3.3). I am uncertain exactly when our hourglass turns over; one could forever consider this question. But the hourglass probably begins to turn over during our late teens and early twenties.

There are several interesting features in our overturned hourglass that we need to consider. We have two different filters through which the sand falls. One is our *hereditary filter* with which we can do very little. For example, you may have inherited a predisposition toward coronary heart disease or some other debilitating condition. Or, you may be able to look at your family history and trace a remarkable record of longevity. As a result, our hereditary filter is going to be either dense, causing the sand to filter through slowly, or widely spaced, causing the sand to flow

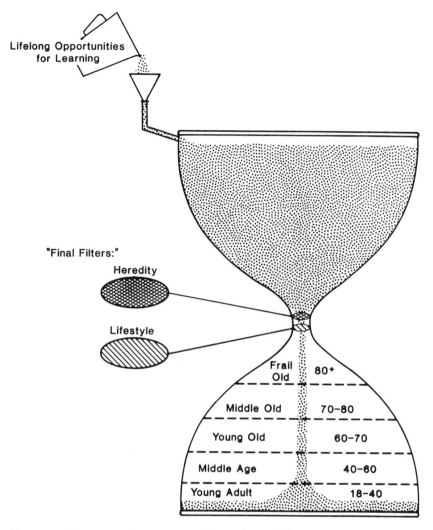

Figure 3.3. Emptying the overturned hourglass of life

through more rapidly. We can never recover sand that has fallen through our hereditary filter, but we have a second, or final, filter through which our sand must fall. This is called the lifestyle filter.

The density of our *lifestyle filter* is determined by such things as our fitness, nutritional status, diet, exercise, and ability to handle stress. Our lifestyle filter is environmentally based, and we have a good deal of control over the rate at which sand falls through this filter. Although we can never stop sand from flowing to the bottom of our hourglass, we can slow down the rate at which it falls. The former Surgeon General of the United States, Dr. C. Everett Koop, stated that, although we cannot stop the aging process, we can control it by up to 40 percent (1980). Think about that. We can control approximately 40 percent of our age process! We can directly influence how fast sand falls through our hourglass. As teachers, coaches, and parents, we have the wonderful opportunity to shovel "sand" into people's "hourglasses." We also have the opportunity and the obligation to help them develop a "lifestyle filter" that will slow the rate at which sand falls to the bottoms of their hourglasses.

It should be noted that sand can still be added to one's hourglass even when it is overturned and the sand is falling to the bottom. Each of us has *lifelong opportunities for learning.* By taking advantage of the numerous opportunities that exist for continued development and an active way of life, we can continually add sand to our hourglass. Unfortunately, we cannot add sand faster than it disappears, therefore claiming immortality. We can, however, have a definite impact on our longevity and the quality of our years on earth by taking advantage of lifelong opportunities for learning and active involvement.

SUMMARY

The development of movement abilities is an extensive process beginning with the early reflexive movements of the newborn and culminating with the refined specialized movements of the adolescent and adult. The process by which an individual progresses from the reflexive movement phase, through the rudimentary and fundamental movement phases, and, finally, to the specialized movements skill phase of development is influenced by both hereditary and environmental factors.

Reflexes and rudimentary movement abilities are largely maturationally based. They appear and disappear in a fairly rigid sequence deviating only in the rate of their appearance. They do, however, form an important base upon which fundamental movement abilities are developed.

Fundamental movement patterns that begin developing around the same time that the child is able to walk independently and move freely through his or her environment. These basic locomotor, manipulative, and stability abilities go through a definite, observable process from immaturity to maturity. A variety of stages within this phase have been identified for a number of fundamental movements; these are initial, elementary, and mature stages. Attainment of the mature level is influenced greatly by opportunities for practice, encouragement, and instruction. All indications are that, given the proper environment, children are capable of performing at the mature stage in the vast majority of fundamental movement abilities by age six. Therefore, the elementary school years may be more properly viewed as a time for fundamental skill refinement rather than for skill acquisition. The fundamental movement abilities of children entering school are too often incompletely developed. So, the primary grades offer an excellent opportunity to develop fundamental movement abilities to their mature level. It is these same fundamental skills that will be elaborated on and refined to form the sport skill abilities so highly valued by our society.

The specialized movement skill phase of development is in essence an elaboration of the fundamental phase. Specialized skills are more precise than fundamental skills. They often involve a combination of fundamental movement abilities and require a greater degree of exactness in performance. Specialized skills have three related stages. The transition stage is typically the level of the girl or boy in grades three through five. At this level, children are involved in their first real application of fundamental movements to sport. If the fundamental abilities used in the particular sport activity are not at the mature level, the child will have to resort to the use of less mature or elementary patterns of movement. It should be obvious that involving children in sport skill refinement prior to achieving a mature level of ability in prerequisite fundamentals is unwise. When this happens, the immature movements found in the basic patterns are carried over to those related sport skills. The child will in fact regress to his or her characteristic pattern. It is important that sensitive teaching and coaching be incorporated at this point. Today, children are often not completely ready motorically when they are thrust into youth sport activities. If these activities are to be of any real benefit to children, the teacher/coach must ensure that the mature fundamental movement pattern is completely developed and that the transition to the sport skill is based on sound teaching and coaching. In defense of this point of view Wickstrom (1983) has stated:

> The major consequences of accelerated progression into sport skills should be considered carefully. If immature movements become a permanent part of a sport skill pattern, premature encounter with the sport is undesirable. However, if immature movements become modified positively by encouragement and the challenge of the more difficult task, the eventual result is beneficial to motor skill development. The question of when to move on to more difficult tasks is an important one with the fate of optimal motor development possibly being in the balance. Unfortunately, a patent answer to the question does not exist. (p. 13)

When we look at the process of motor development we need to look at it first from a theoretical perceptive. Each of us needs to have a theoretical framework to use as the basis for our actions. It is not important that you agree with the theoretical framework presented here. The hourglass model is simply my way of viewing the process of motor development and its implications for life. What is your theoretical framework? How does it influence your teaching/coaching/parenting, and how does it influence you personally?

CHAPTER CONCEPTS

3.1 Few comprehensive theories of motor development exist.

3.2 A theoretical model of motor development should integrate existing facts and stimulate the generation of new facts.

3.3 Development of theoretical models can use inductive or deductive approaches to theory formulation.

3.4 The Phases of Motor Development utilize a deductive means of theory formulation.

3.5 The human organism progresses from simple to the complex and moves from general to specific in the development of movement abilities.

3.6 Four phases of motor development, each containing two or three stages, comprise the hierarchical sequence of motor development.

3.7 Each successfully completed phase and stage of development leads to higher levels of functioning.

3.8 Difficulty in the performance of a specific skill at one stage of development will result in difficulty or inability in progressing to subsequent stages.

3.9 Individuals are often at different stages of development within tasks and between tasks.

3.10 The interaction of a variety of factors with the phases and stages of motor development makes each individual's developmental schedule unique.

3.11 Opportunity for practice, encouragement, and instruction plays a key role in the individual's progress through the phases of motor development.

3.12 Motor development does not cease with the attainment of specialized movement abilities. It is a lifelong process of change affected by both biological and environmental factors.

3.13 The process of aging may be modified through control over one's "lifestyle filter" and by taking advantage of lifelong opportunities for learning.

TERMS TO REMEMBER

Descriptive Theory
Explanatory Theory
Inductive Method
Deductive Method
Stability
Locomotor Movement
Manipulative Movement

Reflexes
Primitive Reflexes
Postural Reflexes
Information Encoding Stage
Information Decoding Stage
Rudimentary Movement Phase
Reflex Inhibition Stage

Precontrol Stage
Fundamental Movement Phase
Initial Stage
Elementary Stage
Mature Stage
Specialized Movement Stage

Transitional Stage
Application Stage
Lifelong Utilization Stage
Hereditary Filter
Lifestyle Filter
Lifelong Opportunities for Learning

CRITICAL READINGS

Lerner, R. M. (1986). *Concepts and Theories in Human Development*. New York: Random House, (Chapter 1).

Roberton, M. A. and Halverson, L. E. (1984). *Developing Children—Their Changing Movement*. Philadelphia: Lea & Febiger, (Pages 1-16).

Seefeldt, V. and Haubenstricker, J. (1982). "Patterns, Phases, or Stages: An Analytic Model for the Study of Developmental Movement," In Kelso, J. A. S., and Clark, J. E. (eds.), *The Development of Movement Control and Coordination*. New York: Wiley.

4

Biological, Environmental, and Physical Factors Affecting Motor Development

CHAPTER COMPETENCIES

Upon Completion of This Chapter You Should Be Able To:

* *Identify genetic and environmental factors influencing growth and biological maturation.*

* *Derive principles of motor development and apply these principles to teaching/learning situations at various points in the life span.*

* *Describe "catch-up" growth and developmental plasticity and the factors affecting each.*

* *Analyze relationships among growth, biological maturation, and physiological changes in motor skill development.*

* *Discuss the effects of environmental deprivation on life span motor development.*

* *Discuss the effects of enrichment, special practice, and teaching on life span motor development.*

* *Define and discuss the concepts of critical and sensitive periods, phylogenetic and ontogenetic skills, and co-twin control.*

* *Identify and order from simple to complex the environmental variables that may influence developmental levels.*

• *Explain the similarities and differences between bonding and imprinting.*

- *Hypothesize about the impact of temperament on the interactive process of development.*

- *Describe differences and similarities implied by the terms "low birth weight" and "young-for-date."*

- *Discuss the long-term effects of prematurity.*

- *Analyze the collective impact of eating disorders, fitness levels, and mechanical laws on motor development.*

The process of motor development is influenced by a number of biological and environmental factors operating both in isolation from and in combination with one another. The individual is the product of the interaction of these factors. Both the process and product of one's movement and physical performance are rooted in his or her unique genetic and experiential background. Any study of motor development would be incomplete without a discussion of several of these influencing factors. This chapter focuses on biological, environmental, and other associated factors that impact on the process of motor development.

BIOLOGICAL FACTORS

The unique genetic inheritance that accounts for our individuality can also account for our similarity in many ways. One of these similarities is the trend for human development to proceed in an orderly, predictable fashion. A number of biological factors affecting motor development seem to emerge from this predictable pattern of development.

Developmental Direction

Developmental direction refers to the orderly, predictable sequence of physical development that proceeds from the head to the feet *cephalocaudal* and from the center of the body to its periphery *proximodistal*.

The cephalocaudal aspect of development refers specifically to the gradual progression of increased control over the musculature, moving from the head to the feet. It may be witnessed in the prenatal stages of fetal development as well as in later postnatal development. In the developing fetus, for example, the head forms first, and the arms form prior to the legs. Likewise, infants exhibit sequential control over the musculature of the head, neck, and trunk, prior to gaining control over the legs. Young children are often thought to be clumsy and to exhibit poor control over the lower extremities. This may be due to incomplete cephalo-caudal development.

The second aspect of developmental direction, known as proximodistal development, refers specifically to the child's progression in control of the musculature from the center of the body to its most distant parts. As with cephalocaudal development, the proximodistal concept of development applies to both growth processes and the acquisition of movement skills. In regard to growth, the trunk and shoulder girdle grow prior to arms and legs, which grow prior to the fingers and toes. In terms of skill acquisition, the young child is able to control the muscles of the trunk and shoulder girdle prior to gaining control over the muscles of the wrist, hand, and fingers. This principle of development is utilized by teachers of primary grade children in the teaching of the less refined elements of manuscript writing prior to the introduction of the more complex and refined movements of cursive writing.

The cephalocaudal and proximodistal process is operational throughout life and has a tendency to reverse itself as one ages. Payne and Isaacs (1987, pp. 10-11), note: "The most currently acquired movements of the lower body or periphery will be the first to exhibit signs of regression. The process of movement regression slowly evolves in a 'tail-to-head' and 'outside-in' direction." Such regression, however, can be forestalled and reduced through an active way of life throughout the entire life cycle.

Rate of Growth

One's *growth rate* follows a characteristic pattern that is universal and resistant to external influence. Even the interruption of the normal pace of growth is compensated for by a still-unexplained self-regulatory process that comes into operation to help the child catch up to his or her age-mates. For example, although severe illness may retard a child's height and weight gain and movement ability, there will be a tendency to catch up with the other children on recovery from the illness. The same phenomenon is seen with the low-birth-weight infant. Despite this low birth weight, there is still a tendency to catch up to the characteristic growth rate of one's age-mates in a few years. Therefore, measures of height, weight, and motor development taken prior to age 2 are generally meaningless for predicting later growth and development.

The self-regulatory process of growth will compensate for minor deviations in the growth pattern, but it is unable to remedy major deviations such as those in the low-birth-weight infant weighing under 3½ pounds. In this case the child often suffers permanent deficits in height, weight, and cognitive and motor abilities and is unable to completely recoup these initial losses.

Restricted opportunity for movement and deprivation of experience have been repeatedly shown to interfere with children's abilities to perform movement tasks that are characteristic of their particular age level. The effects of this deprivation of sensory and motor experience can sometimes be overcome when nearly optimal conditions are established for a child (McGraw, 1939a). The extent to which the child will be able to catch up to his or her peers, however, depends on the duration and severity of deprivation and the age of the child.

Differentiation and Integration

The coordinated and progressive intricate interweaving of neural mechanisms of opposing muscle systems into an increasingly mature relationship is characteristic of the developing child's motor behavior. There are two related processes associated with this increase of functional complexity: differentiation and integration.

Differentiation is associated with the gradual progression from the gross globular (overall) movement patterns of infants to the more refined and functional movements of children and adolescents as they mature.

For example, the manipulative behaviors of the newborn in terms of reaching, grasping, and releasing objects is quite poor. There is little control of movement, but control improves as the child develops and begins to differentiate between various muscle groups. With practice, control improves further until we see precise movements such as those involved in cursive writing, cutting with scissors, block building, and violin playing.

Integration refers to bringing various opposing muscle and sensory systems into coordinated interaction with one another. The young child, for example, progresses gradually from ill-defined corralling movements when attempting to grasp an object to more mature and visually guided reaching and grasping behaviors. This differentiation of movements of the arms, hands, and fingers, followed by integration of the use of the eyes with the movements of the hand to perform eye-hand coordination tasks, is crucial to normal development.

Differentiation and integration tend to be reversible with aging. As one ages and movement abilities begin to regress, the coordinated interaction of sensory and motor mechanisims become inhibited. The extent to which one's coordinated movement abilities regress is determined not merely as a function of age, but is influenced greatly by activity levels and one's attitude toward the aging process.

There is little doubt that differentiation and integration operate simultaneously. The complex abilities of the adult cannot be explained merely in terms of a process of integration of simpler responses. What occurs, instead, is a constant interlacing of both differentiation and integration. The term *reciprocal interweaving* is sometimes used to describe this ever-expanding tapestry of movement behavior.

Readiness

Thorndike, the "grandfather" of learning theory, first proposed the principle of readiness primarily in reference to emotional responses to actions or expected actions. According to his concept, readiness was dependent on the biological maturation model which was popular at the turn of the century. Today's concept of readiness, however, is much broader and refers to readiness for learning. *Readiness* may be defined as conditions within the individual and the environment that make a particular task an appropriate one for an individual to master. The concept of readiness, as used today, extends beyond biological maturation and includes consideration of environmental factors that can be modified or manipulated to encourage or promote learning. There are, therefore, several related factors that, in combination, promote readiness: physical and mental maturation, interacting with motivation, prerequisite learnings, and an enriching environment. At this juncture, we do not know how to determine when one is ready to learn a new movement skill. Research suggests, however, that experience in a movement activity before the individual is ready is likely to have minimal benefits (Magill, 1982).

In recent years, a great deal of attention has been focused on the concept of developing reading readiness in accordance with the types of experiences in which preschool and primary grade children should be involved. Entire educational programs have been built around the notion that children must achieve a certain level of development before they are ready to pursue intellectual tasks such as reading and writing. Readiness training is a part of many preschool and primary grade educational programs. An integral part of these readiness programs has been the use of movement as a means of enhancing basic perceptual-motor qualities (See Chapter 13). The remedial and readiness programs of Frostig (1969), Getman (1952), Kephart (1971) and others have been used to prepare children for learning. Each of these programs use movement as an integral part of readiness training. Although it has not been documented that the inclusion of these perceptual-motor experiences have a direct effect on the attainment of specific skills necessary for success in school, it is safe to assume that they at least have an indirect influence through enhancement of the child's self-esteem and the development of a more positive "I can" attitude. The concept of readiness as it is used today, whether for the learning of cognitive skills or motor skills, is probably best summed up in Bruner's (1965, p. 12) statement that "the foundation of any subject may be taught to anybody at any age in some form." In other words, the burden of being ready is as much the adult's responsibility as the child's. Readiness is a combination of maturational ripeness, environmental openness, and teacher sensitivity.

Critical Learning Periods

The concept of *critical learning periods* is closely aligned with readiness and revolves around the observation that there are certain time frames during which an individual is more sensitive to certain kinds of stimulation. Normal development in later periods may be hindered if the child fails to receive the proper stimulation during a critical period. For example, inadequate nutrition, prolonged stress, inconsistent mothering, or a lack of appropriate learning experiences may have a more negative impact on development if introduced early in life rather than at a later age. The concept of critical periods also has a positive side. It suggests that appropriate intervention during a specific period of time tends to facilitate more positive forms of development at later stages than if the same intervention occurs later.

One should recognize that the trend of the child to follow a critical period pattern is closely linked to the theory of developmental tasks and to a lesser degree linked to the milestone and age-stage views. Havighurst's (1972) theoretical framework of development is actually a critical period hypothesis applied from the perspective of education.

The notion of critical periods of development has been so pervasive in education that an entirely new federally funded educational program was instituted based on this premise. Operation Head Start, begun in the 1960s, viewed the age period of 3 to 5 as critical to children's intellectual development. It was hypothesized that if given a "head start" through a carefully structured environment designed to develop school-oriented skills, deprived children would be able to begin school on a level closer to that of their nondeprived counterparts. The results of Head Start programs did not entirely substantiate the critical period hypothesis. This was probably due to the existence of more than one critical period for intellectual development. In addition, the age period of 3 to 5 may not be as critical as originally assumed. Current views of the critical period hypothesis reject the notion that there are highly specific time frames in which one must develop motor skills (Seefeldt, 1975). There are, however, broad periods during which development of certain skills is most easily accomplished.

It is safe to assume that there are *sensitive periods* or broad time frames for development. The point is that care should be taken that critical or sensitive periods not be too narrowly defined. Failure to account for individual differences and for special environmental circumstances will lead to the conclusion that a sensitive period is a universal point in time that may be described in terms of weeks, months, or a few years. Instead, a notion of sensitive periods as broad, general guidelines susceptible to modification should be adopted and adhered to.

Individual Differences

The tendency to exhibit *individual differences* is crucial. Each person is a unique individual with his or her own timetable for development. This timetable is a combination of a particular individual's heredity and environmental influences, and although the sequence of appearance of developmental characteristics is predictable, the rate of appearance may be quite variable. Although development is age-related, it is not age-dependent. Therefore, strict adherence to a chronological classification of development by age is without support or justification.

The average ages for the acquisition of all sorts of developmental tasks, ranging from learning how to walk (the major developmental task of infancy) to gaining bowel and bladder control (the first restrictions of a civilized society on the child) have been bandied about in the professional literature and the daily conversation of parents and teachers for years. It must be remembered that these average ages are just that and nothing more. They are merely approximations meant to serve as convenient indicators of developmentally appropriate behaviors. It is common to see deviations from the mean of as much as six months to one year in the appearance of numerous movement skills. The tendency to exhibit individual differences is closely linked to the concept of readiness and helps explain why some individuals are ready to learn new skills when others are not.

Phylogeny and Ontogeny

Many of the rudimentary abilities of the infant and the fundamental movement abilities of the young child are considered to be phylogenetic. That is, they tend to appear automatically and in a predictable sequence within the maturing child. *Phylogenetic skills* are resistant to external environmental influences. Such abilities as the rudimentary manipulative tasks of reaching, grasping, and releasing objects; the stability tasks of gaining control of the gross musculature of the body; and the fundamental locomotor abilities of walking, jumping, and running are examples of phylogenetic skills. *Ontogenetic skills*, on the other hand, are those that depend primarily on learning and environmental opportunities. Such skills as swimming, bicycling, and ice-skating are ontogenetic because they do not appear automatically within individuals but require a period of practice and experience and are influenced by one's culture. The entire concept of phylogeny and ontogeny needs to be reevaluated in light of the fact that many skills heretofore considered phylogenetic can be influenced by environmental interaction (Bower et al. 1970; Bower, 1974).

Although there may be a biological tendency for the development of certain abilities due to phylogenetic processes, it is ludicrous to assume that maturation alone will account for motor development. The extent or level to which any voluntary movement ability is mastered depends, in part, on ontogeny or the environment. In other words, practice, instruction, and encouragement contribute significantly to movement skill development, particularly beyond the rudimentary movement phase. There seems to be little solid support for the notion that ontogeny recapitulates phylogeny, although some phylogenetic behaviors are present in humankind (Santrock and Yussen, 1987).

ENVIRONMENTAL FACTORS

Over the past several years there has been considerable speculation and research on the effects of parenting behaviors during infancy and early childhood as they influence the subsequent functioning of the child. Because of the extreme dependence of the human infant on its caregivers and because of the length of this period of dependence, a variety of parental care factors have been shown to influence later development. Among the most crucial are the effects of environmental stimulation and deprivation, the temperament of the child, and the bonding that occurs between parent and child during the early days of life.

Bonding

The study of parent-to-infant attachment, or *bonding* has its roots in the imprinting studies conducted by Lorenz (1952), Hess (1959), and others on birds, ducks, and other animals. Basically, these experiments with animals revealed that the degree to which the newborn would imprint on its mother was directly related to their contact time. This critical period for *imprinting* animals has been shown to be very short. Klopper et al. (1964), for example, has shown that separation of a mother goat from her kid right after birth for little more than an hour will result in the mother's refusal to accept or nurse it.

Although human infants do not imprint in the narrow sense of the word as animals do, there is compelling evidence that there is a sensitive period in which parent-to-infant attachment occurs. If this sensitive period is missed, the parent and child may fail to bond. This may result in later developmental difficulties, particularly in the affective development of the child.

In their excellent review of bonding, Kennell et al. (1979, p. 786) stated:

> Perhaps the parent's attachment to a child is the strongest bond in the human species. The power of this attachment is so great that it enables the mother and father to make the unusual sacrifices necessary for the care of the infant. Early in life the infant becomes attached to one individual, most often it is the mother. The original mother-infant bond is the wellspring for all the infant's subsequent attachments and is the relationship through which the child develops a sense of himself.

The effects of long-term maternal separation on the motor, cognitive, and emotional aspects of the infant's development have been documented by Spitz (1945), Bolby (1958), and A. Freud (1965) on children evacuated from London during World War II. The results of these investigations, according to Kennell et al. (1979, p. 786) "have dramatically altered infant care throughout the world."

Bonding, in essence, is a strong emotional attachment that endures over time, distance, hardship, and desirability. Recent research has shown that this emotional bond begins developing at birth and can fail to develop or be incompletely established with early separation (Kennell et al. 1974; Leifer et al. 1972; Robson, 1967; Winters, 1973). The leading factors contributing to initial separation are prematurity and low birth weight, which result in the incubation of the newborn; mild or severe neonatal problems at birth; and standard hospital operating procedures. Fortunately, the trend is now in favor of promoting early parental contact. Fathers are routinely permitted in the labor and delivery rooms and allowed to take a role in the child-bearing process. Rooming-in is on the increase in many maternity hospitals. Breastfeeding has gained renewed acceptance, and home births are on the rise. Giving birth at home—not always a recommended procedure—is dramatically different from the usual hospital routine. In the home birth, the mother is clearly in command. Instead of being a passive patient, she is an active participant in the birthing process, along with her husband and the midwife.

Early attachment between parent and child appears to influence development. One must question, however, whether or not bonding is *essential* to the welfare of the child. Generations of adopted children will attest to the success of their development even though bonding with mother was delayed by weeks, months, or even years. The reciprocal interaction between parent and child creates a mutually satisfying and rewarding relationship whose importance cannot be minimized. Care must be taken, however, not to define the concept of bonding too narrowly or to overemphasize its importance (Santrock and Yussen, 1987). Further research is necessary to clearly establish its link to the process of development. The reader is referred to the excellent discussion on infant-mother attachment by Lamb et al. (1985).

Stimulation and Deprivation

A great deal of study has been done over the years in an effort to determine the relative merits of *stimulation and deprivation* in the learning of a variety of skills. In fact, there has been considerable controversy among hereditarians and environmentalists over the issue during the past 100 years. Numerous textbooks have recorded the nature versus nurture debates, but little has been settled in the attempt to categorize the effects of each on development. The current trend has been to respect the individual importance of each and to recognize that the influences of both maturation and experience are complexly intertwined.

Students of motor development have recognized the futility of debating the separate merits of maturation and experience and have instead concentrated their research and study on three major questions. The first of these questions deals with the approximate ages at which various skills can be learned most effectively. The research of Bayley (1935), Shirley (1931), and Wellman (1937) in the 1930s represents the first serious attempts to describe the age at which many of the rudimentary and fundamental movement abilities appear. Each of these researchers reported a somewhat different timetable for the appearance of numerous phylogenetic skills. They did, however, show amazing consistency in the order of appearance of these abilities. This factor illustrates the combined effect of both intrinsic, or maturationally determined, influences on behavior and extrinsic, or environmentally influenced, behaviors. Unfortunately, until recently, little has been done to more clearly ascertain the ages at which both phylogenetic and ontogenetic skills can be learned most effectively. The principle of readiness has been viewed as a cornerstone of our educational system, but little more than lip service has been paid to its importance, particularly with regard to developing movement abilities. We know that children can develop many movement abilities early in life, but we still do not know the best time to introduce specific skills. Only recently has this important question come under serious study. The excellent work being done at many colleges and universities represents a first step in answering many of the important questions concerning the age at which fundamental movement patterns can be effectively developed and refined in young children.

The second question being studied deals with the effects of special training on the learning of motor skills. A number of co-twin control studies have been conducted in an effort to ascertain the influence of special practice on early learning. The use of identical twins enables the researcher to ensure identical hereditary backgrounds and characteristics of the subjects. One twin is given advanced opportunities for practice, while the other is restricted from practicing the same skills over a prescribed length of time. The famous studies of Gesell and Thompson (1929), Hilgard (1932), and McGraw (1935) have all demonstrated the inability of early training to hasten development to an appreciable degree. It is important, however, to note that follow-up studies of the co-twin control experiments of both Gesell and McGraw showed that the trained subjects exhibited greater confidence and assurance in the activities in which they had received special training. In other words, special attention and training may not have an influence on the quantity or rate of onset of the movement skills learned, but it may have an effect on the quality of performance of specific skills. Again, we see the complex interrelationship between maturation and experience.

Investigations by Gerber and Dean (1957) recorded the advanced development in Ugandan infants during the first days and months of life. The investigators concluded that the infants' motor superiority over infants raised in the United States was due, in part, to the enriched environmental stimulation that they received. They were carried on their mothers' backs much of the time, were fed on demand, and were constantly the center of attention and affection. But their advanced state at birth (that is, ability to hold head erect, early disappearance of certain reflexes, and so forth) suggests that a genetic factor may also have been the cause of their developmental superiority. Again, we see the interrelatedness of maturation and experience.

With the advent of neonatal intensive care units in the 1970s the survival rate for preterm and low-birth-weight infants has risen dramatically. Of major concern to parents, physicians, and researchers has been the question of the effects of infant stimulation programs on the subsequent development of these high-risk infants. Ulrich (1984, p. 68) in her comprehensive review of the research concluded that:

> Despite difficulties in comparing studies due to the variability of subjects used, and type, intensity, and duration of treatment, the overwhelming evidence indicates beneficial effects.

Such a conclusion is encouraging and leads one to consider, in light of the forgoing discussion, the importance of timing and duration of special training or stimulation. In other words, is there a sensitive period beyond which the benefits of stimulation are minimally beneficial?

The third question being studied is the effect of limited or restricted opportunities for practice on the acquisition of motor skills. Studies of this nature have generally centered on experimentally induced environmental deprivation in animals. Only a few studies have been reported in which children have actually been observed in environments where unusual restrictions of movement or experience have existed.

An investigation conducted by Dennis (1960) examined infants reared at three separate institutions in Iran. The infants in two of the institutions were found to be severely retarded in their motor development. In the third there was little motor retardation. The discrepancy between institutions led Dennis to investigate the life-styles of the children in each institution. The results of his investigation led to the conclusion that lack of handling, blandness of surroundings, and general lack of movement opportunity or experience were causes of motor retardation in the two institutions. Another investigation by Dennis and Najarian (1957) revealed similar findings in a smaller number of crèche infants reared in Beirut, Lebanon. Both of these investigations lend support to the hypothesis that behavioral development cannot be fully accounted for by the maturation hypothesis.

Due to cultural mores, the humanistic virtues of most investigators, and concerned parents, there are few experiments in which the environmental circumstances of infants or young children have been intentionally altered in an attempt to determine whether serious malfunctioning or atypical behavior will result from these practices. The general consensus of the research that does exist is that severe restrictions and lack of experience can delay normal development. We need only to look as far as the school playground and observe the girls jumping rope expertly and the boys throwing and catching balls with great skill. When asked to reverse the activities, however, each tends to revert to less mature patterns of movement. Factors within our culture, unfortunately, often predetermine the types of movement experiences in which boys and girls engage.

Dennis (1935) conducted an investigation in which fraternal twin infant girls were reared in a very sterile nursery environment (that is, they were intentionally given a minimal amount of motor and social stimulation). After 14 months in this environment, their movement behavior was compared with normative data and was found to be retarded beyond the normal limits. Social development, however, was well within the limits of the standard norms, a factor that may suggest a greater need for motor stimulation than for social stimulation of the infant. This investigation, however, represents the only attempt at intentionally limiting the child's environment in order to study the possible consequences on development. Care should be taken in drawing any sweeping conclusions from a single investigation without collaborative support.

The child-rearing practices of the Hopi Indians were the subject of another investigation by Dennis (1940). These Indians have traditionally restricted their infants' movements by binding them to a cradle board that the mother carries on her back. The infants spend nearly all of their time bound in the cradle board for their first three months of life. As they grow older, the number and length of freedom periods is gradually increased. Dennis observed that the movement abilities of these children were not as retarded as expected when compared with the results of the investigations just mentioned. It may be beneficial to consider that motor activity is perhaps not of crucial importance during the first months of life. Being bound securely to the cradle board and feeling the rhythmical movements of the mother carrying the child may have simulated life in the womb. The close physical contact with the mother and an opportunity to begin utilizing perceptual modalities may have been crucial factors in these first months. One may also consider what the infant observed through his or her developing visual sense while bound to the cradle board. While on the board, the infant was generally on the mother's back in a position that permitted viewing of the many new and interesting sights that were going on all around. When not being carried about, the child was generally propped up by a nearby tree or in a corner and able to observe the mother going about her daily chores. In other words, the visual and motor stimulation of the Hopi Indian infants was of considerably higher quality than the sterile environments of the Iranian and Lebanese infants and the two girls investigated by Dennis. This study may point up the close identification of the visual modality with the motor dimension of behavior. It leads one to consider the interrelatedness of perceptual and motor functions and the importance of enriching stimulation.

It becomes impossible to make a case for either maturation or learning as the sole or even primary influence on development. The literature is overwhelmingly in favor of the interaction of one with the other. This compromise view of development is summed up by Carmichael who, as early as 1925, recognized that "Heredity and environment are not antithetical, nor can they expediently be separated; for in all maturation there is learning: in all learning there is hereditary maturation" (p. 260).

Both maturation and learning play important roles in the acquisition of movement abilities. Although experience seems to have little influence on the sequence of their emergence, it does affect the time of appearance of certain movements and the extent of their development.

One of the greatest needs of children is the opportunity to practice skills at a time when they are developmentally ready to benefit the most from them. Special practice prior to maturational readiness is of dubious benefit. The key is to be able to accurately judge the time at which each individual is ripe for learning and then to provide a series of educationally sound and effective movement experiences. All indications are, however, that young children are generally capable of more than we have suspected, and that many of the traditional readiness signposts that we have used may actually be incorrect.

Temperament

Anyone who has been around young children for an extended period is quick to notice the differences in temperament (i.e., disposition) that exist. These individual differences in the responsiveness of children are probably caused by their unique environmental and experiential histories. It is interesting to note, however, that differences in temperament are observable even at birth. Persistent differences in newborns have been documented on a variety of physiological and perceptual-motor dimensions in newborns (Eisenberg, 1966). Differences in cardiac reactions and response intensity have also been observed, along with many other individual differences in reactions to environmental conditions (Lipton et al. 1961; Westman, 1973).

The temperaments of children have been classified in a number of ways. The method utilized by Chess and Thomas (1973) is a popular one. They classify children as (1) the easy child, (2) the difficult child, and (3) the slow-to-warm-up child. Chess and Thomas observed children longitudinally, using a parental report system of data collection. Infants divided into "cuddler" and "noncuddler" classifications exhibited a variety of differences when viewed over time. Noncuddlers were found to sit, stand, and crawl sooner than cuddlers. They were also found to sleep less and to protest more than those identified as cuddlers.

Recent research by Korner (Korner et al. 1975; Korner, 1981; Korner et al. 1982) has highlighted the beneficial effects of rhythmical rocking of babies. Korner's research has shown that premature babies placed on oscillating waterbeds are less irritable, more alert, and more responsive to the human face and voice. Such information may have important implications for premature infants who are routinely placed in an incubator and deprived of normal movement and tactile stimulation. The disorganized movements, fragmented sleep pattern, and excessive irritability of premature babies makes them difficult to care for and is a likely impact on the parent-child bonding and temperament triad. Rhythmical rocking may be an effective means to reduce these risks.

Although the research on the development of temperament is speculative, it seems safe to assume that because temperament tends to remain consistent from birth, it will have an effect on how parents respond to the child (Osofsky and Conners, 1979). The hyperactive child, the chronic crier, or the fussy child may be inadvertently adversely influencing the nurturing responses of his or her caregivers. The ill-tempered child may receive less attention than the even-tempered child and, as a consequence, may be slower to talk and slower to develop mature movement and socialization skills. The epidemic proportions of child battering in our culture may be attributable, in part, to the interaction between the ill-tempered child and the parent who in stressful situations is unable to cope with such a child.

PHYSICAL FACTORS

A number of additional factors have been shown to have an impact on motor development. The influence of culture (Malina, 1980), gender (Branta et al. 1987), birth order (McGillicuddy-Delisi and Sigel, 1982), and ethnic and cultural background (Bril, 1985) have all been shown to have an impact on motor development. Motor development is not a static process. It is not only the product of biological factors but is also influenced by environmental conditions and physical laws. The interaction of both environmental and biological factors modifies the course of motor development during infancy, childhood, adolescence, and adulthood. Premature birth, eating disorders, fitness levels and biomechanical factors all impact in important ways on the lifelong process of motor development.

Prematurity

The normal birth weight of an infant is about 3,300 g (about 7 lb). Formerly, any infant weighing under 2,500 g (about 5½ lb) was classified as premature. Today, however, 2,000g (4½ lb) is often used, unless there is evidence that the gestation period was less than 37 weeks. The practice of labeling a newborn premature based on gestation period or weight alone is for two reasons no longer used. First, it is often difficult to accurately determine the gestational age of the infant, and second, the highest mortality and morbidity rates are present for infants of the very lowest birth weight (Susser et al. 1972). As a result the terms low birth weight and young-for-date have emerged as more accurate indicators of prematurity in the true sense of the word (Kopp and Parmelee, 1979). Prematurity is of major concern because it is closely associated with physical and mental retardation, hyperactivity and infant death. Prevention is generally considered to be the most important factor in improving infant health and survival rates.

Low-birth-weight. Infants whose birth weight is clearly below the expected weight for their gestational age are called low-birth-weight infants. Two standard deviations below the mean for a given gestational age is the generally accepted criterion for low birth weight. (Ounsted and Ounsted, 1973). Therefore, a low-birth-weight infant may be one who is born at term (40 weeks) or preterm (37 weeks or under). Low-birth-weight infants have experienced what Warkany et al. (1961) first termed as "intrauterine growth retardation" and are generally called "small-for-dates."

A variety of prenatal maternal factors have been implicated in low birth weight, including diet, drugs, smoking, infections, and disease (Santrock and Yussen 1987). Other factors such as social class, multiple births, and geographic locale have been shown to influence birthweight (Seifert and Hoffnung, 1987). The long-term effects of low-birth-weight are directly related to the degree of intrauterine growth retardation and gestational age of the child. Kopp and Parmelee (1979, p.59) have stated:

> In summary, it is clear that the infant born with intrauterine growth retardation may have severe medical problems in the neonatal period. Reflexive and behavioral differences may occur in early life, possibly leading to disrupted patterns of parent-infant interaction. The overall outcome for intellectual functioning is relatively positive, even for pre-terms who were small-for-date. Yet, inevitable questions arise. Would the intelligence of this group of children have been higher if they had not been malnourished in utero?

Young-for-date. Children born at the expected birth weight (less than 2 SD below the mean) for their gestational age but before full term (37 weeks or less) are called young-for-date, preterm infants. There is little agreement on the exact causes of preterm birth, but a number of factors have been shown to contribute to its likelihood. Factors such as drug use, smoking, maternal age, excessive weight gain, and adverse social and economic conditions have been shown to contribute to the incidence of young-for-date births (Susser et al. 1972). Until recent years the prognosis for young-for-date infants who were either small-for-date or of normal weight for date was bleak. Their morbidity and mortality rates were abnormally high. Drillien (1970) reported that as many as 40 percent showed evidence of neurological and intellectual damage. Recent advances in neonatal intensive care have, however, done much to reduce this unusually high rate of difficulties.

The preterm infant is still likely to have more learning difficulties, language and social interaction problems, and motor coordination problems than his or her full-term counterpart (Davies and Stewart, 1975). For some unknown reason, boys seem to be more severely affected than girls. The usual treatment of hospital-born premature infants is to put them in a sterile isolette, where temperature, humidity, and oxygen can be precisely controlled. It has been suggested that the absence of normal stimulation from the mother and the surrounding environment contributes to the retardation (Hasselmeyer, 1964). A study by Solkoff et al.

(1969), although tentative, seems to verify this notion. The results of the two-treatment-group study of premature infants in which one group was given routine care and the other was given five extra minutes of handling per hour seem to support the need for early handling. The extra handling group performed better on two measures. The infants were more active and gained weight faster. Seven months later the handled group still performed better on tests of motor performance and appeared more active and healthier.

The long-term effects of prematurity has been a topic of debate. The data are clear that low-birth-weight babies are more likely to die in the first few weeks of life than are normal weight babies. Tremendous strides have been made, however, in reducing their mortality rate. Table 4.1 demonstrates a clearly positive trend since 1960. Still, statistics such as those presented in Table 4.2 reflect that the United States and several other developed countries have a long way to go in the reduction of infant mortality.

The long-term effects of premature birth are not as clear as are the short-term consequences. Both Lubchenco (et al. 1963) and Drillien (1964), however, found that children who were very small at birth (under 3½ lb) tended to weigh less and were shorter than their age-mates. Low-birth-weight children also tend to be delayed in language development (Crawford, 1982, Richman, 1980), and have more visual-motor problems in school (Drillien et al. 1980; Rubin et al. 1973); however, no conclusive data are available regarding the effects of prematurity on later intelligence.

Eating Disorders

We are living today in a world far different from that of our ancestors. Vigorous physical exertion is not a necessary part of the daily life

Table 4.1 Trends in Survival and Degree of Impairment of Low-Birth-weight Infants*

	Low-Birth-weight			Very Low-Birth-weight (under 3½ lb)		
	1960	1970-75	1976	1960	1971-75	1976
Percent Died	72	54	33	92	80.5	50
Percent Severely Abnormal	6.7	4.5	7.6	2.3	2.8	5.7
Percent Moderately Abnormal	14	23.5	10.5	4.0	3.2	7.3
Percent Normal	7.2	17.8	48.6	1.7	13.5	36.5

*Adapted from: Rosenblith, J. F., and Sims-Knight, J. E. (1985). *In the Beginning: Development in the First Two Years.* Monterey, CA: Brooks/Cole.

Table 4.2 Worldwide Infant Mortality

A baby born in the United States is nearly twice as likely to die before its first birthday than one born in Finland. Deaths before age 1 per 1,000 live births:

 1. Finland 6.0
 2. Japan 6.2
 3. Sweden 7.0
 4. Switzerland 7.7
 5. Norway 7.8
 6. Denmark 8.2
 7. Netherlands 8.4
 8. France 9.0
 9. Canada 9.1
10. Belgium... 9.2
11. Spain 9.6
12. West Germany 10.1
13. United Kingdom 10.1
14. Australia... 10.3
15. Ireland... 10.5
16. USA 10.5
17. East Germany 10.7

Source: World Population Data Sheet (1985). Population Reference Bureau.

pattern of most people. Today, most exercise, if it occurs, is planned and is not an integral part of one's existence. In addition to a reduction in the exercise required in our daily lives, we also enjoy, for the present, an abundance of available food. Thus it is possible for an individual to consume a large amount of food while using up little of the energy contained in that food. The maintenance of body weight is relatively simple. It requires maintaining a balance between the number of calories taken into the body in the form of food and the number of calories burned through exercise and other daily activities. If more calories are consumed than are burned over a period of time, obesity is the eventual result.

Obesity. Fat has a number of constructive functions. It is a reserve source of energy; it is a vehicle for fat-soluble vitamins; it provides protection and support for the body parts, insulating the body from the cold; and in proper proportion, it enhances the appearance of the body. To serve these functions, however, the proportion of fat desired in individuals is about 15 percent for males and 22.5 percent for females. The full-term infant has about 16 percent fat, much of which develops during the last two months of the gestation period (Documenta, 1970). Ideally, there is very little change in the percentage of body fat in proportion to total body weight from birth to adulthood. The percentage of body fat, however, may range from a low of about 8 percent (typical of the long-distance, ectomorphic-built, runner) to as high as 50 percent (characteristic of the very obese). It is estimated that there are more than 70 million overweight Americans (Wimore, 1974). In North America the percentage of lean body mass decreases with age and the percentage of body fat is the most important determiner of obesity. A person's weight is less crucial than how much fat compared to lean body mass constitutes his or her body. Body composition is the only valid criterion for determining obesity.

Obesity places additional stress on the circulatory, respiratory, and metabolic systems and may cause, or intensify, disorders in these systems. The mortality rate for obese men and women is higher than for their non-obese counterparts. Several investigations have shown a strong correlation between obesity and the onset of diabetes. In addition, obese individuals, particularly children and adolescents, often suffer ridicule from their peers and discrimination by adults.

The primary causes of obesity in individuals with normal hormonal balances are excessive eating and lack of exercise, or a combination of both, which often results in a vicious cycle of poor eating and exercise habits being formed and carred into adult life. The child who is urged to clean the plate at every meal, yet who is not encouraged to exercise regularly, has the potential for a serious weight problem.

An area of interest to many who study obesity is the activity levels of obese children. A study by Bruch (1940) examined 160 obese children. It was found that 76 percent of the boys and 88 percent of the girls were rated inactive when compared to normal youngsters. Further studies by M. L. Johnson and his colleagues (1956) compared the caloric intake and activity of normal and obese girls. It was found that the obese girls spend less than half as much time at physical activity as the nonobese group. In fact, excessive television watching has been linked to obesity in children (Dietz, 1985; Groves, 1988). These studies indicate that dieting is not the complete, nor even the best, solution to obesity in children. In fact, since their food intake may be normal, dieting may cause serious deficiencies in the nutrients required for proper growth and health. Since a major cause of obesity in children is lack of activity, increases in this area may be the best and most healthful solution to the problem.

Studies show that obesity runs in families, due either to heredity or environmental factors. Mayer (1968) found that the chances of obesity are 10 percent for children with parents of normal weight, 40 percent if one parent is obese, and 70 percent if both parents are obese. Garn (1986) noted that parent-child and sibling correlations in fatness increase during the growing years. However, they tend to decrease as children move into adulthood and no longer live at home. This gives rise to strong speculative evidence that environmental factors play a key role in becoming obese. Again, the cause seems to be lack of regular vigorous activity rather than dietary excesses or hormonal imbalances.

Studies indicate that poor dietary and exercise patterns established early in life may increase the chances of obesity in adulthood due to an increase in the number of fat cells. Oscai (1973) has indicated that exercise in early life may reduce the number of fat cells formed by the body. The exercise habits developed during childhood may have a pronounced influence on the possible development of obesity in later life. Although hereditary, environmental, and nutritional factors play a role, regular, vigorous physical activity may be the most important variable in preventing obesity.

Figure 4.1 depicts the evolution of the typical fat cell. The primitive fat cell has an irregular shape, a central nucleus, and large amounts of cytoplasm surrounding the nucleus. In the first stage, droplets of fat appear mixed with the cytoplasm. In the second stage, these droplets grow. In the third stage, the fat droplets enlarge and finally merge into one large droplet, with the nucleus pushed to the top of the cell. The fat cell has become bloated with fat substances. It has become fat.

As a person becomes obese, the percentage of body fat increases by storing more and more fat substance in the fat cells. It is believed by many that fat cells are difficult to destroy. In theory, when a person loses weight, the amount of fat decreases but the number of fat cells remains constant. The fat cells become thin, but they remain in the body. This, along with differences in metabolic rates, may help explain why some people have great difficulty losing and keeping excess fat off while others have equal difficulty gaining weight. Kaufman (1975, p. 78) states that "there is strong evidence that if an individual is obese as a child, he has a 90 percent chance of being obese as an adult." However, a 16-year longitudinal study carried out by the school of public health at the University of California, Berkeley (1986) in which 185 individuals were tracked from 6 months to 16 years of age tends to dispel aspects of fat cell theory. The results of this study indicated that fat infants are at no greater risk of becoming obese children than are lean infants. However, the data did reveal that fat preschoolers are more likely to become fat teenagers than are lean preschoolers. A growing body of evidence (Stein et al. 1981) implicates obesity as a factor in the development of atherosclerosis and coronary heart disease.

Enos et al. (1955) and McNamera et al. (1971) autopsied teenage soldiers killed in Korea and Vietnam, respectively. The results of their postmortem investigations revealed that coronary and aortic atherosclerosis were present in no less than one third of the soldiers autopsied. One of the major suspected risk factors in the development of atherosclerosis

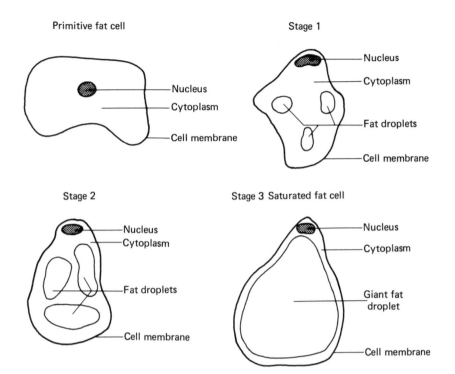

Figure 4.1 Evolution of a fat cell

and subsequent chronic heart disease is the early development of obesity (Stein et al. 1981). It is, however, not yet known whether limiting weight gain during childhood will have any long-term influence on adult weight gain and on reduction of the risk of chronic heart disease (Fisch et al. 1975).

Anorexia Nervosa/Bulimia. A problem as perplexing and potentially dangerous as obesity is *anorexia nervosa*, which is characterized by an aversion to the consumption of food and an obsession with being "too fat" even when clearly underweight. These self-starvers can lose 25 to 50 percent of their normal body weight in the pursuit of thinness. They start dieting and, although emaciated, continue to refuse food because they see themselves as fat. *Bulimia*, another severe eating disorder, is similar in terms of results to anorexia. The bulimic has the same need for thinness but uses a binge-purge process. Bulimics are known to eat enormous quantities of food prior to self-induced vomiting.

The incidence of anorexia nervosa and bulimia is on the rise. It is particularly prevalent among adolescent girls. Bruch (1986) contends that these disorders are increasing so much that probably every family doctor will sooner or later be confronted with an anorectic patient. About 10 percent of all cases of anorexia nervosa are fatal, and many others become chronic invalids (Rothenberg, 1976).

Characteristically, there is no true loss of appetite or awareness of hunger pains corresponding to the body's need for food. Some actually brainwash themselves into believing that the pain actually feels good. In about 25 percent of the cases, food refusal alternates with eating binges (bulimia). Anorectics become obsessed with the whole idea of food. They think about it, talk about it, collect recipes, and often force their family members to overeat (Bruch, 1986; *Physician and Sportsmedicine*, 1985).

In an effort to remove unwanted food from the body, many anorectics resort to self-induced vomiting, or excessive use of enemas, laxatives, and diuretics. All this may result in a serious disturbance of the body's electrolyte balance, which may play a role in cases that end in death (Minuchin et al. 1978).

Anorectics and bulimics usually pursue their goal of thinness not only through food restriction but through exhausting exercise. Many were interested in sports before the illness. Exercise then becomes a solitary activity, a way to burn off calories or show endurance. In spite of their weakness from extreme loss of weight, many display incredible energy and are hyperactive. Anorectics and bulimics drive themselves to unbelievable feats to demonstrate that they can live up to the ideal of mind over body (Bruch, 1986; *Physician and Sportsmedicine*, 1985).

Many anorectics do not want the curves and roundness associated with the developing adolescent body, and they are often terrified of dealing with sexual matters. By starving themselves, they can remain children forever with no menstrual periods or development of secondary sex characteristics.

Anorectics and bulimics are usually described as having been outstandingly good children. They were the pride and joy of their parents and teachers. Psychiatrists have come to recognize the overwhelming sense of ineffectiveness under which the victims operate. They camouflage their self-doubt with perfect, conforming behavior. The extreme control they exercise over their bodies provides them with a sense of accomplishment. Even a slight weight gain may result in depression and self-hatred.

The anorectic child often grows up in a family with highly enmeshed patterns, and close, interpersonal contact becomes important. Loyalty and protection are more valuable to the anorectic than autonomy and self-realization. The individual learns to subordinate the self. The expectation from learning a skill, for example, is not competence, but approval. The reward is love and not knowledge. The family of anorectic children are typically child-oriented. The child grows up protected by parents who over-focus on the child's well-being. Because the child sees family members focusing on his or her actions and commenting on them, an obsessive concern for perfection often develops. The anorectic is both extremely self-conscious and alert to other people's signals. Overinvolvement with the family often creates a developmental lag in dealing with the outside world (Minuchin et al. 1978). Some early warning signals of anorexia nervosa and bulimia are depicted in Table 4.3.

Society is partly to blame for the increase in anorexia nervosa and bulimia. The lean, slender form is glorified by the society in which we live. It propagates the idea that being thin symbolizes beauty, desirability, and self-control and that it is a magic key to a happier life. Educators may be among the first to recognize their eating disorders. They should be able to recognize the early stages of the illness while it is still reversible. Once it has lasted any length of time, it becomes exceedingly difficult to treat.

Fitness Levels

It has been stated repeatedly that the development of one's movement abilities does not occur in a vacuum. A wide variety of factors from all three domains of human behavior influence development. Factors within the psychomotor domain are termed "physical abilities." Physical

Table 4.3 Early Warning Signs of Anorexia Nervosa and Bulimia

Anorexia Nervosa	Bulimia
1. Overidentification with a doctor-prescribed weight-control program.	1. Eating binges
2. Obsession with dieting and talk of food.	2. Irregular weight loss
3. Social isolation accompanying slimness (loner).	3. Long periods in the bathroom after meals
4. No participation in the courting behavior of classmates.	4. Variable performance
5. Sudden increased involvement in athletics, usually of a solitary nature.	5. Loss of tooth enamel
6. Exaggerated concern with achieving high academic grades.	
7. Overconcern with weight.	
8. Failure to consume food, followed by food binges.	
9. Aversion to most foods.	
10. Obsessed with exercise.	

abilities are distinguished from movement abilities in that the health-related fitness and motor fitness components—which make up physical abilities—affect the performance level of one's locomotor, manipulative, and stability movements. Figure 4.2 illustrates this concept.

Health-Related Fitness. The physical development aspects of the motor domain may be divided into *health-related fitness* factors and performance-related fitness factors that influence performance in each of the four phases of motor development. These terms, however, are difficult to define to the mutual satisfaction of experts in the field. Health-related fitness is generally defined in broad terms because the level of fitness required of one individual may not be the same as that required of another. Hence, this form of physical fitness is generally considered to be the health-related aspect of one's existence that influences the ability to perform one's daily tasks at an acceptable level without undue stress. It is also a state in which ample reserves of energy are available for recreational pursuits and emergency needs. Muscular strength, muscular endurance, aerobic endurance, joint flexibility, and body composition are usually considered to be the components of health-related fitness. The extent to which each of these factors is possessed will influence the individual's performance capabilities in movement. For example, how far one can run or ride a bicycle is related to the individual's level of muscular strength and muscular endurance as well as to his or her aerobic endurance.

Motor Fitness. Motor fitness, or motor ability, as it is often erroneously termed, is the performance aspect of fitness. It is also an elusive concept that has been studied extensively over the past several years and is classified as being a part of the global concept of fitness. *Motor fitness* is generally thought of as one's performance capabilities as influenced by factors such as movement, speed, agility, balance, coordination, and power.

The generality and specificity of motor abilities have been debated and researched for years, with the bulk of research evidence in favor of its specificity (Henry, 1960; Henry and Rogers, 1960). For years many physical educators believed that motor abilities were general in nature; as a result, the term "general motor ability" came into vogue. It was assumed that because an individual excelled in a certain sport, corresponding ability would be automatically carried over to other activities. Although this often does occur, it is probably due to the individual's personal motivation, numerous activity experiences, and several specific sport aptitudes, not to the transfer or carryover of skills from one activity to another. One's motor fitness will have a definite effect on the performance of any movement activity that requires quick reactions, speed of

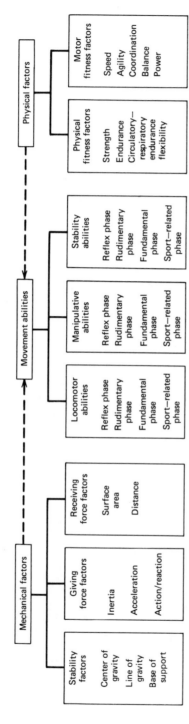

Figure 4.2. Physical and mechanical factors affect the development of movement abilities at all phases of motor development

movement, agility and coordination of movement, and explosive power and balance.

Biomechanics

Before embarking on a detailed discussion of motor development, it will be useful to review some mechanical principles of movement as they relate to stability, locomotion, and manipulation. There are numerous ways in which the human body is capable of moving. At first glance it may appear to be an impossible task to learn all of the skills that are involved in the performance of the numerous game, sport, and dance activities engaged in by children. Closer inspection of the total spectrum of movement will reveal, however, that there are fundamental mechanical laws affecting all human movement. The selected mechanical principles that follow serve as basic preparation for the chapters that follow.

Balance. All masses that are within the gravitational pull of the earth are subjected to the force of gravity. The three primary factors of concern in the study of balance principles are (1) center of gravity, (2) line of gravity, and (3) base of support.

A *center of gravity* exists within all objects. in geometric shapes it is located in the exact center of the object. In asymmetrical objects (e.g., our bodies) it is constantly changing during movement. The center of gravity of our bodies always shifts in the direction of the movement or the additional weight. The center of gravity of a child standing in an erect position is approximately at the top of the hips between the front and the back of the trunk. In activities in which the center of gravity remains in a stable position, as with standing on one foot or performing a headstand, we refer to them as "static balance activities." If the center of gravity is constantly shifting, as with jumping rope, walking, or doing a forward roll, we refer to the activities as "dynamic balance movements" (Figure 4.3).

The *line of gravity* is an imaginary line that extends vertically through the center of gravity to the center of the earth. The interrelationship of the center of gravity and the line of gravity to the base of support determines the degree of stability or instability of the body (Figure 4.4).

The *base of support* is the part of the body that comes into contact with the supporting surface. If the line of gravity falls within the base of support, the body will be in balance. If it falls outside the base, it is out of balance. The wider the base of support, the greater the stability, as can be seen when balancing on two feet as opposed to balancing on one foot. The nearer the base of support to the center of gravity, the greater the stability. This may be readily observed by attempting to push someone off

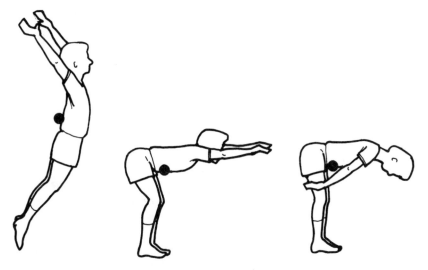

Figure 4.3. The center of gravity shifts as the body changes position

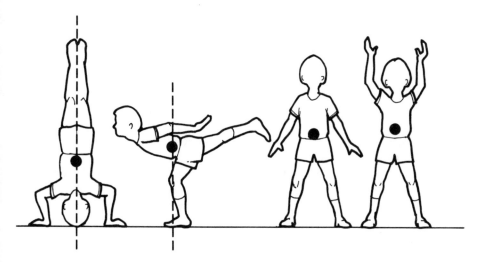

Figure 4.4. The body remains in balance when the center of gravity and line of gravity fall within the base of support

balance from an erect standing position and then repeating the act from the referee's position in wrestling or lineman's stance in football. The nearer the center of gravity to the center of the base of support the greater the stability. A foot position that allows a larger base of support in the direction of the movement gives additional stability. This principle is illustrated by the foot position of a runner who is attempting to stop or of a catcher who is trying to receive and control a heavy object.

Giving Force. *Force* is one of the basic concepts of movement and body mechanics. Force is the instigator of all movement and may be defined as the effort that one mass exerts on another. The result may be (1) movement, (2) cessation of movement, or (3) merely resistance of one body against another. There may be force without motion, as in isometric activities, but motion is impossible without some form of force being applied. Three forces relative to the human body are of concern to us: (1) force produced by muscles, (2) force produced by the gravitational pull of the earth, and (3) momentum. The entire science of force is based on Newton's three laws of motion, namely, the law of inertia, the law of acceleration, and the law of action and reaction.

The *law of inertia* states that a body at rest will remain at rest and a body in motion will remain in motion at the same speed in a straight line unless acted upon by an outside force. In other words, in order for movement to occur, a force must act upon a body sufficiently to overcome that object's inertia. If the applied force is less than the resistance offered by the object, motion will not occur. Large muscles can produce more force than small muscles, as seen in the amount of force generated by the legs as opposed to the arms. Once an object is in motion, it will take less force to maintain its speed and direction (i.e., momentum). This may be readily observed in snow skiing, in the swimming glide, or in rolling a ball. The heavier the object and the faster it moves, the more force is required to overcome its moving inertia or to absorb its momentum, as seen in catching a heavy object as opposed to catching a light object.

The *law of acceleration* states that the change in the velocity of an object is directly proportional to the force producing the velocity and inversely proportional to the object's mass. The heavier an object, the more force is needed to accelerate or decelerate it. This may be observed when throwing a heavy object (shot put) and a light object (softball) a given distance. An increase in speed is proportional to the amount of force applied. The greater the amount of force imparted to an object, the greater the speed at which the object will travel. If the same amount of force is exerted on two bodies with a different mass, greater acceleration will be produced on the lighter or less massive object. The heavier object will, however, have greater momentum once inertia is overcome and will exert a greater force than the lighter object on something that it contacts.

The *law of action and reaction* states that for every action there is an equal and opposite reaction. This principle of counterforce is the basis for all locomotion and may be observed by the depressions left behind while walking in sand. This principle applies to both linear and angular motion. Its application requires that adjustments be made by the individual to sustain the value of the primary forces in any movement. For example, the use of opposition in the running pattern counters the action of one part of the body with that of another.

Receiving Force. In order to stop a moving object body, we absorb the force over the greatest distance possible and with the largest surface area possible. The greater the distance over which the force is absorbed, the less the impact on the part of the body that receives the force. This may be demonstrated by attempting to catch a ball by keeping the arms straight out in front of the body and then repeating the task by bending the arms as the ball is being caught. The same thing may be observed in landing with the legs bent from a jump as opposed to landing with the legs straight. Forces should be absorbed over as large a surface area as possible. In this way the impact is reduced in proportion to the size of the surface area and the likelihood of injury is reduced. For example, keeping the arms extended and trying to absorb the shock of a fall with the hands will probably result in injury because the small surface area of the hand must receive the entire impact. It is far better to let as much of the body as possible absorb the impact.

The final direction of either a moving object or our bodies depends on the magnitude and the direction of all the forces that have been applied. Therefore, whenever we kick, strike, or throw an object, its accuracy and the distance traveled are dependent on the forces acting on it. If we are performing a vertical jump, we must work for a summation of forces in a vertical direction, whereas a good performance in the long jump requires a summation of horizontal and vertical forces so the takeoff is at the appropriate angle.

Separate discussion of the principles of balance, giving force, and receiving forces should not be interpreted that one is used in the absence of the others. Most of our movements combine all three. An element of balance is involved in almost all of our movements, and we both give force to the body and receive force from the body whenever we perform any locomotor or manipulative movement. A gymnast, for example, must maintain his or her equilibrium when performing a tumbling trick such as a front flip, and also must absorb force from the body (on the landing). A handball player must move to a position of readiness (giving to and receiving force from the body), contact the ball (giving force to an object), and maintain balance throughout the act. Although each of the movement patterns and skills discussed in chapters that follow involve a specific sequence of movements, all incorporate the basic mechanics of movement discussed here because these mechanical principles are common to all movement situations.

SUMMARY

Motor development represents one aspect of the total developmental process. It is intricately interrelated with both the cognitive and affective domains of human behavior and is influenced by a variety of factors. The importance of optimal motor development must not be minimized or thought of as secondary in importance to the other developmental areas. The unity of humankind clearly demonstrates the integrated development of the mind and the body and the many subtle interrelationships of each. Common factors affecting motor develpment emerge. These factors illustrate the gradual progression from relatively simple levels of functioning to more complex levels.

Biological, experiential, physical, and mechanical factors influence the development of movement abilities. Developing one's movement abilities contributes markedly to one's physical development. The fitness of today's children and adolescents is of great concern to many because of the frequent lack of opportunity and/or motivation to be physically active. Programs in the home, community, or school must provide ample opportunities for large muscle activities and must strive to increase the level of motivation for vigorous activity. Such programs must also, however, recognize that each individual is unique in his or her development and will progress at a rate determined by both environmental and biological circumstances.

CHAPTER CONCEPTS

4.1 Development of muscular control proceeds from the center of the body to the periphery and from the head toward the feet.

4.2 The rate of growth of children follows a universal pattern.

4.3 The infant can recover from limited amounts of interruption in the normal growth process by a phenomenon called "catch-up growth."

4.4 Restricted opportunity for practice and other forms of deprivation adversely influence the child's ability to perform motor tasks that are characteristic of the child's particular age.

4.5 Children gradually gain mastery over the intricate operation of their bodies through the process of differentiation and integration.

4.6 Readiness for learning involves the combination of biological and environmental processes into a congruent whole.

4.7 The environment may be manipulated or altered in order to promote readiness for learning.

4.8 Taking advantage of an individual's readiness requires maturational ripeness, environmental openness, and teacher sensitivity.

4.9 Some movement abilities are phylogenetically based while others are ontogenetically based.

4.10 There are broadly defined sensitive periods during which the child can learn a new task most efficiently.

4.11 The parent-child bond is probably the strongest of all bonds in nature.

4.12 Proper bonding may have a dramatic effect on parent-child interaction later in life.

4.13 Severe deprivation of experiences will have a debilitating effect on the individual. The degree to which this can be overcome depends on many factors.

4.14 Social class, gender, birth order, and ethnic group all play a role in the child's motor development.

4.15 The infant weighing under 2,500 g at birth (5½ lb.) is not automatically classified as premature.

4.16 The term "prematurity" has been expanded to include low-birth-weight, and young-for-date infants, which more accurately describe the condition of the newborn.

4.17 A wide variety of maternal factors have been associated with prematurity.

4.18 Advanced hospital techniques have done much to reduce the abnormally high mortality rates for preterm infants.

4.19 Obesity is a national health problem that may be counteracted during childhood.

4.20 Poor diet and exercise patterns greatly increase the possibility of obesity. The obese child is likely to be an obese adult.

4.21 Anorexia nervosa and bulimia are emotional problems characterized by an aversion to food and a fear of being fat.

4.22 Anorexia nervosa and bulimia are in our society and may be traced, in part, to society's overconcern with a slim, trim figure or physique.

4.23 A variety of fitness and mechanical factors influence one's motor development as well as motor performance.

4.24 Numerous biomechanical principles influence the actual performance of all movement tasks.

TERMS TO REMEMBER

Developmental Direction
Cephalocaudal
Proximodistal
Growth Rate
Differentiation
Integration
Reciprocal Interweaving
Readiness
Critical Period
Sensitive Period

Individual Differences
Phylogenetic Skill
Ontogenetic Skill
Bonding
Imprinting
Stimulation and Deprivation
Temperament
Premature
Low-birth-weight
Young-for-date

Obesity	Line of Gravity
Anorexia Nervosa	Base of Support
Bulimia	Force
Health-Related Fitness	Law of Inertia
Motor Fitness	Law of Acceleration
Center of Gravity	Law of Action and Reaction

CRITICAL READINGS

Bril, B. (1985). "Motor Development and Cultural Attitudes." In Whiting, H. T. A. and Wade, M. G. (eds.) *Themes in Motor Development*. Dordrecht: The Netherlands: Martinus Nijhoff.

Bruch, H. (1986). "Anorexia Nervosa: The Therapeutic Task." In Brownell, K. D. and Foreyt, J. P (Eds) *Handbook of Eating Disorders*. New York: Basic Books.

Lamb, M. E., et al. (1985). *Infant-Mother Attachment*. Hillsdale, NJ: Lawrence Erilbaum Associates.

Learner, R. M. (1986). *Concepts and Theories of Human Development*. New York: Random House, (Chapters 3-5).

Lustick, M. J. (1985). "Bulimia in Adolescents: A Review." *Pediatrics*, 75, 685-690.

Malina, R. M. (1980). "Environmentally Related Correlates of Motor Development and Performance During Infancy and Childhood." In Corbin, C. (ed.) *A Textbook of Motor Development*. Dubuque, IA: W. C. Brown, (Chapter 24).

Payne, G. V. and Isaacs, L. D. (1987). *Human Motor Development: A Lifespan Approach*. Mountain View, CA: Mayfield, (Chapter 6).

Peck, E. B., and Ullrich, H. D. (1988). "Children and Weight: A Changing Perspective." 1116 Miller Avenue, Berkeley, CA: Nutrition Communication Associates.

Ulrich, B. D. (1984). "The Effects of Stimulation Programs on the Development of High Risk Infants: A Review of Research." *Adapted Physical Activity, Quarterly*, 1, 68-80.

SECTION II
INFANCY

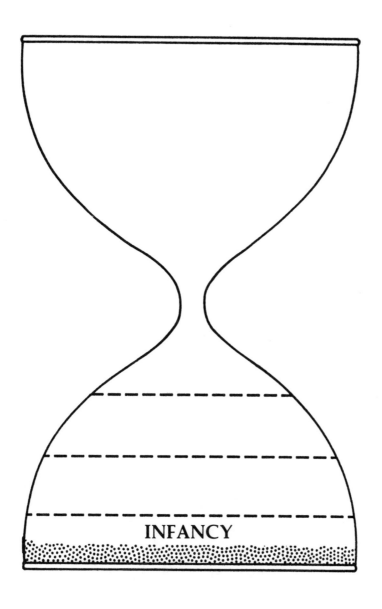

INFANCY

5
Prenatal Factors Affecting Development

CHAPTER COMPETENCIES

Upon Completion of This Chapter You Should Be Able To:

- *Describe the influence of maternal nutrition on later development.*

- *Critically analyze the impact of maternal chemical intake on fetal development.*

- *List and discuss factors to be considered when determining the influence of a drug on an unborn child.*

- *Distinguish between chromosome-based disorders and gene-based disorders.*

- *List and describe the causes and effects of several chromosome and gene-based disorders.*

- *Describe the potential effects of radiation and chemical pollutants on later development.*

- *List and discuss several maternal and fetal medical problems that may affect later development.*

- *Describe the influence of maternal exercise during pregnancy on fetal development.*

- *Demonstrate knowledge of birth process factors that may affect later development.*

- *Critically analyze the prenatal period and describe the interrelated nature of a variety of factors that may influence later development.*

Among the most positive contributions of medical technology are the advances that have been made in reducing infant mortality. As little as two generations ago prenatal and neonatal illness, disease, and death were common in North America. One need only look at less developed cultures throughout the world, and at the poor, deprived, and neglected in our own society, to see that the threat of severely handicapping conditions resulting from a variety of prenatal factors still exists. The current leading cause of severe impairment, among rich and poor, stems from prenatal factors. Birth defects are the most serious child health problem, affecting more than 250,000 babies in the United States each year (March of Dimes, 1984). Although only about 1 percent of the population shows moderate to severe problems in the years before school, Hagberg (1975) estimates that 85 to 90 percent of these intellectual and neurological problems stem from prenatal causes. In a country whose population will exceed 260 million by the year 2,000 (U.S. Bureau of the Census, 1988) it seems important that as many prenatal factors that adversely affect later growth and development as possible be identified and eliminated. It is staggering to contemplate that more than 2 million Americans have severe afflictions because of conditions over which they have no control. It is doubly staggering when we speculate on the number of individuals that have been only moderately or slightly affected by these conditions.

The number of high-risk pregnancies is estimated to be between 20 to 25 percent and the number is increasing due to the increasing number of women over 35 that are becoming pregnant (Freeman, and Pescar, 1982). A *high-risk pregnancy* is one in which the expectant mother has a condition before pregnancy or during pregnancy that increases the chances of her unborn child experiencing either prenatal or postnatal problems. Table 5.1 presents a list of conditions that may put a mother-to-be in the high-risk category. Several of these are described in further detail throughout the chapter.

NUTRITIONAL AND CHEMICAL FACTORS

Whatever the expectant mother ingests will affect the unborn child in some way. Whether these effects are harmful and have lasting consequences depends on a variety of circumstances. The condition of the fetus, degree of nutritional or chemical abuse, amount or dosage, period of pregnancy, and the presence of other influencing factors are but a few of the circumstances that influence the probability of *teratogenic effects*. A teratogen is any substance that may cause the unborn child to develop in an abnormal manner. The fetus is "at risk" when one or more of the following nutritional or chemical factors are present.

Maternal Nutrition

The fetus depends on the mother's blood supply and the osmotic action of the placenta and umbilical cord for its nutrients. Because of this,

Table 5.1 Conditions That May Result in High-Risk Pregnancy

Medical Conditions:	Exposure to:	Use of:	History:
Asthma	Certain Medications	Alcohol	Age ($<$16, $>$35)
Cancer	Chemical Pollutants	Street Drugs	Bleeding
Diabetes	Cytomegalovirus	Tobacco	Heredity
Hypertension	Excessive Radiation		Nutritional Inadequacy
Heart Disease	Rubella		Previous Miscarriage
Kidney Disease	Toxoplasmosis		Seriously over or underweight
Liver Disease			
Maternal Stress			
Thyroid Disorders			
Sexually-Transmitted Diseases			

deficiencies in the mother's diet both prior to and during pregnancy can have a harmful effect on the child. A sound, nutritious diet is absolutely essential for both the mother's health and that of her unborn child.

Although most of us, at least for now, in our Western culture enjoy an abundance of food, *malnourishment* and not *undernourishment* is an area of concern among nutritionists and specialists in child development. Literally millions of women of childbearing age, worldwide, are malnourished. In other words, they are not receiving the proper nutrients through their normal daily intake of food. The mother-to-be who is malnourished may be so for reasons ranging from the potentially easy-to-alter esthetic reasons and the lifelong "junk" food, "fast" food habits of millions, to the more difficult to deal with reasons of poverty, low socioeconomic class, anxiety, stress, and trauma.

The sharpest contrasts in *maternal malnutrition* and normal nutrition are seen between poor and nonpoor mothers. Naeye et al. (1969) studied 252 infants who were either stillborn or died within two days of birth. His survey indicated that infants below the poverty level were 15 percent smaller than nonpoverty infants. Also, a higher percentage of stillborn children were born to impoverished mothers. Maternal malnutrition may account for low socioeconomic families having a higher percentage of children with birth defects than families with higher and generally more adequate nutrition (Hepner, 1958; McGarrity et al. 1958; Eichorn, 1979).

Inadequate nutrition has been shown to be a major factor in low-birth-weight infants. Low-birth-weight babies are much more susceptible to a variety of developmental abnormalities and have a higher mortality rate than normal birth-weight infants. Figure 5.1 shows that the mortality rate for low-birth-weight babies is significantly higher than for those of normal weight.

Lack of vitamins C, B-complex, D, K, and E, as well as protein deficiencies may result in serious physical and mental damage or even death to the unborn child (Litch, 1978). McGowan (1979) indicated that more than 1 million children in the United States suffer from chronic malnutrition to the extent that it interferes with normal brain development. It is difficult to gather experimentally acquired information regarding the effect of specific vitamin and mineral deficiencies in the diet of the expectant mother and mother-to-be. It is unethical to study the effects of malnutrition by purposely depriving expectant mothers. Because of confounding variables such as extreme anxiety, stress, poverty, and poor nutritional habits, it is difficult to compare mothers who have inadequate diets against those who have adequate nutrition.

The amount of weight gained by the expectant mother in the absence of other complications may serve as a general indicator of the unborn child's nutritional status. Chez (1977) reported that 24 to 28 pounds is an ideal amount of maternal weight gain. Table 5.2 shows the proportions of the average weight gain during pregnancy.

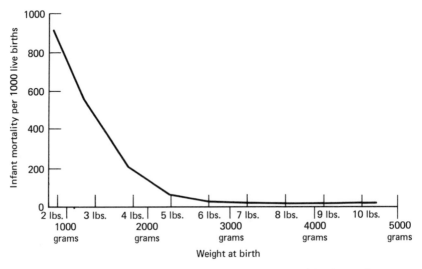

Figure 5.1. The relationship between infant mortality and birth weight

Table 5.2 Distribution of Maternal Weight Gain During Pregnancy (adapted from Samuel, M. D., and Samuel, N. (1979). *The Well Baby Book*. New York: Cummit Books (p. 41).

	Weight Averages
Fetus	7.5 pounds
Placenta	1.0 pounds
Amniotic Fluid	2.0 pounds
Increase in uterus' weight	2.5 pounds
Increase in breasts' weight	3.0 pounds
Increase in the mother's fat (stores needed for energy)	4-8 pounds

Common Maternal Drugs

The wall of the placenta is porous, and chemicals may penetrate it with tragic results to the unborn child. The drugs found in the average person's medicine cabinet are potentially destructive to the fetus. Every drug has side effects. Whether it is a prescription or nonprescription drug and whether the drug has been given to others during pregnancy without serious side effects do not imply that it is safe for all unborn children. The following factors need to be considered whenever the influence of a drug on an unborn child is determined:

1. The time of pregnancy during which the drug is taken
2. The dosage of the drug
3. The length of time the drug is taken
4. The genetic predisposition of the fetus
5. How these four factors interact

There are various ways in which a drug may affect the unborn child. Drugs may interfere with organ growth or cell differentiation and result in deviations from normal development. The penetrability of the placenta may be altered thereby reducing the flow of oxygen and nutrients or magnifying the drug concentration flowing to the fetus. Drugs may impair development and functioning of the liver which balances blood waste products called bilirubin.

The inability of the biliary ducts to excrete bilirubin efficiently results in *jaundice*. Excessive jaundice is called *kernicterus*. Kernicterus can cause permanent and devastating brain damage. Table 5.3 provides a few examples of common drugs taken during pregnancy and the associated risk factors.

Table 5.3 The Effects of Common Drugs on the Unborn Child

Drug	Use	Possible Effects
Coumadin	An anticoagulant used for blood clots	May cause bleeding before or during birth, resulting in brain damage
Diuretics	To treat toxemia, particularly water retention.	Water and salt imbalance. An electrolyte imbalance may result in brain damage
Streptomycin	To treat infection in the mother	Impairment of kidneys, hearing, and balance
Aspirin	For aches, pain, fever. Almost 80% of over-the-counter drugs contain aspirin	Death; congenital deformities; bleeding under the skull, causing brain damage; hemorrhaging during birth
Tetracyclines	For acne	Stunts bone and teeth growth

"Necessary" Maternal Drugs

During pregnancy, the expectant mother may be under the care of a physician because of an illness or disease. Good, consistent medical care is doubly important because the developing fetus inside a mother with a special medical condition may have special needs. The medication prescribed for the mother may have to be modified to protect the unborn child. A mother being treated for epilepsy, for example, should avoid the use of Dilantin and phenobarbital and other drugs used for seizure control. Although she may not be able to completely discontinue the use of medication, the drug should not continue to be taken automatically and the dosage may need modification under medical supervision.

The expectant mother with cancer is at risk when chemotherapy is being used to decrease the rate of malignant cell growth, particularly during the first three months of pregnancy. Also, the use of progesterone to correct menstrual cycle abnormalities and to prevent miscarriage should be avoided in all expectant mothers because of the potentially harmful effects on the newborn.

The unborn child of a diabetic mother-to-be is particularly vulnerable. The severity of the disease and whether the mother is insulin-dependent or non-insulin-dependent has a great deal to do with possible problems for mother and baby. Prior to the development of insulin, diabetic women simply did not have children. After insulin became available (about 1922) more diabetic women were able to give birth. However, the prenatal mortality rate was over 50 percent and many of those who did survive had serious congenital deformities (Freeman and Pescar, 1982). Today, with careful management of the diabetes, utilization of special tests to monitor fetal well-being, and excellent medical care the fetal mortality rate has been sharply reduced. Freeman and Pescar (1982, p. 18) report that: "fetal mortality rates have been dramatically reduced to 3 percent to 4 percent, and nearly all these deaths are due to serious congenital malformations incompatible with survival." Table 5.4 provides a brief overview of some common medical conditions of the expectant mother that may affect later development.

Street Drugs

During the past two decades there has been an alarming increase in the habitual use of mind-altering or *street drugs* by women of childbearing age. The use of opiates (opium, heroin), cocaine, amphetamines ("speed"), lysergic acid diethylamide (LSD), and cannabis (hashish, marijuana) has been of great concern to those interested in the well-being of the unborn

Table 5.4 Common Drugs for Medical Conditions During Pregnancy and the Possible Effects on the Unborn Child

Maternal Condition	Drug	Possible Effects on the Unborn Child
Hypertension	Resperine	Choking, gasping, nasal congestion at birth
Thyroid	Thiouracile Iodides Radioactive iodine	Thyroid abnormalities in child: cretinism (hypothyroidism)
Diabetes	Insulin	Excessive birth weight, prematurity, heart defects, jaundice, low blood sugar, convulsions, mental and physical retardation, deformities
Menstrual abnormality	Progesterone	Gross deformities, masculinization of female organs
Allergy or cold	Antihistamines	Deformities (in animal studies)
Epilepsy	Seizure control drugs	Cleft palate and other malformations

child. Because of legal, moral, and ethical reasons, it is impossible to conduct controlled experiments on the effects of these mind-altering drugs on fetal development. Our knowledge is therefore limited to laboratory settings with animals and retrospective case studies of users. The results of two carefully controlled studies with mice indicated that LSD produced a much higher incidence of birth defects (Alexander et al. 1967) and that cannabis produced a high number of stillbirths (Harbison and Mantilla-Plata, 1972). Houston's (1969) research suggests that hallucinogens produce birth defects when taken early in pregnancy. Persons taking LSD are much more likely to have chromosome abnormalities than are nonusers. Although available research is limited to animals and only correlational in nature, it seems reasonable to assume that mind-altering drugs are likely to adversely affect the unborn child. Table 5.5 provides an overview of the possible effects of some mind-altering drugs on the newborn child.

In regard to the use of marijuana, Hoyt (1981, p. 31) notes that:

The transfer of marijuana's active ingredients through the placenta affects production of testosterone in the fetus, inhibits DNA synthesis in human cells, thus increasing the potential for mutation, and is believed to be a contributing factor in certain cases of spontaneous abortion.

Alcohol and Tobacco

Although alcohol and tobacco are considered by some to be mind- or mood-altering drugs, they have been separated here because of the legality of their usage and to amplify their potential hazards. It has been variously reported that there are more than 1 million alcoholics of childbearing age. The fetus is affected twice as fast as the mother by her alcohol consumption and at the same level of concentration. Until recently, the widespread myth that the fetus will take what it needs from its mother and be uninfluenced by her consumption of foods and beverages caused expectant mothers to be unconcerned about their alcohol consumption. The potential dangers of alcohol to the unborn child were recognized, however, as far back as the Greek era, when newly married couples were forbidden to consume alcohol in order to prevent conception while intoxicated.

In the 1890s, William Sullivan, a physician at a Liverpool, England, prison for women was the first to carefully document the effects of chronic alcoholism on the offspring of 120 alcoholic inmates. This early study revealed a significantly higher morality rate among the 600 offspring and a much greater number of developmental difficulties of the infants (cited in Rossett and Sander, 1979). Further research into the

Table 5.5 Possible Effects of Street Drugs on the Development of the Unborn Child

Drug	Possible Effects on the Unborn Child
Heroin and morphine	Irritable. Sleeps poorly. High-pitched cry. Vomiting and diarrhea. Marked physiological withdrawal symptoms. Decreased oxygen in the blood tissues. Hepatitis from unclean needle. Susceptible to infection. Complications in 40 percent of addicted: 1. Toxemia. 2. Breech birth. 3. Prematurity. 4. Small for date of birth. 5. Premature separation of the placenta. Complications if not treated: 1. Dehydration. 2. Respiratory distress. 3. Shock. 4. Coma. 5. Mineral imbalance.
Amphetamines and barbiturates	Miscarriage. Birth defects.
Tranquilizers	Such drugs as Sominex,® Nytol,® Sleep-Eze® and Compoz® contain two antihistamines that have produced congenital deformities in animals.
LSD (lysergic acid diethylamide)	May cause chromosome damage. Sometimes contaminated with quinine or other materials that may harm the unborn child. A few surveys have found a higher incidence of congenital defects in children of LSD users.

effects of maternal alcoholism lagged in the United States and Great Britain after 1920, following the enactment of Prohibition, although some research continued in France and Germany. It was not until 1970 that the actual "discovery" and labeling of *Fetal Alcohol Syndrome* (FAS) took place (Witti, 1978).

Alcohol is now recognized as the third leading cause of birth defects (Litch, 1978). The other two are Down's syndrome and spina bifida. About one in every 750 babies born has FAS (Centers for Disease Control, 1984). Fetal Alcohol Syndrome is the only birth defect that is completely preventable. Twenty-four to 29 percent of infants born to mothers who are chronic alcoholics (with a consumption level of three or more average-sized drinks per day) or who go on drinking binges are born mentally retarded or with marked physical defects (Cooper, 1987). Table 5.6 summarizes some of the potential dangers of FAS.

Table 5.6 Characteristics of Fetal Alcohol Syndrome

Growth	Growth failure before birth.
	Growth failure after birth.
	Skull that is too small for the brain.
	Small in length compared to weight.
Eyes	Lesions in the eyelids.
	Fold of the skin in the corner of the eye.
	Perceptual problems.
	Narrow eyes.
Face	Low nasal bridge.
	Short, upturned nose.
	Outer ear deformity.
	Underdevelopment of jaw.
Other	Heart defects.
	Hip dislocation.
	Skeletal defects.
	Decrease in joint mobility.
	Motor development delay.
	Abnormal creases in the palm of the hand.
	Female genital defects.
Behavior	Jittery.
	Hyperactive.
	Weak grasp, poor coordination.
	Poor sucking.
	Irregular sleeping.
	Self-stimulator.
Intelligence	Mentally retarded: borderline to moderate.

Alcohol in the mother's blood is passed directly through the placenta to the fetus. The fetus does not have any ethanol-oxidizing or alcohol dehydrogenasic abilities, and therefore the alcohol is fed directly into its system (Brown et al. 1979). Evidence on the exact amounts of alcohol harmful to the fetus and on the critical periods during which it should be avoided is unclear. But, a recent study by Vingan et al. (1986) revealed that consumption of large quantities of alcohol is likely to result in central nervous system damage, growth and mental retardation, distinct facial abnormalities, and that moderate to small doses of alcohol may have the same results. Although social drinking during pregnancy has not been conclusively associated with an increase in risk, Witti (1978, p. 23) suggests that "until the answers are in on the key questions of exactly how much or when alcohol is safe to drink during pregnancy, medical authorities agree that it is wise to be cautious." The March of Dimes Birth Defects Foundation (1985) is even stronger in their recommendation. They state that: "The best decision is not to have any [alcohol] while you are pregnant." Pawlak-Frazier (1978) concluded that there is no risk of FAS if alcohol consumption has been stopped before pregnancy.

Smoking has been implicated in numerous studies as a cause of low birth weight in infants (Meredith, 1975; Pasamanuck and Knoblach, 1966). Stevenson (1977, p. 116) notes that the single unquestionable effect of maternal cigarette smoking is growth retardation. The March of Dimes Birth Defects Foundation (1985) has indicated that women who smoke a pack of cigarettes or more a day tend to have low-birth-weight babies and almost double their chances of miscarriages or stillbirths. Maternal smoking speeds up the fetal heart rate and has an adverse effect on central nervous system integration of the newborn. Furthermore, surveys of children born to nicotine-addicted mothers showed that they tend to rate lower on behavior assessment scales than other newborns. They tend to be more fretful, less coordinated, less alert, and less responsive to cuddling (Strauss et al. 1975). Butler et al. (1972), however, found that women who stop smoking before the fourth month of pregnancy are no more likely than nonsmoking mothers to have a low-birth-weight baby. Therefore, there may be cause for cautious optimism in that the effects of smoking may not be cumulative and their impact on the unborn child may be negligible if smoking ceases early in pregnancy. Smoking, according to the March of Dimes Birth Defects Foundation (1985) is most harmful to a baby's growth during the second half of a pregnancy.

HEREDITARY FACTORS

Until relatively recently, the study of heredity through the science of genetics was only a matter of theory and speculation. Today, however, we have more precise and experimentally verifiable knowledge of heredity. Since it is impossible to discuss it in detail within the confines of this chapter, we will concern ourselves with the potential impact of various hereditary factors on later development.

The union of a sperm with an egg begins the process of development. The sperm carries 23 chromosomes which contain all of the hereditary material that the father contributes. The egg also contains 23 chromosomes, the mother's contribution to the child's heredity. The new fetus, therefore, contains a total of 46 chromosomes (23 pairs). Each chromosome, by the process of cell division (*mitosis*) has a replica in every cell of the body. Genes are found on each chromosome. It has been estimated that each chromosome may contain up to 20,000 genes (Whithurst and Varta, 1977). The genes determine the vast variety of individual characteristics such as gender, hair and eye color, body size and structure.

Under most conditions the chromosomes and genes remain unaltered throughout the prenatal period. (There is growing speculation that certain chemical substances may cause chromosomal damage after conception.) But, a variety of genetic factors prior to conception have been shown to alter the normal process of development.

Chromosome-Based Disorders

It has been estimated that between 3 and 6 percent of all conceptions show evidence of *chromosome damage* and that, of these, about 90 percent will be spontaneously aborted (Ford, 1973). Most chromosome variations are so potent that they are rarely seen in surviving newborns, but fully 1 percent of live infants show evidence of chromosomal damage, according to Ford (1973).

Probably the most common chromosomal alteration is that of *Down's syndrome*. Down's syndrome is the result of an error in which 47 chromosomes are present rather than the standard 46. This cause of Down's syndrome is called trisomy 21 because of three #21 chromosomes. Trisomy 21 accounts for 95 percent of all Down's syndrome (March of Dimes, 1984). Down's syndrome occurs in approximately 1 out of every 500 to 700 live births (Thompson and Thompson, 1973). The rate of incidence seems to be age-related and shows dramatic increases in births occurring in women over 45 years of age. In fact, the frequency of women age 30 is about 1 in 885, while women at 49 years of age have a 1-in-17 chance of giving birth to a child with Down's syndrome (Freeman and Pescar, 1982).

Down's syndrome children are often born prematurely. Their rate of growth is slower than normal, often resulting in shorter stature. The nose, chin, and ears tend to be small, along with poor development of the teeth and poor eyesight. Poor balance, hypotonus, short arms and legs, and nonelastic skin are other characteristics of the Down's child. Cardiovascular defects resulting in frequent respiratory ailments are common, along with limited intellectual functioning. Language and conceptualization skills are generally poor. Motor development proceeds in the same manner as it does in the normal infant but at a slower rate.

Chromosome-linked disorders other than Down's syndrome sometimes occur. Fortunately, conditions such as Patau's syndrome and Edward's syndrome are rare. Little is known about them other than that they are also associated with an extra chromosome and that they result in severe deformities, retardation, and early mortality (Kopp and Parmelee, 1979). The risk of chromosomal abnormalities increases from 2.5 per 1,000 live births for women age 30 to 4.5 for women 35, and to 3.7 for 40-year-old women (Freeman and Pescar, 1982). Certainly, age is a factor to consider when deciding to become pregnant.

Gene-Based Disorders

Genetic defects vary widely in their consequences. The severity of the defect is dependent on whether the mutant gene is on an autosomal or on a sex-linked chromosome and whether it is on a single gene or also on its mate. Delay and retardation in motor and cognitive functioning are not usually present in autosomal dominant mutations. Autosomal recessive mutations, however, are often associated with mental retardation and problems in motor development. Nora and Fraser (1974) list 61 *autosomal syndromes*, one third of which are associated with mental retardation and other developmental abnormalities that interfere with the normal process of motor development. Among the more common autosomal mutations that affect later motor development are clubfoot, sickle cell anemia, Tay-Sachs disease, phenylketonuria (PKU), and spina bifida.

Clubfoot is one of the most common birth defects and historically has been one of the major orthopedic problems of children. About one in 400 babies born in the United States each year have clubfoot, and boys are twice as likely to have this condition as girls (March of Dimes, 1984). There are three major forms of culbfoot; equinovarus, calcaneal valgus, and metatarsus varus. With *Equinovarus* the foot is twisted inward and downward. The Achilles' tendon is generally very tight, making it impossible to bring the foot into normal alignment. *Calcaneal valgus* is the most common form of clubfoot. The foot is sharply angled at the heel, with the foot pointing up and outward. This condition is less severe than equinovarus and easier to correct. *Metatarsus varus* is the mildest form of clubfoot. The front part of the foot is turned inward and is often not diagnosed until the baby is a few months old. With all forms of clubfoot,

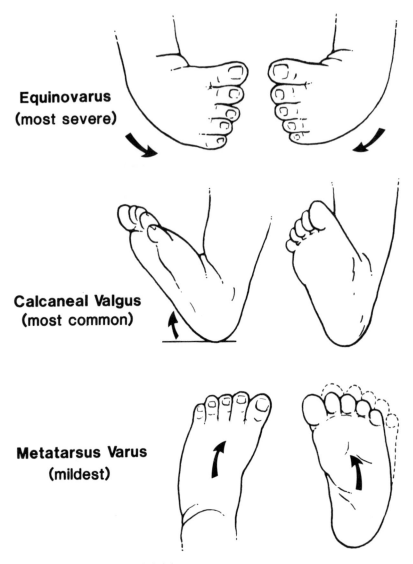

Equinovarus (most severe)

Calcaneal Valgus (most common)

Metatarsus Varus (mildest)

Figure 5.2. Three forms of clubfoot

early, persistent treatment will maximize the individual's chances of leading a normal active life. Left untreated until late in childhood, clubfoot will be a major limiting factor in normal upright locomotion. Figure 5.2 depicts the three types of clubfoot.

Sickle cell anemia is a relatively common gene-based disorder occurring in every 400 to 600 blacks and in one in every 1,000 to 1,500 Hispanics.

One in 10 blacks carry the sickle cell gene, and there is a one-in-four chance that a child of a gene carrier will develop the disease (March of Dimes, 1984). As an inherited blood disease, anemia, pain, damage to vital organs, and death in childhood or early adulthood are possible. The effects of the disease vary greatly from person to person. The growth and motor development of individuals with sickle cell disease are often adversely affected. Also, patients tend to tire easily and are frequently short of breath. The sickle cell trait or disease can be easily tested for through a simple blood test called *hemoglobin electrophoresis*. A prenatal test to determine if the fetus will either carry the trait, be normal, or develop the disease is also available.

Tay-Sachs Disease is a gene-based disorder typical of descendants of Central and Eastern European Jews. Nearly one out of every 25 American Jews carries the Tay-Sachs gene (March of Dimes, 1984). If both parents carry the Tay-Sachs gene there is a one-in-four chance that any of their children will develop Tay-Sachs disease or become carriers of the disease. If only one parent carries the gene, none of the children can have the disease, but there is a one-in-two chance of becoming a carrier. There is no known cure for Tay-Sachs disease, and it is always fatal. It first appears in infancy with the baby losing motor control. Blindness and paralysis follow with death resulting around age 3 or 4. Tay-Sachs disease can be diagnosed through amniocentesis prior to birth. A simple blood test prior to pregnancy will determine if one is a carrier.

Phenylketonuria (PKU) is the only gene-based disorder completely treatable if detected early enough. PKU, a metabolic disorder, is the result of a recessive gene that causes failure to produce phenylalanine hydroxylase which is necessary to convert the amino acid phenylalanine to tyrosine. Treatment simply consists of restricting foods which contain phenylalanine from the diet. It is interesting to note that the can of diet cola you may be consuming right now contains phenylalanine with a warning on the label. Untreated, PKU will result in severe mental retardation. If detected (about 1 week after birth), however, and if proper dietary precautions are heeded, the devastating results of PKU can be entirely avoided.

Spina bifida is a birth defect of the spinal column. According to the March of Dimes Defects Foundation (1984), about one in every 2,000 babies born each year has spina bifida ("open spine"). Spina bifida follows no particular law of inheritance, although it does appear to run in certain families. Families with one affected child have about a one-in-forty chance of having a second with spina bifida. Families with two affected children have about a one-in-twenty chance (March of Dines, 1984). Spina bifida may take three forms. The first may be so slight that only an x-ray of the spinal column will detect its presence. This form rarely bothers the child. In the second form, a lump or cyst which contains the spinal cord pokes through the open part of the spine. The lump may be surgically removed, permitting the baby to grow normally. In the third and most severe form of spina bifida the cyst holds deeper nerve roots of the spinal cord. Little or no skin protects the lump and spinal fluid may leak out. The site of this cyst is generally in the lower spine resulting in paralysis and loss of sensation to the legs, a permanent condition. Table 5.7 summarizes a variety of gene-based birth defects.

ENVIRONMENTAL FACTORS

In recent years greater concern has focused on the effects of the general environment on prenatal development. The influence of radiation and chemical pollutants are areas of particular concern to parents of an unborn child.

Radiation

The environment's influence on development is no more clearly indicated than when we consider the effects of high doses of radiation. Radiation dosage is measured in units called *rads*. An exposure to the developing fetus of more than 25 rads would be considered a high dosage. The fetus is most vulnerable during the first trimester of pregnancy. Excessive radiation has been implicated in *microcephaly* (small head and brain) and mental retardation. Therefore, exposure to x-rays early in pregnancy, especially repeated x-rays of the pelvic region, may put the developing fetus at risk (March of Dimes, 1984). Radiation prior to preg-

Table 5.7 Common Gene-Based Birth Defects

Genetic Defect	Condition
Clubfoot	Equinovarus Calcaneal Valgus Metatarsus Varus
Sickle Cell Anemia	Anemia, pain, damage to vital organs, slow growth and motor development, possible death
Tay-Sachs Disease	Loss of motor control, blindness, paralysis, certain death
Phenylketonuria (PKU)	Severe mental retardation
Spina Bifida	Paralysis in legs, poor bladder and bowel control

nancy is also an area of concern. Freeman and Pescar (1982) report that a few studies suggest a relationship between ovarian radiation and chromosomal defects and the build-up of rads over the years and genetic damage.

Chemical Pollutants

It is difficult to establish a direct causal link between *chemical pollutants*, the pregnant mother, and later developmental abnormalities in her offspring. A number of other variables may account for, or interact with, chemical pollutants to cause birth defects. But lead and mercury have been conclusively linked to birth defects in humans (March of Dimes, 1984). Other pollutants such as acid rain, PCB contamination, and exposure to chemicals such as Agent Orange have speculative evidence (a casual relationship) of contributing to an increased incidence of birth defects.

MEDICAL PROBLEMS

The causes and effects of developmental difficulties in the offspring of mothers with various sexually transmitted diseases, maternal infections, hormonal and chemical imbalances, Rh incompatibility, and severe maternal stress are being researched. These conditions play a significant role in placing the unborn child at risk.

Sexually Transmitted Diseases

In recent years there has been a growing awareness and concern over a variety of sexually transmitted diseases. The ravages of genital herpes, chlamydia, gonorrhea, syphilis, and acquired immunodeficiency syndrome (AIDS) are a direct threat to the unborn child. Yarber (1987, p. 8) notes that: "Sexually transmitted diseases (STD), of which AIDS is one, impair the health of more teenagers than do all other communicable diseases combined." Moreover, Yarber notes that the National Research Council has estimated that, by age 19, about 63 percent of all American females and 78 percent of all American males have had at least one coital experience. Teens and young adults who are sexually active are at risk. The risks are great and the consequences to the developing fetus of a mother with a sexually transmitted disease are even greater.

Genital herpes has become a serious health problem with an estimated 5 to 25 million sufferers in the United States (March of Dimes, 1986). A pregnant woman with an active case of genital herpes may infect her baby resulting in permanent brain damage or death. The baby may be protected through a caesarean delivery rather than a conventional vaginal birth (Yarber, 1985).

Chlamydia is a highly contagious sexually transmitted disease that may be passed on to the baby during a vaginal delivery. Although curable with certain antibiotics, it is difficult to diagnose. Untreated, chlamydia may result in sterility, premature and still births, infant pneumonia, eye infections, and blindness (Yarber, 1985).

Gonorrhea is reported by Yarber (1985) to be the number one reportable communicable disease in the United States with more than 2 million new cases each year. Although curable with antibiotics, some strains of the bacteria have become resistant to treatment. Gonorrhea may result in ectopic pregnancies and eye damage to the newborn (Yarber, 1985).

Maternal syphilis is easily cured with antibiotics if detected in the early stage. The newborn with congenital syphilis is likely to be born dead or displaying severe illnesses. The long-term effects of maternal syphilis are still unclear, but preliminary data indicate a greater incidence of prematurity and, later, motor, sensory, and cognitive disabilities.

Acquired Immunodeficiency Syndrome (AIDS) is the newest and most feared of the various sexually transmitted diseases. AIDS is a virus that attacks the body's immune system. It is transmitted through sexual contact, contaminated needles, and transfusions. Mothers with the AIDS virus are at risk of transmitting the virus during pregnancy or childbirth. Also, the virus may be transmitted by breast-feeding (Yarber, 1987). Although only about 1 percent of all AIDS cases in the United States occur in children, women with a positive AIDS antibody test should not become pregnant. Table 5.8 summarizes the possible effects of sexually transmitted diseases.

Maternal Infections

Perhaps the most significant diseases contracted by the mother that adversely affect the fetus are cytomegalovirus (CMV), and rubella contracted during the first trimester of pregnancy. Both of these diseases pass through the placenta to the fetus and can have serious debilitating effects.

CMV is a common infectious cause of birth defects including blindness, deafness, and mental retardation. Very little is known about this virus and its effects. It is still unclear whether the virus is introduced into the fetus by a primary infection to the mother during pregnancy or whether it may already be present genetically but in latent form (Marx, 1975).

Rubella, sometimes called the "three-day measles," is a mild, contagious virus. It is not the same as regular measles, which is called "rubeola." Vaccination against rubella has been possible since 1969 and has greatly reduced the incidence of birth defects due to this virus. Vaccina-

Table 5.8 Sexually Transmitted Diseases and Their Possible Effects

Sexually Transmitted Disease	Possible Effects on the Newborn Child
Acquired Immunodeficiency Syndrome (AIDS)	Fever, weight loss, lethargy, diarrhea, pneumonia, death
Chlamydia	Prematurity, still births, pneumonia, eye infections, blindness
Genital Herpes	Brain damage, death
Gonorrhea	Ectopic pregnancies, eye damage
Syphilis	Severe illnesses, nervous system damage, death

tion should occur during childhood and not during pregnancy. Also, a simple blood test called a "rubella titer" is available to determine whether a person has had rubella or is immune. Figure 5.3 depicts the decline in infectious rubella since 1969 (March of Dimes, 1985). The child born of a mother who has had rubella during the first trimester of pregnancy is likely to be deaf, blind, or mentally retarded due to interference with sensory and/or cognitive development during the embryonic, or early fetal, period (Alford et al. 1983).

Hormonal and Chemical and Imbalances

An inadequate hormonal or chemical environment in the thyroid patient, for example, can result in congenital hypothyroidism and cretinism in the infant, due to a lack of thyroxine in the mother's blood during the early months of pregnancy.

Diabetes in the expectant mother is a chronic chemical imbalance that may adversely affect later development in the child. The inadequate production of insulin prevents the proper metabolizing of sugar and other carbohydrates. Untreated diabetes can result in mental retardation, circulatory and respiratory problems in the infant, or even death.

Rh Incompatibility

Rh incompatibility results from the incompatibility of blood types between mother and child. Although there is no direct link between the bloodstream of the infant and that of the mother, there may be some seepage of blood from the fetus to the mother during the later stages of pregnancy. If the expectant Rh-negative mother is carrying her first Rh-positive child, this seepage to the mother will cause her to produce antibodies in her blood. The production of antibodies generally has no effect on the first child. The time lag between the first and subsequent children,

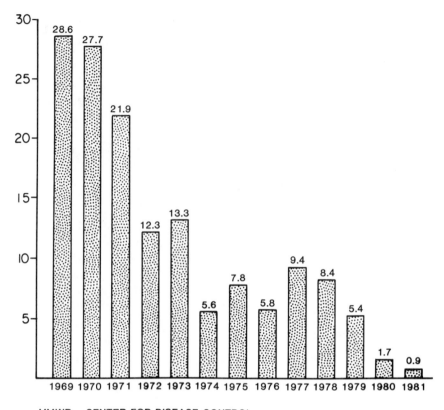

MMWR – CENTER FOR DISEASE CONTROL
RATE PER 100,000 POPULATION

Figure 5.3. Incidence of infectious rubella

however, provides ample opportunity for the production of antibodies in the mother. These antibodies can have a devastating effect on future pregnancies by destroying the fetal red corpuscles. *Erythroblastosis fetalis* is the name given to this condition, which is characterized by anemia and jaundice (Winchester, 1979).

Rh incompatibility occurs only in cases where the father is Rh positive and the mother is Rh negative. Eckert (1987) reports that approximately 12 percent of all marriages result in Rh incompatibility. Routine blood tests and a *rhogam* injection immediately after birth of the first child will prevent the formation of antibodies. Rhogam is the gamma globulin component of blood obtained from an Rh-negative person previously sensitized to the Rh factor. The rhogam neutralizes the Rh factor in the mother and prevents her buildup of antibodies. A rhogam injection must be given with each Rh-positive pregnancy.

Maternal Emotional Stress

Some research has raised concern over the effects of severe prolonged maternal emotional stress on the unborn child. Severe stress factors such as death of a loved one and marital problems have been associated with complications during pregnancy and fetal abnormalities (Davids et al. 1961). Although there is no direct link between the nervous system of the mother and the fetus, the mother's emotional state can influence development. Because the nervous system and the endocrine system communicate through the blood, the emotional trauma experienced by the mother is transferred from the cerebral cortex to the thalamus and hypothalamus. The autonomic nervous system acts on the endocrine system which empties into the bloodstream. The mother's bloodstream then transports the endocrine secretions to the placenta through which some are passed into the fetal bloodstream and finally to its nervous system (Montague, 1962; Rosenblith, and Sims-Knight, 1985). This hypothesis is speculative, but it is clear that prolonged maternal stress may have detrimental effects. Children born of emotionally stressed mothers tend to be more prone to a variety of illnesses and physical problems thoughout life (Bee, 1985). Rosenblith and Sims-Knight (1985, p. 140), conclude that: "Considering both the relatively well-controlled animal research and the human studies with their varifying methodological problems, it seems likely that babies of women who feel stressed during pregnancy are adversely affected."

Teenage Pregnancy

In the United States alone, more than a half million girls give birth each year. Babies born to teen mothers have a much higher risk of serious health problems than do children born of a fully mature mother (Cabrera, 1980). Teenage mothers as a group are more likely to bear small-for-date, or young-for-date infants. Low-birth-weight babies are statistically more likely to suffer from a variety of developmental abnormalities including mental retardation, immature organ systems, thermoregulatory difficulties, and death (March of Dimes, 1984). Furthermore, the maternal death rate from complications in pregnancy is much higher among girls under age 15 who give birth than among older mothers.

Additional risk factors often found in teenage pregnancies include psychological stress, low socioeconomic status, inadequate parenting behavior, maternal drug and alcohol abuse, and poor or nonexistent medical care (Parron and Eisenberg, 1982). The complexity of the risks involved in teenage pregnancies necessitates investigation into a number of areas so that appropriate intervention strategies may be devised.

Toxoplasmosis

Besides all of the infections, diseases, and special conditions already discussed as high-risk considerations, expectant parents need to be aware of *toxoplasmosis* so they can protect their unborn child against the offending protozoan. Toxoplasmosis is amazingly prevalent. It has been estimated that 1 in every 1,000 infants and 1 in every 500 pregnant women are infected by it (Litch, 1978). Infected children, although often small-for-date at birth, may appear normal and even through when the toxoplasma cysts rupture, releasing thousands of parasites that attack the eyes, heart, and other internal organs, and the central nervous system.

Toxoplasmosis is a more prevalent health problem than either rubella or PKU, but its devastation to the unborn child has had little publicity. Parents of an unborn child, however, can do some very specific things to protect their child from this infection. All beef, pork, and lamb should be cooked until well done; the protozoan cysts exist in the muscle of meat. Because the toxoplasma organisms are transmitted through cat feces, it is wise to avoid contact with cats during pregnancy.

The natural reservoir of the toxoplasma gondii sporozoan is the mouse, and most cats come in contact with mice. The spores passed in the feces of infected cats can be inhaled or ingested. The symptoms of infection in humans are similar to the flu, yet many times there are no symptoms at all. Persons who have been infected carry antibodies against toxoplasmosis. The fetus, however, does not have the ability to make such antibodies and takes the effects of the infection with full force. About 10 percent of the 3,000 infants infected with toxoplasmosis each year are severely brain damaged and suffer a variety of sensory and motor disabilities (Alford et al. 1975).

PRENATAL DIAGNOSIS

In recent years a variety of prenatal diagnostic procedures have become available and are frequently used to detect the presence of fetal developmental abnormalities. Among the most frequently used techniques are amniocentesis, ultrasound, and fetoscopy.

Amniocentesis is a technique whereby a hollow needle is inserted into the pregnant's woman's abdomen. It is a nearly painless procedure. A small amount of amniotic fluid (containing fetal cells) is withdrawn through the needle and analyzed. Amniotic fluid can be analyzed to detect any form of chromosomal abnormality, nearly 100 metabolic disorders, and some structural defects (March of Dimes, 1984). Even so, Payne (1987, p. 96) warns that:

Before a woman is subjected to this procedure, she should be given a full account of its limitations and benefits. Only a small number of abnormalities can be tested for, and if abnormalities are not detectable, this still does not guarantee a normal child.

Amniocentesis is generally performed between the 14th and 16th weeks of pregnancy. It can, however, be performed late in the pregnancy as a means of determining fetal maturity and the severity of Rh disease. Amniocentesis is an invasive procedure that should only be used for specific medical purposes and not for determining gender.

Ultrasound is another prenatal diagnostic technique. It uses high-frequency sound waves to determine the size and structure of the fetus and provides visual information about its position in the womb. Ultrasound is frequently used in conjunction with amniocentesis as a means of guiding the physician when inserting the needle through the abdomen and into the uterus.

Fetoscopy is a third fetal diagnostic procedure. It is the most recent of the three prenatal diagnostic procedures and involves inserting an instrument directly into the womb to enable physicians to view the fetus and take blood samples. Fetoscopy is frequently used after amniocentesis and ultrasound for diagnosis of still-suspected blood diseases and fetal malformations.

VIGOROUS ACTIVITY DURING PREGNANCY

Along with the fundamental societal changes regarding vigorous exercise and the quest for fitness have come several important questions concerning vigorous physical activity during pregnancy. Among them are: how will maternal exercise affect fetal development? will maternal exercise help or hinder delivery? and will maternal exercise influence infant development? Conclusive answers to each of these questions are not yet available, but a growing body of research has begun to shed some light on each.

A number of recent studies have examined the influence of vigorous activity on fetal development. Bonds and Delivoria-Papadopoulos (1985) reviewed a number of animal and human studies on the fetal effects of exercise and reported no negative findings. Lotgering et al. (1985, p. 30) reported that, in contrast to rather significant physiological changes in the exercising mother and despite reduced uterine blood flow during maternal exercise, physiological changes to the fetus are small. They state that: "Acute exercise normally does not represent a major stress for the fetus." Cohen et al. (1989, p. 87) concluded that: "strenuous anaerobic exercise during pregnancy is not harmful, [but] more studies are needed to determine if these cases are isolated."

Furthermore, Pijpers et al. (1984) in their paper "Effect of Short-Term Maternal Exercise on Maternal and Fetal Cardiovascular Dynamics" found no significant changes in fetal heart rate and no signs of fetal stress at the conclusion of moderate, short-term maternal exercise. But, Collings et al. (1983) found small but significant increases in fetal heart rates measured during a maternal aerobic exercise program, but no differences in Apgar scores or fetal growth when compared to a nonexercising control group. Thus far, the data tend to be overwhelmingly in support of exercise during pregnancy in terms of both fetal and maternal responses. Several questions regarding how much exercise, what types of exercise, and contraindications for maternal exercise during pregnancy still need clarification. Guidelines for exercise during pregnancy are available from the American College of Obstetricians and Gynecologists (1985) and should be followed until these questions are resolved (see Table 5.9).

The concern over the effects on fetal delivery of strenuous exercise during pregnancy has little basis for support. Historically, there have been two distinct opinions about delivery in female athletes. One opinion held that extensive sport activity made the muscles of the pelvic floor rigid and led to difficulty during labor. The other opinion denied this supposition and emphasized the positive effect of increased abdominal strength particularly during the second stage of labor (Erdelyi, 1962). No differences between fitness levels and labor duration have been found (Erkkola, 1976; Collings et al. 1983).

In regard to the effects of maternal exercise on later infant development, Clapp and Dickstein (1984) found that women who continued endurance exercise at or near their preconceptual levels gained less weight, delivered earlier, and had lighter-weight babies than their matched counterparts who stopped exercising prior to the 28th week of their pregnancy. Furthermore, Lotgering et al. (1984), in their excellent review, report a number of studies that have clearly linked maternal exercise to low-birth-weight. They state that several studies have reported decreases in birthweight of as much as 400 grams. They do note, however, that this may reflect poorer nutritional status of these women rather than the effect of physical activity itself. Further study is needed before any conclusive link can be established between exercise intensity and low birth weight.

BIRTH PROCESS FACTORS

The average length of intrauterine life is 279 days—from the day of conception to the day of birth. Two-thirds of all expectant mothers give birth within 279 days plus or minus two weeks. The beginning of labor is

Table 5.9 American College of Obstetricians and Gynecologists Guidelines for Exercise During Pregnancy and Postpartum

1. Regular exercise (at least three times per week) is preferable to intermittent activity. Competitive activities should be discouraged.

2. Vigorous exercise should not be performed in hot, humid weather or during a period of febrile illness.

3. Ballistic movements (jerky, bouncy motions) should be avoided. Exercise should be done on a wooden floor or a tightly carpeted surface to reduce shock and provide a sure footing.

4. Deep flexion of extension of joints should be avoided because of connective tissue laxity. Activities that require jumping, jarring motions, or rapid changes in direction should be avoided because of joint instability.

5. Vigorous exercise should be preceded by a five-minute period of muscle warm-up. This can be accomplished by slow walking or stationary cycling with low resistance.

6. Vigorous exercise should be followed by a period of gradually declining activity that includes gentle stationary stretching. Be-

cause connective tissue laxity increase risk of joint injury, stretches should not be taken to the point of maximum resistance.

7. Heart rate should be measured at times of peak activity. Target heart rates and limits established in consultation with the physician should not be exceeded.

8. Care should be taken to gradually rise from the floor to avoid orthostatic hypotension. Some form of activity involving the legs should be continued for a brief period.

9. Liquids should be taken liberally before and after exercise to prevent dehydration. If necessary, activity should be interrupted to replenish fluids.

10. Women who have led sedentary life-styles should begin with physical activity of very low intensity and advance activity levels very gradually.

11. Activity should be stopped and the physician consulted if any unusual symptoms appear.

Pregnancy only

1. Maternal heart rate should not exceed 140 beats $\cdot$ min^{-1}.

2. Strenuous activities should not exceed 15 minutes in duration.

3. No exercise should be performed in the supine position after the fourth month of gestation is the completed.

4. Exercises that employ the Valsalva maneuver should be avoided.

5. Calorie intake should be adequate to meet not only the extra energy needs of pregnancy, but also of the exercise performed.

6. Maternal core temperatures should not exceed 38 C.

Source: American College of Obstetricians and Gynecologists (1985). "Exercise During Pregnancy and the Postnatal Period" (*American College of Obstetricians and Gynecologists Home Exercise Programs.*) Washington, DC, ACOG.

marked by the passage of blood and amniotic fluid from the ruptured amniotic sac through the vagina and the onset of labor pains. There are three distinguishable stages of labor. In the first stage, the neck of the uterus (the cervix) dilates to about 4 cm in diameter. Dilation is responsible for labor pains and may last for only a few hours or up to several hours. Labor is generally longer with the first child (*primiparas*) than for subsequent children (*multiparas*). When the cervix reaches 2 cm, full labor begins. It is at this point that the amniotic sac breaks and the fluid flows out of the mother. Complete dilation marks the onset of the second stage of labor: the expulsion period. During this stage the baby, through the continued increase in uterine pressure, is forced down the birth canal. This phase takes an average of 90 minutes for the first child and about half as long for subsequent children. The third stage of labors begins after the baby has emerged and continues until after the umbilical cord and *placenta* (afterbirth) have been delivered. During any stage of the birth process, a number of obstetrical medications and obstetrical procedures may influence later development of the child.

Obstetrical Medication

One of the most controversial issues today among obstetricians and infant researchers is the effects of obstetrical medication commonly used during the birth process. The paper published by Brackbill (1979) which elicited sensational attention from the popular press and the subsequent rebuttal of her findings by many, has done much to add fuel to this already heated debate. Basically, the argument is as follows: Due to both the structural and functional immaturity of the nervous system at birth and the rapid absorption rate across the placenta, drugs given during the birth process will have an adverse effect on the newborn and its subsequent development. It is estimated, based on a variety of surveys, that 90 to 95 percent of all hospital births involve the use of some form of medication (Brackbill, 1979; Standley, 1974). Table 5.10 lists common types of predelivery, general, and local anesthetics used during delivery. These medications are used to initiate or augment labor (*oxytocics*), relieve pain (*analgesics*) and relieve anxiety (*sedatives*).

The results of several studies point to a relationship between drug use during labor and later development. There is compelling evidence that muscular strength and motor coordination are impaired as measured on infant development scales (Brackbill, 1970; Conway and Brackbill, 1970). Muller et al. (1971) and Goldstein et al. (1976) have found a relationship between obstetrical drugs and lowered IQ scores. Brackbill (1979) contends that obstetrical drug use has had a significant effect on lowering the IQ of most Americans. This is due to the increased risk of

Table 5.10 Function of Common Types of Predelivery and Delivery Drugs

Predelivery Drugs	Delivery Drugs

Oxytocics (premedication agents)
  Induce labor
  Augment labor
  Increase uterine tonus
	General anesthetics (inhalants, intra-
	  venous injections)
	  Relieve fetal distress
	  Speed up delivery
	  Mother emotionally unsuited to re-
	    main awake
	  Multiple births

Sedatives (Demerol, meperidine)
  Reduce anxiety
  Reduce excitement
  Slow down labor
	Local anesthetics (lumbar, spinal,
	  caudal)
	  Pain relief
	  Relaxation

anoxia and delay in organization of the central nervous system. The extent of these influences is open to considerable debate and is dependent on a variety of factors, including type and combination of drugs, amount administered, and the time lag between administration and birth. It is safe, however, to say that drugs taken during the birth process put the newborn at risk. The extent and certainty of this risk is unclear, but it seems reasonable to assume that a drug-free birth, or at least the judicious use of drugs during labor, would do much to reduce the risk of later developmental difficulties.

Birth Entry

A variety of birth entry factors also have been shown to put the infant at risk. Among them are malpresentation, the use of forceps, and Caesarean section.

About 4 in every 100 babies are born buttocks first, or feet first (*breech birth*) and 1 out of 100 are in a crosswise position (*transverse presentation*) (Travers, 1977). These presentations can sometimes be altered by the attending physician or midwife. The danger in malpresentation, as with drug-assisted labor and umbilical cord difficulties, is anoxia. In fact, anoxia has been described as the major cause of perinatal death and has been implicated as the cause of mental retardation, learning disabilities, and cerebral palsy (Bonica, 1967).

Forceps are occasionally used to withdraw the baby from the birth canal. Today, the use of forceps is limited largely to emergency situations, but they were used routinely in obstetrics until the 1940s. Forceps are used to speed delivery when the mother is displaying uncontrollable pushing, when the infant has a weak heartbeat, when the umbilical cord emerges before the head endangering the baby's oxygen supply, or when there is a premature separation of the placenta (Milinaire, 1974). Forceps have played, and continue to play, a vital role in obstetrics as a lifesaving device, but their overuse and misuse have had debilitating and lethal effects on both mothers and children.

A *Caesarean section* involves surgical delivery of the baby. The survey conducted by Jones (1976), based on more than 72,000 births over a period of 35 years, showed a definite increase in the number of Caesarean operations. In 1970 Caesarean deliveries comprised 5.5 percent of births. By 1978 that figure had risen to 15.2 percent (Freeman and Pescar, 1982). The reasons for this seem to be associated with planning the exact delivery date, avoidance of pain (a general anesthetic is usually given), the advent of newer incision techniques leaving a smaller and less noticeable scar, and the desire to spare the fetus any distress. A Caesarean section is a major operation and in the past was considered only in cases of necessity in that it was performed due to malpresentation, fetal distress, and failed use of forceps. Recently, however, Caesarean section has become an operation of choice, but most obstetricians still recommend that it be used only when there are extenuating circumstances.

SUMMARY

A wide variety of factors have been shown to adversely influence the process of later development. There is a growing realization among many prospective parents that they can do something to reduce the chances of putting their offspring at risk. Many now realize that their choice of what they ingest (nutrients, alcohol, tobacco, and other drugs) can have an impact on the unborn child. Many are now sensitive to the possible harmful effects of caffeine, saccharin, overexposure to radiation and noxious chemicals, and obstetrical medication. As a result there has been a resurgence of interest in natural childbirth techniques, rooming-in, and home births, and a return to a more responsible attitude about giving birth. A greater number of mothers are asserting their rights for a drug-free pregnancy and are working knowledgeably with concerned obstetricians to produce the healthiest offspring possible.

The birth process can be an important beginning in the three-way bonding of mother, infant, and father. Because of this, parents should be granted the right to choose the method in which they wish to introduce their offspring into the world. The Lamaze (1970) and the Le Boyer (1975) methods of childbirth are two procedures from which prospective parents can choose. The Lamaze method centers on the mother and father. It is a conscious relaxation technique that incorporates rhythmical breathing to block the sensations of pain and a complete knowledge of what to expect during labor and delivery. The Le Boyer method focuses almost entirely on the infant. The aim is to simulate the conditions of the womb as closely as possible. Delivery occurs in a dimly-lit, quiet room. The baby is immediately immersed in a warm fluid solution and gradually, but gently, introduced into the world. Furthermore, many hospitals have more dramatic changes in their birthing procedures. Birthing rooms, birthing chairs, and rooming-in are all presently popular procedures that reflect greater concern for the health and comfort of both mother and child.

The prenatal period is too important to be left to chance. An intelligent pregnancy and delivery, although not a guarantee, can do much to reduce the risk involved to both mother and child.

CHAPTER CONCEPTS

5.1 Growth and motor development begin at conception and are influenced by numerous factors.

5.2 Malnourishment is a problem in many developed as well as developing countries and has been shown to have a negative impact on the unborn child.

5.3 Children born to malnourished and undernourished mothers tend to be smaller, have a higher number of developmental difficulties, and have a higher mortality rate than children born to properly nourished mothers.

5.4 Maternal malnutrition cuts across all socioeconomic classes, ethnic and racial backgrounds.

5.5 Many nonprescription drugs routinely taken during pregnancy have a negative effect on the developing fetus.

5.6 Several commonly prescribed drugs for special maternal conditions have a negative effect on the developing fetus.

5.7 Street drugs have been shown to have a negative effect on the development of the fetus and infant.

5.8 The dosage, duration, time during pregnancy, and genetic predisposition of the fetus determine whether the unborn child will be adversely affected by improper nutrition or chemical substances.

5.9 The regular use of alcohol and tobacco by the expectant mother has been shown to increase the risk of damage to the fetus.

5.10 The genetic inheritance of the fetus will control the upper and lower limits of its functioning.

5.11 Several chromosome-based factors may adversely affect the development of the fetus and infant.

5.12 Gene-linked abnormalities have been shown to adversely influence development.

5.13 A variety of maternal medical conditions may adversely influence development.

5.14 Maternal infections and the buildup of antibodies may adversely affect development.

5.15 Severe maternal stress has been associated with fetal abnormalities and complications during pregnancy.

5.16 A variety of prenatal diagnostic techniques are available for detecting suspected fetal developmental difficulties.

5.17 Vigorous physical activity can be engaged in by the mother-to-be throughout the pregnancy on the advice of her physician.

5.18 The use of drugs and medication during the birth process has been shown to affect later development.

5.19 The use of certain birthing techniques and procedures has been shown to affect later development.

5.20 The mother- and father-to-be have an obligation to their unborn child to ensure its normal development by monitoring the factors over which they exercise more control.

TERMS TO REMEMBER

Teratogenic Effects
High-Risk Pregnancy
Malnourishment
Undernourishment
Maternal Malnutrition
Jaundice
Kernicterus
Street Drugs
Fetal Alcohol Syndrome
Mitosis
Chromosome Damage
Down Syndrome
Genetic Defect
Autosomal Syndrome
Clubfoot
Equinovarus
Calcaneal Valgus
Metatarsus
Sickle Cell Anemia
Hemoglobin Electrophoresis
Tay-Sachs Disease
Phenylketonuria (PKU)
Spina Bifida
Rads
Microcephaly

Caesarean Section
Chemical Pollutants
Genital Herpes
Chylamydia
Gonorrhea
Maternal Syphilis
Acquired Immunodeficiency Syndrome (AIDS)
Cytomegalovirus (CMV)
Rubella
Rh Incompatability
Erythroblastosis Fetalis
Rhogam
Toxoplasmosis
Amniocentesis
Ultrasound
Fetoscopy
Primiparas
Multiparas
Placenta
Oxytocics
Analgesics
Sedatives
Breech Birth
Forceps
Transverse Presentation

CRITICAL READINGS

Beregin, N. (1980). *The Gentle Birth Book*. New York: Simon and Schuster.
Brackbill, Y. (1979). "Obstetrical Medication and Infant Behavior," In, Osofsky, J. D. (ed.), *The Handbook of Infant Development*. New York: Wiley.

Cooper, S. (1987). "The Fetal Alcohol Syndrome." *Journal of Child Psychology and Psychiatry*, 49, 1, 223-227.

Eckert, H. (1987). *Motor Development*. Indianapolis: Benchmark Press. (Chapter 2.).

Freeman, R. K. and Pescar, S. C. (1982). *Safe Delivery Protecting Your Baby During High Risk Pregnancy*. New York: McGraw-Hill.

Seifert, K. L. and Hoffnung, R. J. (1987). *Child and Adolescent Development*. Boston: Houghton Mifflin, (Chapter 4).

Streissguth, A., et al. (1985). "Natural History of the Fetal Alcohol Syndrome: A 10-Year Follow Up of Eleven Patients." *Lancet*, 2, 85-91.

6

Prenatal and Infant Growth

CHAPTER COMPETENCIES

Upon Completion of This Chapter You Should Be Able To:

* *Discuss embryonic and fetal growth and biological maturation.*

* *Describe and interpret the normal displacement and velocity graphs of infant growth.*

* *Discuss proportional changes in segmental length from birth through childhood.*

● *Speculate on prenatal time periods that are critical to normal growth.*

● *Describe the process of prenatal growth from conception to birth.*

This chapter will focus on the process of normal growth from conception through infancy. It is important for the student of motor development to have a reference point from which to view the normal growth process. The approach taken here provides that reference point from the standpoint of the mythically "average" child. In other words, heights, weights, and other growth statistics are presented in terms of averages. There may be considerably normal variation from these figures. This variation may be thought of as the result of the interaction between both biological and environmental processes on the child.

PRENATAL GROWTH

Growth begins at the moment of conception and follows an orderly sequence throughout the prenatal period. Prechtl's (1986) and Hooker's (1952) studies of the motor development of the fetus demonstrated that prenatal movement and growth patterns are just as predictable during the fetal period as they are throughout infancy. The uniting of a mature sperm and ovum marks the beginning of this process. The ovum is one of the largest cells in the female body. It is about 0.004 in. in diameter and is just barely visible to the naked eye. The sperm, on the other hand, is microscopic and one of the smallest cells in the male body. Fertilization occurs if one of the approximately 20 million sperm released from the male during intercourse meets and penetrates the ovum in the Fallopian tube. Once the sperm cell penetrates the outer membrane of the egg, fertilization occurs. Each parent contributes 23 chromosomes (barlike structures in cells that carry all of our genetic information). The two cell nuclei lie side by side for a few hours before they merge to form a *zygote* (the fertilized egg with 46 chromosomes). It is at this instant that one's genetic potential is determined. Realization of this potential will depend on many environmental and hereditary factors. The genetic inheritances of both mother and father are transferred to this single cell and the pattern for a variety of traits is now established, including eye and hair color, general body shape, and complexion. During the germinal period, the zygote splits into two cells through a process called *mitosis*. The two cells form four cells, and the four cells form eight. Three days after conception the ovum has grown into 32 cells, and after four days it consists of about 90 cells. Because all cells have the same genetic setup except for sex cells, the division of cells is not simultaneous, and odd numbers of cells have been observed in some early life stages (Sundberg and Wirsen, 1977). After the first three or four days of mitotic cell division, the zygote travels down the Fallopian tube to the uterus where it attaches itself to the uterine wall. This implantation process marks the true onset of pregnancy, although the days of pregnancy are counted from the first day of the last menstrual bleeding. The ovum is normally fertilized within a day of ovulation, near the fourteenth day of the cycle. Therefore, during the first two weeks of what is considered pregnancy, the woman is not actually pregnant. Implantation generally occurs by the end of the first week after fertilization.

Zygotic Period (Conception-1st week)

During the first week (period of the *zygote*) the fertilized egg remains practically unchanged in size. It lives off its own yoke and receives little outside nourishment. By the end of the first week the zygote is only a small round disk about 0.01 in. wide. The situation for the zygote is especially precarious during this time. Although the mother-to-be may be unaware of the pregnancy, her system will automatically attempt to slough off this foreign body, as it would any foreign body. Also, the expectant mother may continue to ingest a variety of chemical substances (drugs, alcohol, and tobacco) that may prove damaging, if not lethal, to the zygote.

Embryonic Period (2nd week–2nd month)

The differentiation of embryonic cells into layers marks the end of the period of the zygote and the beginning of the period of the *embryo*. By the end of the first month there is a definite formation of three layers of cells. The *ectoderm*, from which the sense organs and nervous system develop, begins to form. The *mesoderm* accounts for the formation of the muscular, skeletal, and circulatory systems. The *endoderm* eventually accounts for the formation of the digestive, respiratory and glandular systems (see Table 6.1). Every part of the body develops from these three kinds of cells. Special cells form the *placenta*, through which nutritive substances will be carried and wastes removed. Another special layer of cells begins formation of the *amnion* which will enclose the embryo except at the umbilical cord throughout the prenatal period.

By the end of the first month the embryo is about one quarter of an inch long and weighs about 1 ounce. It is crescent-shaped, with small bumps on its sides (limb buds) and has a tail and tiny ridges along the neck. These gill-like ridges mark the beginning of a primitive mouth opening, heart, face, and throat. By the end of the first month the embryo has a rudimentary circulatory system, and the heart begins to beat. Growth accelerates toward the end of the first month. The organism grows about one quarter of an inch each week. By the end of the second month the embryo is about 1½ in. long. The beginnings of the face, neck, fingers, and toes develop, and the embryo starts to take on a more human appearance. The limb buds lengthen, the muscles enlarge, and the sex organs begin to form. Brain development is rapid and is represented by a very large head in comparison to the rest of the body (Figure 6.1). The embryo is now firmly implanted in the uterine wall and receives nourishment through the placenta and the umbilical cord. This marks the end of the embryonic period and the beginning of the fetal period of prenatal life.

Table 6.1 Systems That Develop From Three Layers of Cells

Layer	Systems
Endoderm (inner layer)	Digestive system
	Respiratory system
	Glandular system
Mesoderm (middle layer)	Muscular system
	Skeletal system
	Circulatory system
	Reproductive system
	Central nervous system
	Sensory end-organs
Ectoderm (outer covering)	Peripheral nervous system
	Skin, hair, nails

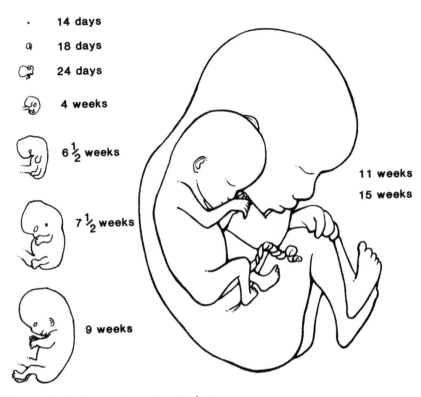

	14 days
	18 days
	24 days
	4 weeks
	6 ½ weeks
	7 ½ weeks
	9 weeks
	11 weeks
	15 weeks

Figure 6.1. Embryos drawn to actual size

Early Fetal Period (3rd-6th month)

The period of the *fetus* begins around the third month and continues until delivery. This is a critical time for the fetus, which is easily influenced by a variety of factors over which it has no control. During the third month the fetus continues to grow rapidly. It is about 3 inches long by the end of the third month. Sexual differentiation continues, buds for the teeth emerge, the stomach and kidneys begin to function, and the vocal cords appear. By the beginning of the third month the first reflex actions begin to be felt (DeVries, 1982). The fetus opens and closes its mouth, swallows, clenches its fist, and can even reflexively suck its thumb. The growth rate during the fourth month is the most rapid for the fetus. During this period it doubles in length to about 6 to 8 inches and weighs about 4 ounces. The hands are fully shaped, and the transparent cartilaginous skeleton begins to turn into bony tissue, starting in the middle of each skeletal bone and progressing toward the ends. The lower limbs, which had been lagging behind in their development, now catch up with the rest of the body. By the beginning of the fifth month the fetus has reached half of its birth length but only 10 percent of its birth weight. The fetus is now sloughing off skin and respiratory cells and replacing them with new ones. Sloughed off cells remain in the amniotic fluid, thus providing a basis for amniocentesis. (Refer to Chapter 5 for a discussion of this technique.)

At the beginning of the fifth month the fetus is about 8 to 10 inches long and weighs about ½ pound. Skin, hair, and nails appear. The internal organs continue to grow and assume their proper anatomical positions. The entire body of the fetus is temporarily covered with a very fine, soft hair called *lanugo*. The lanugo on the head and eyebrows becomes more marked by the end of the fifth month and is replaced by pigmented hair. The lanugo is generally shed before birth, although some may still remain. The larger size and cramped quarters of the rapidly developing fetus generally result in considerable reflexive movement during the fifth month.

By the sixth month the fetus is about 13 inches long and weighs over a pound. During this month the eyelids, which have been fused shut since the third month, reopen and are completed. The *vernix caseosa* forms from skin cells. It is a fatty secretion that protects the thin, delicate skin of the fetus. There is little in the way of subcutaneous fat at this point, and the fetus appears red and wrinkled, resembling someone old and frail. An infant born prematurely during the sixth month has a very poor chance of survival even with the most sophisticated technology available. Although it can cry weakly and move about, it cannot perform the more basic functions of spontaneous breathing and temperature regulation. By the end of the sixth month the fetus weighs approximately 2 pounds and is about 14 inches long. It is structurally complete but needs additional time for functional maturity of the various systems of the body.

Later Fetal Period (7th-9th month)

From the seventh month to term, the fetus triples its weight (Figure 6.2). A layer of adipose tissue begins to form under the skin and serves as both an insulator and food supplier. The lanugo hair is shed, along with much of the vernix fluid, and the nails often grow beyond the ends of the fingers and toes, necessitating an immediate manicure after birth to prevent scratching. During the seventh month the fetus is often quiet for long periods of time as if resting up for the "big event." The fetal brain becomes more active and takes increasing control over the body systems. More than 70 percent of fetuses born at the end of the seventh month survive, although most require special handling during the early months after birth (Rogers, 1977).

During the eighth and ninth months the fetus becomes more active. The cramped quarters result in frequent changes in position, kicking, and

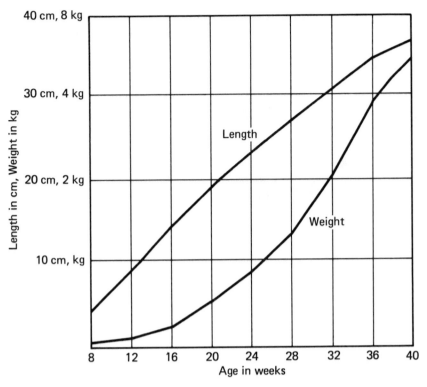

12. Sex distinguishable. Eyelids sealed shut. Buds for deciduous teeth. Vocal cords. Digestive tract. Kidneys, and liver secrete.

16. Head about one third of total length. Nose plugged. Lips visible. Fine hair on body. Pads on hands and feet. Skin dark red, loose, wrinkled.

20. Body axis straightens. Vernix caseosa covers skin as skin glands develop. Internal organs move toward mature positions.

24–28 Eyes open. Taste buds present. If born, can breathe, cry, and live for a few hours.

28–40 Fat deposited. Rapid brain growth. Nails develop. Permanent tooth. Testes descend. Becomes viable.

Figure 6.2. Summary of development during the fetal period

thrusting of the legs and arms. During these last two months the red coloration disappears as fatty deposits become more evenly distributed. The birth process is initiated by both the placenta and contraction of the uterine musculature, not by the fetus. At birth the normal-term infant is about 19 to 21 inches long and weighs between 6 and 8 pounds. (Please refer to Table 6.2 for a summary of development during the fetal period.)

INFANT GROWTH

The growth process during the first two years of life is truly amazing. The infant progresses from a tiny, helpless, horizontal, sedentary creature to a considerably larger, autonomous, vertical, active child. The physical growth of the infant has a very definite influence on its motor development. The size of the head, for example, will influence the child's developing balance abilities. Hand size will influence the mode of contact with different-size objects, and strength development will influence the onset of locomotion.

Table 6.2 Highlights of the Prenatal Growth Period

Age	Length	Weight	Major Events
Conception	1 cell	Less than 1 g	Genetic inheritance determined
1 week	0.01 in.	Less than 1 g	Germinal period, period of rapid cell differentiation
2 weeks	0.05 in.	1.5 g	Implantation in the uterus
1 month	0.25 in.	1 oz	Endoderm, mesoderm, and ectoderm formed; growth organized & differentiated
2 months	1.5 in.	2 oz	Rapid growth period, begins to take on human form, weak, reflex activity
3 months	3 in.	3 oz	Sexual differentiation, stomach and kidney function, eyelids fuse shut
4 months	6 to 8 in.	6 oz	Rapid growth period, first reflexive movements felt, bone formation begins
5 months	8 to 10 in.	8 oz	Half birth height, internal organ completion, hair over entire body
6 months	15 in.	1 to 2 lb	Eyes reopen, vernix caseosa forms, structurally complete but functionally immature
7 months	14 to 16 in.	2 to 4 lb	Rapid weight gain, adipose tissue deposited
8 months	16 to 18 in.	4 to 6 lb	Active period, fatty deposits distributed
9 months	19 to 21 in.	6 to 8 lb	Uterine contractions, labor and delivery

Neonatal Period (Birth-4 Weeks)

The neonatal period is generally considered to comprise the first 2 to 4 weeks of life. It is an "adjustive time period to being born" (Krogman, 1980, p. 9). The typical full-term newborn is 19 to 21 inches long, but the head accounts for one fourth of that length. This large size, when compared to adult head size (one seventh of total length), makes it difficult to gain and maintain equilibrium. The remaining body length is taken up with a 4-to-3 ratio of trunk to lower-limb length. The eyes are about half their adult size, and the body is about one twentieth its eventual adult dimension (Figure 6.3).

There is considerably normal variation in the weight of newborns, which may be accounted for by a variety of environmental and hereditary factors. Birth weight is closely related to the socioeconomic and nutritional status of the mother (Eichorn, 1968; Meredith, 1952). The birth weight of male infants is about 4 percent higher than females. Optimal growth requires proper nutrition, a positive state of health, and a nurturing environment. It is interesting to note, however, that low-birthweight babies and young-for-date babies have a definite tendency to catch up to their age-mates if their retarded condition of development is not too severe. J. M. Tanner (1978), a physician who has devoted much time to the study of the growth characteristics of the infant, notes that an individual's ultimate growth seems to be determined early in life and may be amended under limited conditions if prematurity, illness, or malnutrition deflects the child from his or her normal growth curve. Growth will accelerate (or catch up) to the normal trajectory on resumption of an adequate diet or termination of the illness, and then slow down again when it

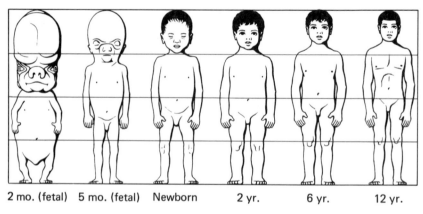

| 2 mo. (fetal) | 5 mo. (fetal) | Newborn | 2 yr. | 6 yr. | 12 yr. |

Figure 6.3. Changes in body form and proportion before and after birth

reaches its goal. Under most conditions, therefore, we see infants and children fitting into broadly determined ranges for height and weight with little in the way of extremes at either end of the developmental continuum. It should be noted, however, that although the trajectory approximates the normal curve, low-birthweight children usually remain somewhat smaller throughout life than full-term children.

Figures 6.4 through 6.7 provide graphical representations of the changes in height and weight of both boys and girls from birth to age 3.

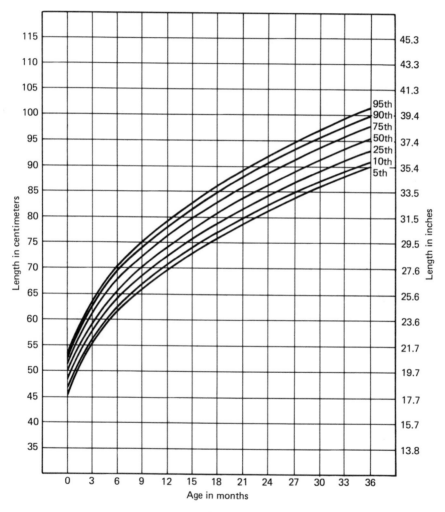

Figure 6.4. Female length by age percentiles: birth to 36 months

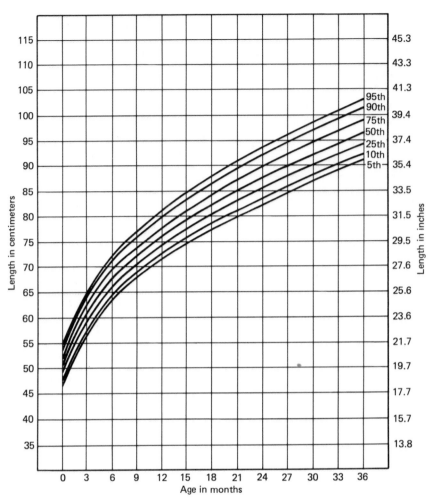

Figure 6.5. Male length by age percentiles: birth to 36 months

These growth charts from the National Center for Health Statistics (1976) indicate by age percentiles the growth patterns of infants. Although height is genetically influenced, there is little relationship between birth length and attained adult height. By the second year, however, the correlation raises to the mid-to-high 70s (Tanner, 1978).

Early Infancy (4 Weeks-1 Year)

During the first year of life there are rapid gains in both weight and length. Growth during the first six months is mainly a filling out process,

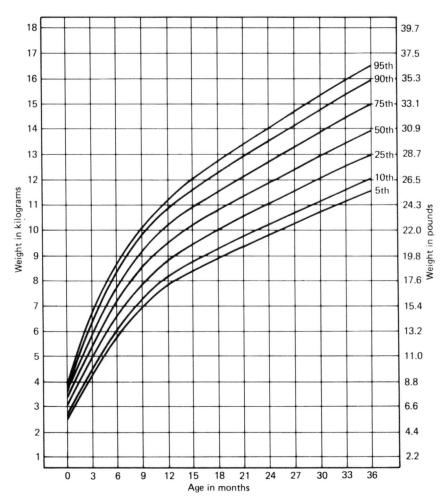

Figure 6.6. Female weight by age percentiles: birth to 36 months

with only a slight change in body proportions. In fact, the chubby "new-borns" often pictured in advertisements are actually 2 or 3 months old, not reddish, wrinkled, actual newborns. Birth weight is doubled by the fifth month, almost tripled by the end of the first year, and quadrupled by 30 months of age. Length increases to about 30 inches by the first birthday. By age 2 boys have attained about 50 percent of their adult height and girls about 53 percent (Krogman, 1980). After 6 months of age the thoracic region is larger than the head in normal children and increases with age. Infants suffering from malnutrition will have a weight deficit but will have a head size larger than the thorax (Dean, 1965).

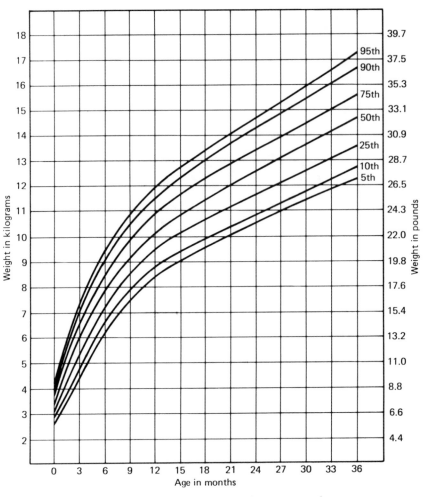

Figure 6.7. Male weight by age percentiles: birth to 36 months

Later Infancy (1 Year-2 Years)

Physical growth during the second year of life continues at a rapid pace but at a slower rate than during the first year. By age 2 the height of the average boy is about 35 inches. Girls are about 34 inches tall and weigh about 31 pounds, whereas boys average 32 pounds (National Center for Health Statistics, 1976). Height and weight have about a .60 correlation, showing a moderate degree of relationship between these two indices of physique. Because growth follows a directional trend (i.e., proximodistal and cephalocaudal), increase in size of the body parts is uneven. Upper arm growth precedes lower arm growth and hand growth. Therefore, from infancy to puberty the greatest amount of growth takes place in the distal portions of the limbs. Head growth slows from infancy onward, trunk growth proceeds at a moderate rate, limb growth is faster, and growth of the hands and feet is most rapid.

SUMMARY

Throughout the prenatal period a variety of environmental factors may influence and dramatically alter later development. The relationship between the unborn child and the mother is essentially one of parasite and host. The fetus uses the mother to supply all of its vital needs, including the intake of oxygen and nutrients and the expulsion of carbon dioxide and other wastes. These nutrients are "screened" by the mother in that they are found in her bloodstream. As a result, the condition and content of the circulatory systems of both mother and fetus are crucial to future growth and development.

The normal process of prenatal and infant growth is crucial to the motor development of the child. The height, weight, physique, and maturational level of the child plays an important role in his or her acquisition and performance of movement abilities. The prenatal period and infancy set the stage for what is to come in the development of the child's repertoire of movement and physical abilities.

CHAPTER CONCEPTS

6.1 Prenatal growth patterns are predictable and can be charted from the moment of conception.

6.2 The union of an ovum and a sperm marks the point of conception and the determination of one's genetic inheritance.

6.3 Implantation of the zygote in the uterine wall marks the true beginning of pregnancy.

6.4 The period of the zygote from conception to the fourth week is especially precarious because the expectant mother is often unaware that she is pregnant.

6.5 The period of the embryo marks the formation of the endoderm, mesoderm, and ectoderm, the three layers of cells that will eventually form the various systems of the body.

6.6 Growth proceeds at a more rapid pace by the end of the first month in utero.

6.7 The fetal period begins during the third month and is marked by the very first reflexive movements.

6.8 Growth is rapid during most of the fetal period, and there is considerable movement felt by the mother-to-be.

6.9 The fetus triples its weight from the seventh to the ninth month.

6.10 The seventh month is generally quiet, with increasing activity during the eighth and ninth months.

6.11 The head of the newborn makes up about one fourth of its entire length. Other body parts are in less dramatic proportional deviation.

6.12 Birth weight is related to a variety of factors, including the nutritional status of the mother.

6.13 Early infancy is characterized by rapid growth in length and an increase in subcutaneous tissue.

6.14 Growth during later infancy is less rapid than during the first year.

6.15 Increases in body proportions are uneven and based on the principles of proximodistal and cephalocaudal development.

TERMS TO REMEMBER

Zygote
Mitosis
Embryo
Ectoderm
Mesoderm
Endoderm
Placenta
Amnion
Fetus
Lanugo
Vernix Caseosa

CRITICAL READINGS

Caplan, F. (1981). *The First Twelve Months of Life.* New York: Bantam.
Oppenheimer, S. B. (1980). *Introduction to Embryonic Development.* Boston: Allyn and Bacon. (Chapters 1 and 2).
Rosenblith, J. F. and Sims-Knight, J. E. (1985). *In the Beginning: Development in the First Two Years.* Monterey, CA: Brooks/Cole.
Sundberg, A. I. and Wirsen, C. (1977). *A Child is Born: The Drama of Life Before Birth.* New York: Delacorte.
Tanner, J. M. (1978). *Fetus into Man.* Cambridge, MA.: Harvard University Press.

7

Infant Reflexes &
Rhythmical Stereotypies

CHAPTER COMPETENCIES

Upon Completion of This Chapter You Should Be Able To:

* *Describe primitive reflexes that are inhibited, and postural reactions that appear, before either birth or the first year of life and explain the neural development that goes with these changes.*

* *Relate inhibition of specific reflexes and appearance of specific reactions to development of particular voluntary motor skills.*

• *Distinguish between "primitive reflexes" and "postural reflexes."*

• *Speculate on the relationship of reflexes and rhythmical stereotypies to later voluntary movement behavior.*

• *Identify and discuss several rhythmical stereotypies present in the human infant.*

• *Speculate on the purpose and role of rhythmical stereotypies.*

• *Devise your own infant reflex/stereotypy observational assessment instrument.*

Reflex movements are evidenced in all fetuses, neonates, and infants to a greater or lesser degree, depending on their age and neurological makeup. Reflex movements are involuntary reactions of the body to various forms of external stimulation. They are subcortical in that they are controlled by the lower brain center, which is also responsible for numerous involuntary life-sustaining processes, such as breathing. Voluntary motor control in the normal child is a function of the mature cerebral cortex. Movements that are consciously controlled result from nerve impulses transmitted from the cerebral cortex along motor neurons. In the developing fetus and newborn infant, the cortex, more specifically, the motor area of the cortex, is generally considered to be nonfunctional (Wyke, 1975). Thus, movement is thought to be largely of a reflexive or involuntary nature.

Many early reflexes are related to infant survival (primitive reflexes), while others are precursors of voluntary movements that will appear between the ninth and fifteenth months after birth (postural reflexes). Reflexive walking, swimming, crawling, and climbing movements were reported by Shirley (1931), McGraw (1939b), and Ames (1937). These reflexes are inhibited prior to the appearance of their voluntary counterparts, but their mere presence is an indication of how deeply locomotor activities are rooted within the nervous system. The investigations by Hooker (1952) lend further support to the influence of genetics on motor behavior. He indicated that the voluntary movements of the postnatal period develop in the same sequence in which they are elicited as reflexes during fetal life.

From about the fourth month of fetal life until about the fourth month of infancy, movement is controlled largely, but not entirely, by involuntary reactions to changes in pressure, sight, sound, and tactile stimulation. These stimuli and resultant responses form the basis for the *information encoding and decoding stages* of the reflexive movement phase. Reflexes, at this point in the child's life, serve as his or her primary information gathering device for information storage in the developing cortex. As higher brain centers gain greater control of the sensorimotor apparatus, the memory trace that has been established through repeated performance of various postural reflex actions enables the infant to process information more efficiently (Hebb, 1949). This information processing period parallels Piaget's first three stages within his sensorimotor phase of development, namely, the use of reflexes, primary circular reactions, and secondary circular reactions.

REFLEXIVE BEHAVIOR AND VOLUNTARY MOVEMENT

As *primitive reflexes* are examined, two of their main functions are revealed to be nourishment seeking and protection. It is within these categories that primitive reflexes relate to the movement patterns of the lower primates. The palmar and plantar grasping reflexes, for example, have been related to arboreal primates, as have the various righting reflexes that have frequently been associated with the amphibious behavior of the lower life forms. The swimming reflex, which occurs during the second week after birth, provides what appears to be a fascinating link with the past. A coordinated swimming movement is elicited in the infant when held in or over water. One's creative mind may play with each of the reflexes and fit its occurrence into a lower order of life.

Several reflexes exist during early infancy that resemble later voluntary movements. These *postural reflexes*, as they are sometimes called, have been a topic of considerable debate over the past several years. It has been hypothesized and demonstrated that these reflex movements form the basis for later voluntary movement (Bower, 1976; McGraw, 1954; Thelen, 1980; Zelazo, 1976). As the cortex gradually matures, it assumes control over the postural reflexes of walking, climbing, swimming, and the like. In fact, Zelazo (1976, p. 88) questions the dualistic position of the anatomists in favor of a hierarchical view, stating:

> Indeed, current behavioral and neurological research with infants challenges the validity and generality of the hypothesized independence between early reflexive and later instrumental behavior. An alternative hypothesis holds that the newborn's reflexes do not disappear but retain their identity within a heirarcy of controlled behavior.

Anatomists and neurologists, on the other hand, argue that there is a recognizable gap of up to several months between the inhibition of a postural reflex and the onset of voluntary movement (Kessen et al. 1970; Prechtl and Beintema, 1964; Pontius, 1973; Wyke, 1975). Therefore, the foregoing view has been heavily criticized. This time lag, they contend, clearly indicates that there is no direct link between postural reflexes and later voluntary movement. Furthermore, it is argued that the performance of reflexive movements and voluntary movements are controlled by entirely different brain centers. Bower (1976, p. 40), however, contends that: "Such results pointed to the possibility that the reason abilities disappear is that they are not exercised."

From these statements, and from the anatomists' research, it appears there is little basis for assuming that the infant's first reflexive movements prepare him or her for later voluntary movement in a direct way. We know, however, that the results of early reflexive activity of the infant are internalized and that this information is stored for future use when he or she is neurologically ready to attempt similar voluntary movements (Zelazo, 1976). Thelen et al. (1987) further argues in support of this point of view, stating that studies do, in fact, demonstrate that there is a continuous link between reflexive and voluntary walking. She contends, as does Bower (1976), that the period of inhibition need not be present if the reflex is exercised. Thelen argues, however, that the reflex disappears because leg mass increases. Perseveration of the reflex strengthens the leg and lower body thus permitting the infant to continue the movement with little or no lag between the locomotor reflex and its voluntary counterpart. Explanations such as this account for at least an indirect link between the infant's postural reflexes and later voluntary movement. It is, therefore, important for those interested in the study of movement to have a clearer understanding of the very first forms of movement behavior.

The *neuromaturational theory* of motor development (Eckert, 1987) holds that as the cortex develops, it inhibits some of the functions of the subcortical layers and assumes ever-increasing neuromuscular control. The cortex joins in its ability to store information that is received by way of sensory neurons. This phenomenon is evidenced in the phasing-out of reflex behaviors and the assumption of voluntary movements by the infant. Concurrent formation of myelin prepares the body for the mature neuromuscular state. Movements become more localized as functional neural pathways serve isolated regions of the body with greater precision and accuracy.

However, more recent explanations of infant motor development (Thelen, 1986; Thelen et al., 1987) subscribe to what is termed a *dynamical systems* point of view. This theory contends that neuromaturation is only one of many rate-limiters to development, and that the dynamics of the system (i.e., affordances) shape the movement. In other words, (Whitehall, 1988) "movements [are] *not* prescribed but emerge from interaction between body, task, and environment with little central input." A *rate-limiter* is something which prevents a movement from occurring, such as body proportions, weight, or a host of environmental conditions.

DIAGNOSING CENTRAL NERVOUS SYSTEM DISORDERS

It is common procedure for the pediatrician to attempt to elicit primitive and postural reflexes in the neonate and young infant. If a reflex is absent, irregular, or uneven in strength, neurological dysfunction is suspected. The failure of normal reflexive movements to develop, or the prolonged continuation of various reflexes beyond their normal period, may also cause the physician to suspect neurological impairment.

The use of developmental reflexes as a tool for diagnosing central nervous system damage has been widespread. Over the years scientists have compiled an approximate timetable for the appearance and inhibition of neonatal and infant behaviors. Prechtl and Beintema (1964) have noted that the resting posture of the newborn is the flexed position. The flexors, in fact, are dominant over the extensors in the early part of life. But cortical control soon permits the normal neonate to raise its head from the prone position. Prechtl notes that:

An absence of the head-lifting response at the third day or later was highly correlated with other signs of neurological abnormalities. We may conclude, therefore, that normal babies are able to lift their chins when they are in the prone position. (p. 83)

Several other meaningful examples of this principle exist. The doll-eye movements of the neonate permit it to maintain constancy of the retinal image. When the head is tilted back, the eyes look toward the chin, and when the head is tilted forward, the eyes look toward the forehead. This response is almost always seen in premature infants and during the first day of life in the normal neonate, after which it is replaced by voluntary eye movements. Perseveration of this reflex could indicate delayed cortical maturation.

One means of diagnosing possible central nervous system disorders, therefore, is through perseverating reflexes. It must be noted that complete absence of a reflex is usually less significant than a reflex that remains too long. Other evidence of possible damage may be seen in a reflex that is too strong or too weak. A reflex that elicits a stronger response on one side of the body than on the other may also indicate central nervous system dysfunction. An asymmetrical tonic neck reflex, for example, which shows full arm extension on one side of the body and only weak extensor tone when the other side is stimulated, may also provide evidence of damage.

Examination of reflexive behaviors in the neonate has provided the physician with a primary means of diagnosing central nervous system integrity in full-term, premature, and at-risk infants. Neurological dysfunction may be suspected when any one of the following conditions appear (Egen et al. 1969).

1. Perseveration of a reflex beyond the age at which it should have been inhibited by cortical control
2. Complete absence of a reflex
3. Unequal bilateral reflex responses
4. Responses that are too strong or too weak

PRIMITIVE REFLEXES

Primitive reflexes are closely associated with the obtainment of nourishment and the protection of the infant. They first appear during fetal life and persist well into the first year. The following is a partial list of the numerous primitive reflexes exhibited by the fetus and the neonate. Their approximate times of appearance and inhibition are found in Table 7.1.

Table 7.1 Developmental Sequence for Appearance and Inhibition of Selected Primitive and Postural Reflexes

Primitive Reflexes	Month												
	0	1	2	3	4	5	6	7	8	9	10	11	12
Moro	X	X	X	X	X	X	X						
Startle	X	X	X	X				X	X	X	X	X	X
Search	X	X	X	X				X	X	X	X	X	X
Sucking	X	X	X	X									
Palmar-mental	X	X	X										
Palmar-mandibular	X	X	X	X									
Palmar grasp	X	X	X	X									
Babinski	X	X	X	X									
Plantar grasp	X	X	X		X	X	X	X	X	X	X	X	X
Tonic neck	X	X	X	X	X	X	X	X					
Postural Reflexes													
Labyrinthine righting			X	X	X	X	X	X	X	X	X	X	X
Pull-up				X				X	X	X	X	X	X
Parachute and propping					X	X	X	X	X	X	X	X	X
Neck and body righting			X	X	X	X	X						
Crawling	X	X	X	X									
Stepping	X	X	X	X	X								
Swimming	X	X	X	X	X								

Moro and Startle Reflexes

The Moro and startle reflexes may be elicited in the infant by placing it in a supine position and tapping on the abdomen, or by producing a feeling of insecurity of support (possibly by allowing the head to drop sharply backward a short distance). It may even be self-induced by a loud noise or by the infant's own cough or sneeze. In the *Moro reflex* there is a sudden extension and bowing of the arms and spreading of the fingers. The legs and toes perform the same action but less vigorously. The limbs then return to a normal flexed position against the body. The startle reflex is similar in all ways to the Moro reflex except that it involves flexion of the limbs without prior extension (Figure 7.1).

The Moro reflex is present at birth and during the first three months of life. It has been one of the most widely used tools in the neurological examination of the young infant (Bench et al. 1972). The reaction is most pronounced during the infant's first few weeks. The intensity of the response gradually decreases until it is finally characterized by a simple jerking motion of the body in response to the stimulus (*startle reflex*). Persistence of the reflex beyond the sixth month may be an indication of neurological dysfunction. An asymmetrical Moro reflex may indicate Erb's palsy or an injury to a limb.

Search and Sucking Reflexes

The search and sucking reflexes enable the newborn to obtain nourishment from its mother. Stimulation of the area around the mouth (*search reflex*) will result in the infant's turning its head toward the source of stimulation. The search reflex is strongest during the first 3 weeks of life and gradually gives way to a directed head turning response that becomes quite refined and appears to be a purposeful behavior to bring the mouth into contact with the stimulus (Prechtl, 1964). The search reflex is most easily obtained when the infant is either hungry, sleeping, or in his or her normal feeding position. Stimulation of the lips, gums, tongue, or hard palate will cause a sucking motion (*sucking reflex*) attempt to ingest nourishment. The sucking action is usually rhythmically repetitive. If it isn't, gentle movement of the object within the mouth will produce sucking. The sucking reflex actually has two phases, the expressive phase and the suction phase (Sameroff, 1968). During the expressive phase the nipple is squeezed between the tongue and palate. During the suction phase negative pressure is produced in the mouth cavity. Leonard et al. (1980) studied the nutritive sucking of high-risk neonates in a neonatal intensive care unit of a large hospital to determine if stimulation of the area around the mouth (*perioral stimulation*) would facilitate the searching, sucking, and swallowing reflexes. The results

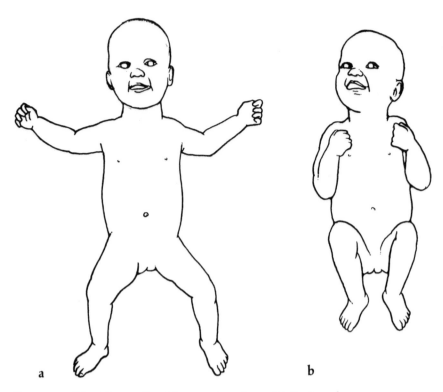

Figure 7.1 The Moro reflex (a) extension phase, (b) flexion phase

were positive, clearly indicating that producing such stimulation prior to feeding would reduce the need for intravenous feeding of high-risk newborns.

Both of these reflexes are present in all normal newborns. The search reflex may persist until the end of the first year of life; the sucking movement generally disappears as a reflex by the end of the third month but persists as a voluntary response.

Hand-Mouth Reflexes

Two hand-mouth reflexes are found in the newborn and relate to the neonate's ancestry. The *palmar-mental reflex*, elicited by scratching the base of the palm, causes contraction of the chin muscles, which lift the chin up. This reflex has been observed in newborns but disappears early in life.

The *palmar-mandibular reflex*, or Babkin reflex, as it is sometimes called, is elicited by applying pressure to the palms of both hands. The responses usually include mouth opening, closing of eyes, and flexing the head forward. This reflex begins decreasing during the first month after birth and usually is not visible after the third month (von Bernuth and Prechtl, 1968).

Palmar Grasping Reflex

The *grasping reflex* is normally present at birth and persists during the first four months of life. The intensity of the response tends to increase during the first month and slowly diminishes after that. Weak grasping or persistence of the reflex after the first year may be a sign of delay in motor development, or of hemiplegia, if it occurs on only one side.

During the first two months of life the infant usually has its hands closed tightly. Upon stimulation of the palm, the hand will close strongly around the object without use of the thumb. The grip tightens when force is exerted against the encircling fingers. The grip is often so strong that the infant is able to support his or her own weight when suspended (See Figure 7.2). Also, the grip with the left hand is generally stronger than the right-hand grip. Grasping is also increased during sucking (von Bernuth and Prechtl, 1968).

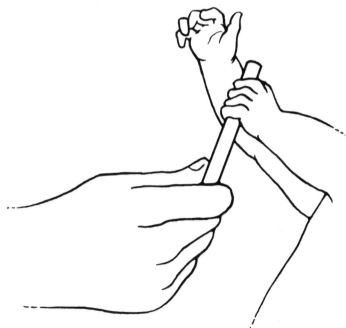

Figure 7.2. The palmar grasp reflex

Babinski and Plantar Grasp Reflexes

The *Babinski reflex* is normally present at birth but gives way to the plantar grasp reflex around the fourth month and may persist until about the twelfth month. The *plantar grasp reflex* is most easily elicited by pressing the thumbs against the ball of the infant's foot. Persistence of the Babinski reflex beyond the sixth month may be an indication of a developmental lag.

In the newborn, the Babinski reflex is elicited by a stroke on the sole of the foot. The pressure causes an extension of the toes. As the neuromuscular system matures, the Babinski reflex gives way to the plantar reflex, which is a contraction of the toes upon stimulation of the sole of the foot (Figure 7.3).

Asymmetrical and Symmetrical Tonic Neck Reflexes

To elicit an *asymmetrical tonic neck reflex*, the infant is placed in a supine position and the neck is turned so that the head is facing toward either side. The arms assume a position similar to the fencer's "on guard." That is, the arm extends on the side of the body that is facing the head and the other arm assumes an acute flexed position. The lower limbs assume a position similar to the arms. The *symmetrical tonic neck reflex* may be

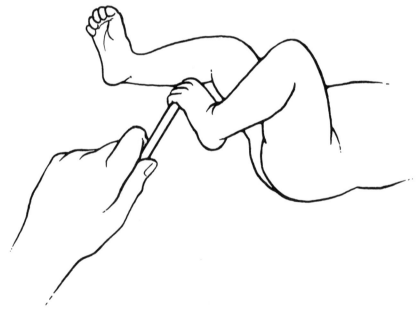

Figure 7.3. The plantar grasp reflex

elicited from a supported sitting position. Extension of the head and neck will produce extension of the arm and flexion of the legs. If the head and neck are flexed, the arms flex and the legs extend (Figure 7.4).

Both tonic neck reflexes may be observed in most premature infants, but they are not an obligatory response in newborns, that is, they do not occur each time the infant's head is turned. The 3- or 4-month-old infant, however, assumes the asymmetrical position about 50 percent of the time before this response begins gradually to disappear (Mehlman, 1940). Persistence beyond the sixth month may be an indication of lack of control over lower brain centers by higher ones (Fiorentino, 1963).

Swartz and Allen (1975) indicate that vestiges of the asymmetical tonic neck reflex are apparent in some older children and that this reflex can affect head position in the breaststroke of young swimmers. They further contend that reflexes do not totally disappear but are "integrated into the central nervous system largely through inhibition" (p. 311). If these reflexes are not properly inhibited, they may result in inadequate muscle tone, lack of independent movement of the head and extremities, midline problems, and difficulty in learning swimming strokes (Swartz and Allen, 1975).

POSTURAL REFLEXES

Postural reflexes are those that resemble later voluntary movements. Postural reflexes automatically provide maintenance of an up-

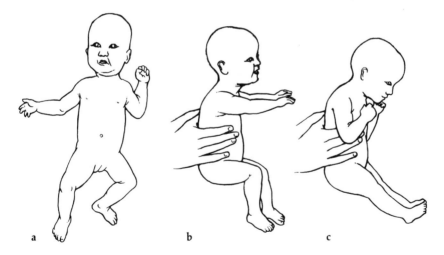

Figure 7.4. (a) The asymmetrical tonic neck reflex, (b & c) the symmetrical tonic neck reflex

right position of the individual in relation to his or her environment (Twitchell, 1965). They are found in all normal infants during the early months of life and may, in a few cases, persist through the first year. The following sections discuss postural reflexes that are of particular interest to the student of motor development. These reflexes are associated with later voluntary movement behavior and should be carefully studied by all concerned with the development of voluntary patterns of movement. The approximate times of appearance and inhibition of these reflexes are found in Table 7.1.

Labyrinthine Righting Reflex

The *labyrinthine righting reflex* may be elicited when the infant is held in an upright position and is tilted forward, backward, or to the side. The child will respond by attempting to maintain the upright position of the head by moving it in the direction opposite the one in which its trunk is moved (Figure 7.5). Impulses arising in the otoliths of the labyrinth cause the head to be maintained in proper alignment to the environment even when other sensory channels (vision and touch) are excluded (Twitchell, 1965).

The labyrinthine righting reflex makes its first appearance around the second month and becomes stronger around the middle of the first year (Fiorentino 1963). It is a major factor in the infant's obtaining and maintaining an upright head and body posture and contributes to the infant's forward movement near the end of the first year.

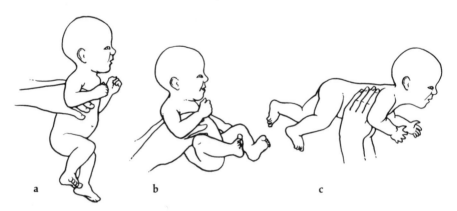

Figure 7.5. The labyrinthine righting reflexes from three positions: (a) upright, (b) tilted backward, and (c) prone

Pull-Up Reflex

The *pull-up reflex* of the arms is an involuntary attempt on the part of the infant to maintain an upright position. When the infant is in an upright position and held by one or both hands, it will flex its arms in an attempt to remain upright when tipped backward. It will do the same thing when tipped forward. The reflexive pull-up reaction of the arms usually appears around the third or fourth month and often continues through the first year (Figure 7.6).

Parachute and Propping Reflexes

The *parachute* and *propping reflexes* are protective reactions of the limbs in the direction of the displacing force. These reflexive movements occur in response to a sudden displacing force or when balance can no longer be maintained. Protective reflexes are dependent upon visual stimulation and so do not occur in the dark. These reflexes may, in fact, be a form of startle reflex.

The forward parachute reaction may be observed when the infant is held vertically in the air and then tilted toward the ground. In an apparent attempt to cushion the anticipated fall, the infant will extend the arms (Figure 7-7). The downward parachute reactions may be observed when the baby is held in an upright position and rapidly lowered toward the ground. The lower limbs extend, tense, and abduct. Propping reflexes may be elicited by pushing the infant off balance from a sitting position either forward or backward.

The forward and downward parachute reactions begin to occur around the fourth month. The sideways propping reaction is first elicited around the sixth month. The backward reaction is first seen between the tenth and twelfth months. Each of these reactions tends to persist beyond the first year and is necessary before the infant can learn to walk.

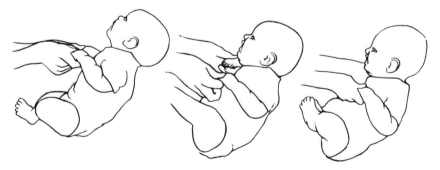

Figure 7.6. The pull-up reflex

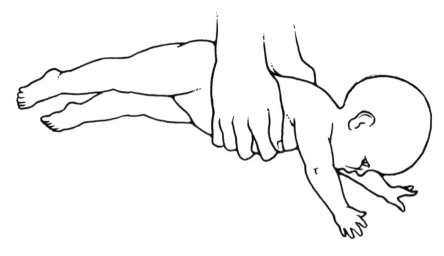

Figure 7.7. The parachute reflex

Neck and Body Righting Reflexes

When the infant is placed in a prone position with the head turned to one side, the remainder of the body moves reflexively in the same direction. First the hips and legs turn into alignment, followed by the trunk (*neck righting reflex*). From a side-lying position the reverse occurs (*body righting reflex*). When the legs and trunk are turned in one direction, the head will turn reflexively in the same direction and right the body in a prone position (Twitchell, 1965) (Figure 7.8).

The neck and body righting reflexes disappear around the sixth month (Fiorentino, 1963). These reflexes form the basis for voluntary rolling that occurs from about the fifth month onward.

Crawling Reflex

The *crawling reflex* can be seen when the infant is placed in a prone position and pressure is applied to the sole of one foot. The infant will reflexively crawl, using both its upper and lower limbs. Pressure on the soles of both feet will elicit a return in pressure by the infant. Pressure on the sole of one foot produces returned pressure and an extensor thrust of the opposite leg (von Bernuth and Prechtl, 1968).

The crawling reflex is generally present at birth and disappears around the third or fourth month. There is a lag between reflexive crawling and voluntary crawling, which appears around the seventh month (Figure 7.9).

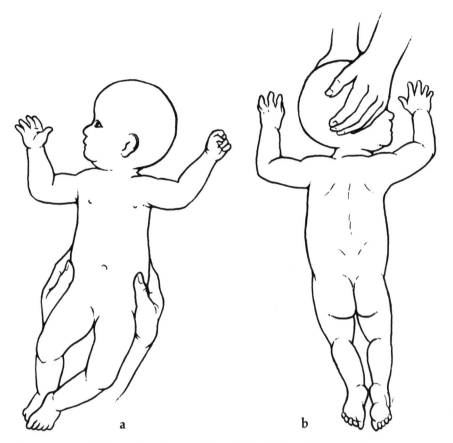

Figure 7.8. (a) The neck righting reflex (b) The body righting reflex

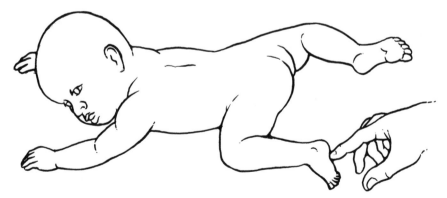

Figure 7.9. The crawling reflex

Primary Stepping Reflex

The *primary stepping reflex* is normally present during the first six weeks and disappears by the fifth month (Figure 7.10). When the infant is held erect with its body weight placed forward on a flat surface, it will respond by "walking" forward. This walking movement involves the legs only.

Zelazo (1976) and Bower (1976) studied the effects of early and persistent practice of the primary stepping reflex on the onset of voluntary walking behavior. The results of these investigations revealed that the age of independent walking was accelerated through conditioning of the stepping reflex in the experimental group; the control group did not show accelerated development. The implications of this important finding are enormous, but further research is necessary before it can be unequivocally stated *why* perseverating a reflex through persistent exercise accelerates the onset of voluntary behavior. An alternative hypothesis

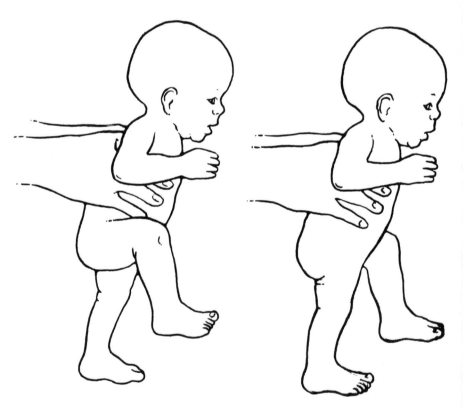

Figure 7.10. The primary stepping reflex

has been presented by Thelen (1983) that needs further testing. Essentially, she purports that conditioning of a reflex actually improves strength in the limbs exercised and that this becomes the key to early voluntary walking rather than an improved memory trace.

Swimming Reflex

When placed in a prone position in or over water, the infant will exhibit rhythmical extensor and flexor swimming movements of the arms and legs (*swimming reflex*). The movements are well organized and appear more advanced than any of the other locomotor reflexes. McGraw (1939b) filmed reflexive swimming movements in the human infant as early as the eleventh day of life. These involuntary movements generally disappear by the fifth month. McGraw discovered that a breath-holding reflex is elicited when the infant's face is placed in the water and that the swimming movements are more pronounced from this position. McGraw (1954, p. 360) has since speculated on the theory that the infant's swimming reflex is a precursor to walking. She stated: "Basically, the neuromuscular mechanisms which mediate the reflexive swimming movements may be essentially the same as those activated in the reflexive crawling and stepping movements of the infant" (p. 360).

It is interesting to speculate on the relationship between the crawling, stepping, and swimming reflexes. Gordon (1981, p. 48) makes this perceptive statement: "If the swimming reflex is a pattern from which later swimming or walking can build, its practice offers a legitimate reason for the existence of infant swim programs."

RHYTHMICAL STEREOTYPIES

Researchers have been interested for several decades in the many intriguing questions concerning infant reflexes. This research has had, and will continue to have, important implications for the diagnosis of central nervous system disorders and for the physical therapist working with individuals who display various pathological conditions. Furthermore, the study of the origin of reflexes and their relationship to later voluntary behaviors is forgoing new inroads into learning theory and how the human organism organizes itself for the learning of new movement skills.

Only recently have investigators gone beyond cataloging and describing infant reflexive behaviors to explain what is going on. The work of Esther Thelen is among the first attempts at answering the many questions raised by the stereotypical behaviors of the infant. Thelen (1979) studied *rhythmical stereotypies* in normal human infants in an attempt to classify these movements *and* to provide an explanation for their occurrence. Stereotypies are rhythmical behaviors performed over and over for their own sake. In children and adults they are generally considered evidence of abnormal behavior, but in infants they are quite normal. Thelen (1979, 1981) observed and cataloged the rhythmical stereotypies of normal infants from four weeks to one year of age. Her observations revealed 47 stereotypical behaviors which have been subdivided into four groups: (1) movements of the legs and feet, (2) movements of the torso, (3) movements of the arms, hands, and fingers, and (4) movements of the head and face. According to Thelen (1979, p. 699): "These behaviors showed developmental regularities as well as constancy of form and distribution. Groups of stereotypies involving particular parts of the body or postures had characteristic ages of onset, peak performance, and decline." Rhythmic movements of given body systems tend to increase just prior to the infant's gaining voluntary control of that system. Therefore, the maturational level of the infant appears to be the determiner of rhythmical stereotypies. Recently, Thelen and her colleagues (Thelen, 1981; Thelen, Kelso, and Fogel, 1987) have argued that the presence of stereotypical behaviors in normal human infants is evidence of a self-organizing central motor program in control of infant motor development.

Legs and Feet

Rhythmical kicking movements of the legs and feet were found by Thelen (1979) to be the earliest stereotypies observed. The majority of rhythmical kicking took place in either a prone or supine position. The supine position afforded infants the greatest amount of freedom with flexibility at both the hip and knee joints. When kicking from this back-lying position, the baby's legs are bent slightly at the hips, knees, and ankles with moderate outward rotation at the hip. From this position the infant is able to alternately kick the legs in what resembles a bicycling action. From the prone position alternate leg kicking is more restricted and occurs only from the knee joint. Thelen noted that stereotypies of the legs and feet began earlier than other forms (around the 4 week of age) and reached their peak occurrence between 24 and 32 months of age. Other kicking forms discovered were foot-rubbing from a seated position and single-leg-kicking from both prone and supine positions.

Torso

Thelen (1979) observed several rhythmical stereotypies of the torso. The most common was from a prone position. The infant arches the back, lifts the arms and legs from the supporting surface, and rhythmically rocks back and forth from an airplane-like position. Another frequently observed stereotypie of the torso occurs from a hands-and-knee prone creeping position. From this position the infant moves the body forward by extending the upper position of the leg and while keeping the lower leg stationary. The arms remain extended throughout but move forward on the backward thrust of the legs.

Other common, but less frequently observed, rhythmical stereotypies of the torso were reported by Thelen to include rhythmical actions from sitting, kneeling, and standing postures. From either a supported or unsupported sitting position the infant rhythmically rocks the torso forward and back. Rhythmical stereotypies from a kneeling position include rocking back and forth, side to side, and up and down. Standing stereotypies are quite common and generally occur from a support-standing position. The infant bends at the knees and performs a rhythmical up-and-down bouncing movement. Infants may also be observed to rhythmically rock forward and back and from side to side.

Arms, Hands, and Fingers

Rhythmical stereotypies of the arms, hands, and fingers were observed in all of the infants sampled by Thelen (1979). Waving (actions without an object) and banging (actions with an object in the infant's grasp) were the most frequently observed. Both are actually the same motor pattern and involve rhythmical movement in a vertical action from the shoulder. Banging differs from waving only in that the infant makes contact with the surface on the downward action. Rhythmical clapping of the hands in front of the body is another common stereotypie, as is arm sway. The arm sway stereotypie is elicited, however, only when the infant is grasping an object and involves shoulder-initiated action across the front of the body.

Head and Face

Rhythmical stereotypies of the head and face, according to Thelen (1979), are much less frequent. They involve actions such as rhythmical head shaking from side to side ("no") and up and down ("yes"). Rhythmical sticking out of the tongue and drawing it back may be observed along with non-nutritive sucking behaviors.

Of the 47 rhythmical stereotypes observed by Thelen, movements of the legs and feet were the most common, began the earliest, and peaked between 24 to 32 weeks of age. Arm and hand stereotypies are also very common but peak somewhat later, between 34 to 42 weeks. Torso stereotypies, although common, are less frequent. Furthermore, torso stereotypies from a sitting, kneeling, or standing posture tend to peak later than the others.

SUMMARY

Primitive reflexes, which are under the control of subcortical brain layers, are observed in the fetus from about the eighteenth week of gestation. Generally, reflexes serve the double function of helping the neonate secure nourishment and protection. Many of the movements, however, are more closely related to functions in lower primates, indicating a possible phylogenetic link of the human with other forms of life.

As neurological development proceeds in the normal fetus, and later in the normal neonate, reflexes appear and disappear on a fairly standard, though informal, schedule. The presence of a primitive or postural reflex is evidence of subcortical control over some neuromuscular functions. This is indicated through voluntary control of a movement by the infant, reflecting operations at the cortical level. The function of the subcortex is not completely inhibited. Throughout life, it maintains control over such activities as coughing, sneezing, and yawning, as well as over the involuntary life processes. The cortex mediates more purposive behavior, whereas subcortical behavior is limited and stereotyped.

Although it is not yet possible to determine whether there is a direct relationship between reflexive behavior and later voluntary movement, it is safe to assume that there is at least an indirect link. This link may be associated with the ability of the developing cortex to store information received from the sensory end-organs regarding the actual performance of the involuntary movement. Or, it may be due to improved strength in the involuntarily (reflexively) exercised body part.

CHAPTER CONCEPTS

7.1   Reflexive activity is the first form of movement engaged in by the fetus and the newborn.

7.2   Some reflexes are related to the performance of later voluntary movements.

7.3   Reflexive movements are subcortically controlled and are present in all fetuses and newborns.

7.4   The cerebral cortex of the newborn is not fully developed, and reflexive movements are predominant over the crude, ill-defined voluntary movements of the neonate.

7.5   Reflex actions serve as the primary information gathering source for the very young infant.

7.6   Changes in pressure, sight, sound, and tactile stimulation produce primitive and postural reflexes.

7.7   Primitive reflexes are nourishment-seeking and protective actions.

7.8   Postural reflexes resemble later voluntary movements and may be related in some manner.

7.9   Reflexive behaviors are observed in the early diagnosis of central nervous system disorder.

7.10 Reflexes appear and are inhibited on a standard schedule, indicating increased cortical control over movement.

7.11 The subcortex plays an important role throughout life by sustaining the involuntary life processes and controlling such behavior as coughing, sneezing, and yawning.

7.12 Early and regular stimulation of a postural reflex may hasten onset of the corresponding voluntary movement.

7.13 Rhythmical stereotypies are repetitive movements performed for their own sake.

7.14 Rhythmical stereotypies provide evidence for a self-organizing central motor program that controls infant motor development.

7.15 The utilization of stereotypical behaviors and reflexive movements in the quest for voluntary motor control provides the basis for a dynamical systems theory of early motor development.

TERMS TO REMEMBER

Information Encoding Stage
Information Decoding Stage
Primitive Reflexes
Postural Reflexes
Neuromaturational Theory
Dynamical Systems
Rate-Limiter
Affordances
Moro Reflex
Startle Reflex
Search Reflex
Sucking Reflex
Perioral Stimulation
Palmar-Mental Reflex
Palmar-Mandibular Reflex

Palmar Grasping Reflex
Babinski Reflex
Plantar Grasp Reflex
Asymmetrical Tonic Neck Reflex
Symmetrical Tonic Neck Reflex
Labyrinthine Righting Reflex
Pull-Up Reflex
Parachute Reflex
Propping Reflex
Neck Righting Reflex
Body Righting Reflex
Crawling Reflex
Primary Stepping Reflex
Swimming Reflex
Rhythmical Stereotypies

CRITICAL READINGS

Easton, T. A. "On the Normal Use of Reflexes," *American Scientist* 60, 591-599, 1972.

Kessen, W., et al. (1970). Human Infancy: A Bibliography and Guide," in Mussen, P. H. (ed.), *Manual of Child Psychology*, New York: Wiley, (pages 311-329).

Payne, G. (1985). "Infant Reflexes in Human Motor Development." Lawren Productions: Box 666 Mendocino, CA 95460 (video tape).

Prechtl, H. F. R. (1986). "Prenatal Motor Development." In Wade, M. G. and Whiting, H. T. A. (eds.) *Motor Development in Children: Aspects of Coordination and Control.* Dordrecht, The Netherlands: Martinus Nijhoff.

Thelen, E. (1979). "Rhythmical Stereotypies in Normal Human Infants." *Animal Behavior*, 27, 699-715.

Thelen, E. (1981). "Rhythmical Behavior in Infancy: An Ethological Perspective." *Developmental Psychology*, 17, 237-257.

Thelen, E., Kelso, J. A. S. and Fogel, A. (1987). "Self Organizing Systems and Infant Motor Development." *Developmental Review*, 7, 39-65.

8

Rudimentary Movement Abilities

CHAPTER COMPETENCIES

Upon Completion of This Chapter You Should Be Able To:

* *Describe intertask "motor milestones" that lead to upright locomotion and visually guided reaching.*

• *Distinguish between the reflex inhibition and the precontrol stages within the rudimentary movement phase of development.*

• *Discuss historical and contemporary study of infant motor development.*

• *List and describe the developmental sequence of acquisition of rudimentary stability, locomotor, and manipulative abilities.*

• *Distinguish between "creeping" and "crawling" and describe the developmental process of each.*

• *Discuss the interaction between maturation and experience on the acquisition of rudimentary movement abilities.*

• *Devise your own rudimentary movement infant observational assessment instrument.*

Preschool and elementary school children are products of a specific genetic structure and all of the experiences that they have had since conception. Children are not a tabula rasa, ready to be molded and shaped to either our whims or a precut pattern. Current research is making it clear that infants are able to process a great deal more information than previously thought. Infants think. They use movement as a purposeful, though initially imprecise, way of gaining information about their environment. Each child is an individual and no two individuals respond in exactly the same manner. The child's hereditary and experiential backgrounds have a profound effect on the development of movement abilities. It is important that we study the child, beginning with the early movement experiences of infancy, in order to gain a better understanding of the development that has taken place before he or she enters the nursery or elementary school. It is also important to study infant motor development in order to gain a better understanding of the developmental concern of how humans learn to move.

Gaining control over one's musculature, learning to cope with the force of gravity, and achieving controlled movement through space are the major developmental tasks facing the infant. During the neonatal period movement is random, ill-defined, and primarily reflexive. As higher brain centers take over, however, these reflexes are gradually inhibited. The *reflex inhibition stage* is a period stretching throughout most of the first year of life. The infant gradually moves toward controlled rudimentary movement that represents a monumental accomplishment in suppressing reflexes and integrating the sensory and motor apparatuses.

As the primitive and postural reflexes of the previous phase begin to fade, higher brain centers take over many of the skeletal muscle functions of lower brain centers. The reflex inhibition stage essentially begins at birth. From the moment of birth the newborn is bombarded by sight, sound, smell, and tactile and kinesthetic stimulation. The task is to bring order to this sensory stimulation. Initial reflexive responses are gradually inhibited throughout the first year until about the first birthday when the infant is seen to have made remarkable progress and to have brought a semblance of order out of apparent chaos.

The period from about 12 months to between 18 and 24 months represents a time for practice and mastery of the many rudimentary tasks initiated during the first year. The infant brings his or her movements under control during this precontrol stage. The *precontrol stage* spans roughly the period between the first and second birthdays. During this stage the infant begins to gain greater control and precision in movement. Differentiation and integration of sensory and motor processes become more highly developed.

Changes in the nervous system are rapid during this period. The brain of the 2-year-old, according to Kessen et al. (1970, p. 290), "is hardly discriminable in histological characteristics from the adult brain". Myelinization in neural development has progressed significantly by the end of the first year to render the child ready for development and refinement of a vast array of rudimentary stability, locomotor, and manipulative tasks (Eckert, 1987). The infant makes crude but purposeful attempts at a variety of movement tasks. These early attempts should be encouraged, and a home environment that stimulates their practice may prove beneficial in hastening their mature development. During this stage, however, the infant is primarily involved in gaining control and mastery over the rudimentary stability, locomotor, and manipulative tasks that will be discussed in this chapter.

STUDY OF INFANT MOTOR DEVELOPMENT

Study of the rudimentary movement abilities of infancy received its impetus in the 1930s and 1940s when a wealth of information was obtained from the observations of child psychologists. Many of these studies have become classics and have withstood the test of time because of their careful controls and thoroughness. The works of Halverson, Shirley, Bayley, and Gesell are particularly noteworthy.

The work by H. M. Halverson (1937) is probably the best ever completed on the sequence of emergence of voluntary grasping behavior during infancy. Through film analysis of infants from 16 to 52 weeks of age, he described three distinct stages of approach toward a cube and the development of the use of fingers-thumb opposition in grasping behavior.

Shirley's (1931) extensive study of 25 infants from birth to age 2 enabled her to describe a sequential developmental progression of activities leading to upright posture and a walking gait. Shirley noted that "each separate stage was a fundamental step in development" and that "every baby advanced from stage to stage in the same order" (p.98). She also noted that, although the sequence was fixed, individual differences were expressed in differences in the rates of development between infants.

Bayley (1935) conducted an extensive study similar to that of Shirley. As a result of her observations of infants, Bayley was able to describe a developmental series of emerging locomotor abilities progressing from reflexive crawling to walking down a flight of stairs using an alternate foot pattern. Based on this information, Bayley was able to develop a cumulative scale of infant motor development that has been widely used as a diagnostic tool to determine an infant's developmental status.

Gesell (1945) conducted extensive studies of infant motor development. He viewed posture (i.e., stability) as the basis of all forms of movement. Therefore, according to Gesell, any form of locomotion or infant manipulation is actually a closely related series of sequential postural adjustments.

The sequence of motor development is predetermined by innate biological factors that cut across all social, cultural, ethnic, and racial boundaries. This common base of motor development during the early years of life has caused many to speculate that some voluntary movements (particularly locomotor movements) are phylogenetic (Eckert 1973) and that, because these movements are maturationally based, they are not actually under voluntary developmental control (Hellebrandt et al., 1961). This has often led to the erroneous assumption that infants and particularly young children acquire their movement abilities at about the same chronological age solely by the action of maturation and with little dependence on experience. The fact is that, although the sequence of skill acquisition is resistant to change during infancy and childhood, the rate of acquisition differs from child to child due to his or her experiential base.

From the moment of birth the infant is in a constant struggle to gain mastery over the environment in order to survive. During the earliest stages of development, the infant's primary interaction with the environment is through the medium of movement. There are three primary categories of movement that the infant must begin to master for survival as well as for effective and efficient interaction and with the world. First, the infant must establish and maintain the relationship of the body to the force of gravity in order to obtain an upright sitting posture and an erect standing posture (*stability*). Second, the child must develop basic abilities in order to move through the environment (*locomotion*). Third, the infant must develop the rudimentary abilities of reach, grasp, and release in order that meaningful contact with objects may be made (*manipulation*).

The establishment of rudimentary abilities in the infant forms the building blocks for more extensive development of the fundamental movement abilities in early childhood and adolescence. These so-called rudimentary movement abilities are highly involved tasks for the infant. The importance of their development must not be overlooked or minimized. The question that arises is: Can factors in the environment enhance the development of those movement abilities? The answer is an unqualified yes. They are not maturationally determined to the point where they are not susceptible to modification. Early enrichment does seem to influence later development, but further information is needed about timing, degree, and duration.

STABILITY

The infant is involved in a constant struggle against the force of gravity in the attempts to obtain and maintain an upright posture. Establishing control over the musculature in opposition to gravity is a process that follows a predictable sequence in all infants. The events leading to an erect standing posture begin with gaining control over the head and neck and proceed down to the trunk and the legs. Operation of the cephalocaudal principle of development is apparent in the infant's sequential progress from a lying position to a sitting posture and eventually to an erect standing posture. Table 8.1 provides a summary of the developmental sequence and the approximate age of onset of rudimentary stability abilities.

Control of the Head and the Neck

At birth the infant has little control over the head and neck muscles. If held erect at the trunk, the head will drop forward. Around the end of the first month, control is gained over these muscles and the infant is able to hold the head erect when supported at the base of the neck. By the end of the first month the infant should be able to lift the chin off the crib when lying in a prone position. By the fifth month the infant should be able to lift the head off the crib when lying in a supine position.

Control of the Trunk

After infants have gained mastery of the head and neck muscles, they begin to gain control of the muscles in the thoracic and lumbar regions of the trunk. The development of trunk control begins around the second month of life. Control of the trunk muscles may be observed by holding the infant off the ground by the waist and noting the ability to make postural adjustments necessary to maintain an erect position.

By the end of the second month, infants should be capable of lifting

Table 8.1 Developmental Sequence and Approximate Age of Onset of Rudimentary Stability Abilities

Control of head and neck	Turns to one side	Birth
	Turns to both sides	1 week
	Held with support	First month
	Chin off contact surface	Second month
	Good prone control	Third month
	Good supine control	Fifth month
Control of trunk	Lifts head and chest	Second month
	Attempts supine-to-prone position	Third month
	Success in supine-to-prone roll	Sixth month
	Prone to supine roll	Eight month
Sitting	Sits with support	Third month
	Sits with self-support	Sixth month
	Sits alone	Eighth month
	Stands with support	Sixth month
Standing	Supports with handholds	Tenth month
	Pulls to supported stand	Eleventh month
	Stands alone	Twelfth month

the chest off the floor when placed in a prone position. After infants are able to lift the chest, they begin to draw the knees up toward the chest and then kick them out suddenly as if swimming. This usually occurs by the sixth month. Another indication of gaining control over the muscles of the trunk is the ability to turn over from a supine to a prone position. This is generally accomplished around the sixth month and is easily done by flexing the hips and stretching out the legs at right angles to the trunk. Mastery of the roll from a prone to a supine position usually occurs somewhat later.

Sitting

Sitting alone is an accomplishment that requires complete control over the entire trunk. The infant of 4 months is generally able to sit with support. This support comes in the lumbar region. The infant has control over the upper trunk but not the lower portion. During the next month or two the infant gradually gains control over the lower trunk. The first efforts at stting alone are characterized by an exaggerated forward lean. This is an attempt to gain added support for the lumbar region. Gradually, the ability to sit erect with a limited amount of support develops. By the seventh month the infant is generally able to sit alone completely unsupported. At this juncture he or she has now gained control over the upper half of the body. At the same time the infant is learning to sit alone, he or she is developing control over the arms and hands: a further example of the cephalocaudal and proximodistal principles of development in operation (Figure 8.1).

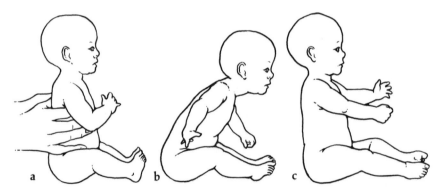

Figure 8.1. The stages of achieving independent sitting: (a) third month, (b) sixth month, and (c) eighth month

Standing

Achievement of an erect standing posture represents a developmental milestone in the infant's quest for stability. It is an indication that control over the musculature has been gained to the extent that the force of gravity can no longer place such demanding restraints on movement. The infant is now on the verge of achieving upright locomotion (walking), a feat that is heralded by parents and pediatricians alike as the infant's most spectacular task of motor development.

The first voluntary attempts at standing occur around the fifth month. When held under the armpits and brought in contact with a supporting surface, the infant will voluntarily extend at the hip, straighten and tense the muscles of the legs, and maintain a standing position with considerable outside support. Around the ninth or tenth month the infant is able to stand beside furniture and support himself for a considerable period of time. Gradually, the infant begins to lean less heavily on the supporting object and can often be seen testing balance completely unsupported for a brief instant. Between the eleventh and twelfth months the infant learns to pull to a stand by first getting to the knees and then pushing with the legs while upward-extended arms pull down. Standing alone for extended periods of time generally accompanies walking alone and does not appear separately in most babies. The onset of an erect standing posture normally occurs somewhere between 11 and 13 months (Figure 8.2).

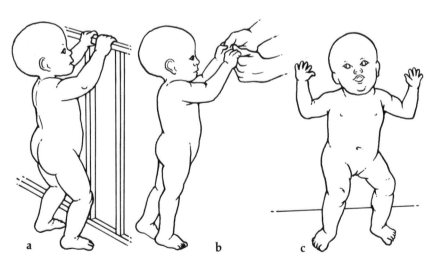

Figure 8.2. Three stages of gaining a standing posture: (a) sixth month, (b) tenth month, and (c) twelfth month

At this point the infant has gained considerable control over the musculature. He is able to accomplish the difficult task of rising from a lying position to a standing position completely unaided.

LOCOMOTION

The infant's movement through space is dependent on emerging abilities to cope with the force of gravity. Locomotion does not develop independently of stability; it relies heavily on it. The infant will not be able to move about freely until the rudimentary developmental tasks of stability (presented in the previous section) are mastered. Following are discussions of the most frequent forms of locomotion engaged in by the infant while learning how to cope with the force of gravity. These forms of locomotion are also summarized in Table 8.2.

Crawling

The crawling movements of the infant are the first attempts at purposive locomotion. *Crawling* evolves as the infant gains control of the muscles of the head, neck, and trunk. While in a prone position, the infant may reach for an object in front of him. In doing so, he raises his head and chest off the floor. On coming back down, the outstretched arms pull the back toward the feet. The result of this combined effort is a slight sliding movement forward (Figure 8.3). The legs are usually not used in these early attempts at crawling. Crawling generally appears in the infant by the sixth month. It may appear, however, as early as the fourth month.

Creeping

Creeping evolves from crawling and often develops into a highly efficient form of locomotion for the infant. *Creeping* differs from crawling in that the legs and arms are used in opposition to one another from a

Table 8.2 Developmental Sequence and Approximate Age of Onset of Rudimentary Locomotor Abilities

Horizontal movements	Scooting	Third month
	Crawling	Sixth month
	Creeping	Ninth month
	Walking on all fours	Eleventh month
Upright gait	Walks with support	Sixth month
	Walks with handholds	Tenth month
	Walks with lead	Eleventh month
	Walks alone (hands high)	Twelfth month
	Walks alone (hands low)	Thirteenth month

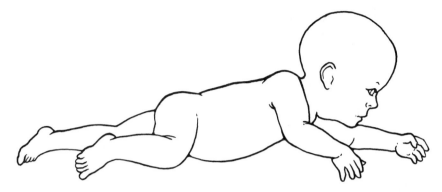

Figure 8.3. Crawling

hands-and-knees position. The infant's first attempts at creeping are characterized by very deliberate movements of one limb at a time. As the infant's proficiency increases, movements become synchronous and more rapid. Most efficient creepers utilize a *contralateral pattern* (right arm and left leg) (Figure 8.4).

There has been considerable speculation in the past two decades concerning the importance of creeping in the infant's motor development and the proper method of creeping. The neurological organization ration-

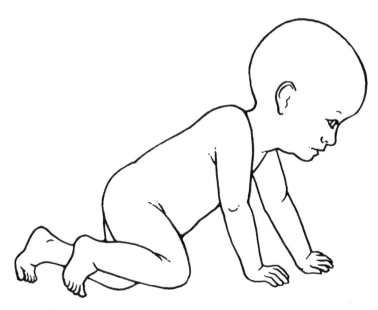

Figure 8.4. Creeping

ale of Carl Delacato (1966a) has placed considerable importance on proper creeping and crawling techniques as a necessary stage in achieving cortical hemispherical dominance. Dominance of one side of the cortex is necessary, according to Delacato, for proper neurological organization. Faulty organization, it is hypothesized, will lead to motor, perceptual, and language problems in the child and adult. This hypothesis has come under considerable attack by neurologists, pediatricians, and researchers in the area of child development. Careful evaluation of the pros and cons of Delacato's rationale is necessary before making any definite conclusions.

Upright Gait

Achievement of upright locomotion depends on the achievement of stability in the infant. The infant must first be able to control the body in a standing position before attention can be turned to the dynamic postural shifts required of upright locomotion. An infant's first attempts at independent walking generally occur somewhere between the tenth and fifteenth months and are characterized by a wide base of support, the feet turned outward, and the knees slightly flexed. These first walking movements are not synchronous and fluid; they are irregular and hesitant and are not accompanied by reciprocal arm movements. In fact, they only vaguely resemble the mature walking pattern of early childhood. The advent of walking and other forms of upright locomotion is influenced primarily by maturation but may also be influenced by environmental factors. A child cannot move through space until developmentally ready. Special training prior to readiness is not likely to accelerate learning. If, however, the child's nervous system and musculature are developed to the point of readiness, we may expect to witness slight acceleration in the advent of upright locomotion when the infant receives the benefit of additional environmental supports (that is, encouragement and assistance of parents and furniture handholds). Physique, heredity, and environmental factors interact to determine the onset of independent walking in the child.

Shirley (1931, p. 18) identified four stages that the infant passes through in learning how to walk unaided. These are: "(a) an early period of stepping in which slight forward progress is made (3-6 months); (b) a period of standing with help (6-10 months); (c) a period of walking when led (9-12 months); (d) a period of walking alone (12-15 months)." As the infant passes through each of these stages and progresses toward a mature walking pattern, several changes occur. First, the speed of walking accelerates and length of the step increases. Second, the width of the step increases until independent walking is well established, and then decreases slightly. Third, the eversion of the foot gradually decreases until the feet are pointing straight ahead. Fourth, the upright walking gait gradually smooths out, the length of the step becomes regular, and the movements of the body become synchronous. Shortly after independent walking has been achieved, the toddler will experiment with walking sideways and backward (Eckert, 1973) and on the tiptoes (Bayley, 1935).

MANIPULATION

As in stability and locomotion, the manipulative abilities of the infant evolve through a series of stages. In this section, only the most basic aspects of manipulation (reach, grasp, and release) will be considered. As with stability and locomotion, the manipulative abilities of the infant may be susceptible to early appearance even though the process is influenced greatly by maturation. If the child is maturationally ready, he will benefit from early opportunities to practice and perfect rudimentary manipulative abilities. Mussen et al. (1969, p. 178) have pointed out:

> The child can be helped to master skills earlier than he ordinarily would through enrichment, but the timing of the enrichment is important. It is almost as bad to present enriching experiences before the child is ready to use them effectively as it is to deprive the child of these stimulations entirely.

The following are the three general steps in which the infant engages during the acquisition of rudimentary manipulative abilities. Table 8.3 provides a summary of the developmental sequence and approximate age of onset of rudimentary manipulative abilities.

Table 8.3 Developmental Sequence and Approximate Age of Onset of Rudimentary Manipulative Abilities

Reaching	Globular ineffective	First to third month
	Definite corralling	Fourth month
	Controlled	Sixth month
Grasping	Reflexive	Birth
	Voluntary	Third month
	Two-hand palmar grasp	Third month
	One-hand palmar grasp	Fifth month
	Pincer grasp	Ninth month
	Controlled grasping	Fourteenth month
	Eats without assistance	Eighteenth month
Releasing	Basic	Twelfth to fourteenth month
	Controlled	Eighteenth month

Reaching

During the first four months of life, the infant does not make definite reaching movements toward objects, although she may attend closely to them visually and make globular encircling motions in the general direction of the object (Bower, 1970). Around the fourth month the infant begins to make the fine eye and hand adjustments necessary for contact with the object. Often the infant can be observed making alternating glances between the two. The movements are slow and awkward, involving primarily the shoulder and elbow. Later the wrist and the hand become more directly involved. By the end of the fifth month, the child's aim is nearly perfect, and she is now able to reach for and make tactual contact with objects in the environment. This accomplishment is necessary before being able to take hold of the object and grasp it in the hand.

Grasping

The newborn will grasp an object when it is placed in the palm of the hand. This action, however, is entirely reflexive until about the fourth month. Voluntary grasping must wait until the sensorimotor mechanism has developed to the extent that efficient reaching and meaningful contact can take place. Halverson (1937) identified several stages in the development of prehension. Briefly, they are: (1) The 4-month-old infant makes no real voluntary effort at tactual contact with object. (2) The infant of 5 months is capable of reaching for and making contact with the object. He is able to grasp the object with the entire hand but not firmly. (3) The child's movements are gradually refined so that by the seventh month the palm and fingers are coordinated. The child is still unable to effectively use the thumb and fingers. (4) By the ninth month the child begins use of the forefinger in grasping. By 10 months, reaching and grasping are coordinated into one continuous movement. (5) Efficient use of the thumb and forefinger comes into play at about 12 months. (6) By the time the child is 14 months old, its prehension abilities are very much like those of adults.

The developmental progression of reaching and grasping is complex. Landreth (1958) stated that six component coordinates appear to be involved in the development of prehension. Eckert (1987, pp. 122-123) has summed up these six developmental acts in the following statement:

> These acts involve transitions and include: (1) the transition from visually locating an object to attempting to reach for the object. Other transitions involve: (2) simple eye-hand coordination to progressive independence of visual effort with its ultimate expression in activities such as piano playing and typing; (3) initial maximal involvement of body musculature to a minimum involvement and

greater economy of effort; (4) proximal large muscle activity of the arms and shoulders to distal fine muscle activity of the fingers; (5) early crude raking movements in manipulating objects with the hands to the later pincer-like precision of control with the opposing thumb and forefinger; and (6) initial bilateral reaching and manipulation to ultimate use of the preferred hand.

Releasing

The frantic shaking of a rattle is a familiar sight when observing a 6-month-old infant at play. This is a learning activity that is generally accompanied by a great deal of smiling, babbling, and glee. Minutes later, however, the same infant may be observed shaking the rattle with obvious frustration and rage. This abrupt shift in moods may be attributed to the infant at 6 months of age not having yet mastered the art of releasing an object from grasp. The child has succeeded in reaching for and grasping the handle of the rattle but is not maturationally able to command the flexor muscles of the fingers to relax their grip on the object on command. Learning to fill a bottle with stones, building a block tower, hurling a ball, and turning the pages of a book are seemingly simple examples of the young child's attempt to cope with the problem of release. But when compared with earlier attempts at reaching and grasping, these are indeed remarkable advances. By the time the child is 14 months old, he has mastered the rudimentary elements of releasing objects from her grasp. The 18-month-old has well-coordinated control of all aspects of reach, grasp, and release (Halverson, 1937).

As the infant's mastery of the rudimentary abilities of manipulation (reach, grasp, and release) are developing, the reasons for handling objects are revised. Instead of learning to manipulate objects simply to touch, feel, or mouth them, the child now becomes involved in the process of manipulating objects in order to learn more about the world in which he lives. The manipulation of objects becomes directed by appropriate perceptions in order to achieve meaningful goals (Figure 8.5).

SPECIAL PROGRAMS FOR INFANTS

In recent years considerable attention has been given to the potential benefits that result from early intervention in the motor development of infants. Infant stimulation programs for at-risk babies have become increasingly popular due to the dramatic reduction in their mortality rates. Similarly, but for different reasons, infant aquatic programs have steadily gained popularity as have land-based baby exercise programs. Care must be taken to separate fact from fiction and to carefully catalog what

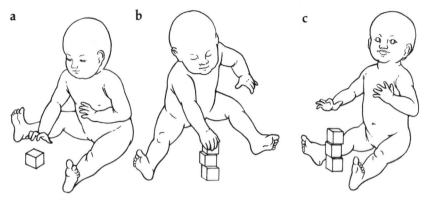

Figure 8.5. (a) Reach (b) Grasp (c) Release

we know about each of these programs on the motor development of the infant.

Infant Stimulation Programs

Infant stimulation is a form of intervention for high-risk infants in which their environment is manipulated in a way that provides enrichment through the various sensory modalities. This is done in an attempt to counteract existing conditions which may interfere with one's ability to have a full and productive life (Denhoff, 1981). These programs are implemented in order to prevent postnatal factors associated with high risk infants from seriously impairing later development.

Studies concerning postnatal factors affecting motor development tend to center around the influences of the postnatal environment, found in the neonatal intensive care unit, on subsequent development. Many researchers believe that the surroundings in which a high-risk infant is placed may actually increase the risk of further developmental deficits. The bright lights, noises, blandness, and restricted handling found in the neonatal intensive care unit may be both sensory-bombarding and sensory-depriving (Ulrich, 1984). Infant development is largely dependent upon learning from and interacting with the environment, and a hospital environment may not allow or restrict these processes.

Infant stimulation, as a treatment for high-risk infants, is based on a number of assumptions concerning infant development and behavior. In the long run the success of these programs will depend upon the validity of the theories underlying these assumptions and the ability of programs to provide appropriate services. The following is a list of some basic assumptions involved in infant stimulation taken from Denhoff (1981), Kopp (1982), and Ulrich (1984):

1. Infancy is a crucial period and intervention will be effective only if started early in life.
2. Appropriate maternal and infant behavior is contingent upon interactions between mother and child.
3. Physical abilities can impinge upon, but do not necessarily interfere with, development when emotional and social growth are maintained as normally as possible.
4. Multiple caretakers in the early months may interfere with infant-parent attachment.
5. A disabled infant must be managed as a total person, with equal emphasis on physical, mental, and social-emotional elements.
6. The environment of the neonatal intensive care unit is different from the intrauterine environment and thus deprives the preterm infant of kinesthetic, tactile and auditory stimulation it would have received in the third trimester.
7. The neonatal intensive care unit does not provide high-risk infants with the nurturing environment the newborn needs during early postnatal growth and development.

The preceding assumptions place considerable emphasis on the infant-parent relationship and stress the need for parental involvement in early intervention in order to enhance the overall development of a child. Because so much of an infant's development is dependent upon family interaction, virtually all programs of infant stimulation utilize parents as primary providers of treatment.

Ulrich (1984) reported the outcomes of a number of studies in which high-risk infants were provided stimulation in the form of rocking, stroking, talking, and increased handling. Some of the improvements produced were increased weight gain, better motor and visual functioning, and improved performance on developmental tests of mental functioning. Ottenbacher (1983) reported similar results and further stated that most clinical studies indicate that stimulation, in a variety of forms, can have positive effects on arousal level, visual exploratory behavior, motor development, and reflex integration in early human development. Some of the research reviewed reported no significant changes occurring as the result of stimulation, but none reported negative effects. According to what we presently know, it seems that the benefits derived from the types of sensory stimulation studied outweigh negative consequences that may exist.

Infant Aquatic Programs

Infant aquatic programs have become increasingly popular over the past 30 years. Most communities offering swimming facilities also have some form of aquatic program for babies (Hicks-Hughs, and Langendorfer, 1986). Parents enroll their children in infant swimming programs for varying reasons. Some want to "drownproof" their child. Others want their baby to learn how to swim during what they believe to be a critical period for developing swimming skills. Still others enroll their babies for the sheer pleasure of interacting in a different medium and enhancing the bonding process. Although each of these reasons may have merit, considerable care needs to be taken with aquatic programs for infants.

Langendorfer (1987, p. 3) points out that "regardless of age or skill, *no* person is completely water safe!" Parents who attempt to drownproof their children need to be alerted that this is impossible and that constant vigilence is necessary when their baby is in a water environment. Langendorfer further indicates that there is no evidence to suggest that infant swimming enhances later development. The notion of a narrowly defined critical period for learning how to swim is not supported by available research.

Other problems associated with infant swim programs are hyponatremia (or infant water intoxication), and Giardia. *Hyponatremia* is a rare but serious condition activated by swallowing excessive amounts of water, thus reducing the body's serum sodium level. Symptoms, as reported by Burd (1986), range from lethargy, disorientation, and weakness to nausea, vomiting, seizures, coma, and death. *Giardia*, a problem much more common to infant swimming classes, is an intestinal parasite that causes severe and prolonged diarrhea that may be transmitted between infants.

As a result of the misinformation about infant aquatics and the potential problems that may arise both the YMCA Division of Aquatics (1984) and the American Academy of Pediatrics (1985) published guidelines prohibiting total submersion of the infant and recommending the limitation of organized aquatic programs to children over 3 years old. Infant aquatic programs that follow the guidelines outlined by the YMCA and the American Academy of Pediatrics can be beneficial to babies. The interaction between parent and child in an atmosphere of fun, enjoyment, and mutual trust can enhance the bonding process. It can also provide parent and child with a time together during which to learn new skills and explore a novel environment. Water adjustment activities can be a part of the life of the infant, but the benefits or detriments of such programs are not completely known and await further study.

SUMMARY

The development of locomotor, stability, and manipulative movement abilities in infants is influenced by both maturation and environment. These two facets of development are interrelated, and it is through this interaction that the infant develops and refines rudimentary movement abilities. These movement abilities are necessary steppingstones to the development of fundamental movement patterns and specialized movement abilities.

During infancy the child's primary concerns are with self-gratification. Primitive reflexes serve the infant well in meeting basic survival needs, but as the child develops, other needs emerge. Among them is the characteristic need to know. The principle of cephalocaudal and proximodistal development governs activity as control is gained first over head and trunk and then over the limbs. Sitting enables the infant to more effectively use the arms for exploration. Manipulative skills including mouthing allow use of the sensorimotor mechanism to gain information. Because language is limited, movements become the symbols of the child's thought process.

The motor activities of the human infant are genetically determined, and the order of the developmental sequence is relatively fixed. The only real room for variation is in the rate of development. Neuromuscular maturation, cognitive development, and other factors must occur for the infant to progress to movements characteristic of the higher developmental levels. Several factors determine this rate. Environments that provide stimulation and opportunities for exploration encourage early acquisition of rudimentary movement patterns. Crawling, for example, is often the outgrowth of an ocular following pattern, while standing and upright gait are encouraged by the presence of handholds in the child's environment.

The argument over relative roles of maturation, learning, and rate-limiters in the development of movement abilities during the first year continues. Motor programming theories and natural history studies suggest that during infancy maturation may be the overriding factor affecting development. But even the best generic specimen will not thrive or develop optimally in an unfavorable environment. Other factors within the organism and within the environment might be equally important (Thelen et al., 1987).

CHAPTER CONCEPTS

8.1 The first two years of life are important determiners of future functioning.
8.2 The developing movement abilities of the infant are highly involved, complicated tasks that require ever-greater movement control.
8.3 Developing the rudimentary movement abilities of infancy is a process regulated by both maturation and experience.
8.4 Maturation determines the sequential emergence of movement abilities.

8.5 The rate of appearance of rudimentary movement abilities is influenced by factors within the environment and the individual.

8.6 The sequence of emergence of stability, locomotor, and manipulative abilities in infancy is predictable and, in general, resistant to change.

8.7 The extent of the development of rudimentary movement abilities is influenced by opportunities for practice.

8.8 Rudimentary stability abilities are the most basic of the three forms of rudimentary movements. Their development is essential to the proper development of locomotor and manipulative abilities.

8.9 The development of rudimentary locomotor movement abilities provides the infant with the means for exploring his or her environment.

8.10 The development of rudimentary manipulative abilities provides the infant with the means for the first meaningful contact with objects in the environment.

8.11 Stimulation programs for at-risk infants may enhance development.

8.12 Infant aquatic programs may be beneficial in terms of parent-child attachment, but have not been shown to enhance motor development.

TERMS TO REMEMBER

Reflex Inhibition Stage

Precontrol Stage

Locomotion

Manipulation

Stability

Crawling

Creeping

Contralateral Pattern

Infant Stimulation

Infant Aquatic Program

Hyponatremia

Giardia

CRITICAL READINGS

Bailey, R. A. and Burton, E. C. (1982). *The Dynamic Self: Activities To Enhance Infant Development*. St. Louis: Mosby (Chapters 1-2).

Campos, J. J. et al. (1982). "The Emergence of Self-Produced Locomotion." In Brecker, D. D. (ed.) *Intervention With At-Risk and Handicapped Infants*. Baltimore: University Park Press.

Nelson, C. (1988). "Infant Movement: Normal and Abnormal Development." *Journal of Physical Education, Recreation and Dance*, 59(7), 43-46.

Ridenour, M. V. (1978). "Programs to Optimize Infant Motor Development." In Ridenour (ed.), *Motor Development: Issues and Applications*. Princeton, NJ: Princeton.

Thelen, E. (1986). "Development of Coordinated Movement. Implications for Early Human Development." In Wade, M. G., and Whiting, H. T. A. (eds.) *Motor Development in Children: Aspects of Coordination and Control*. Dordrecht, The Netherlands: Martinus Nijhoff.

Thelen, E. et al. (1987) "Self-Organizing Systems and Infant Motor Development." *Development Review*, 7, 39-65.

9

Infant Perception

From the moment of birth, the infant begins the process of learning how to interact with the environment. This interaction is a perceptual as well as a motor process. The term *perception* refers to "any process by which we gain immediate awareness of what is happening outside ourselves" (Bower, 1977, p. 1). In order to gain immediate information about the outside world, we must rely on our various senses. Newborns receive all sorts of sensory stimulation (visual, auditory, olfactory, gustatory, tactual, and kinesthetic) through the various sense modalities. They make responses to these stimuli, but these responses have limited utility. Newborns are unable to integrate the sensory impressions that impinge on the cortex with stored information in order for meaning to be attached to them. Only when sensory stimuli can be integrated with stored information do these sensations take on meaning for the infant and truly warrant being called perceptions.

Newborns attach little meaning to sensory stimuli. The ability to integrate stored data with incoming data is limited. For example, light rays impinging on the eyes register on the retinas and are transmitted to appropriate nerve centers in the sensory areas of the cortex. The newborn's reaction is simple (*sensation*); if the light is dim, the pupils dilate; if the light is bright, the pupils constrict and some of the stimulation is shut off (*consensual pupillary reflex*). Soon the neonate blinks as the stimulus approaches. These simple reflex actions persist throughout life, but in a very short time the infant begins to attach meaning to the visual stimuli received. Soon a certain face becomes "mother." An object is identified as having either three or four sides. The infant now attends to certain stimuli and begins to apply basic meaning to them. The powers of visual perception are now developing.

As in the development of movement abilities in the infant, the development of perceptual skills is a matter of both experience and maturation. Maturation plays an important role in the development of increased acuity of perception, but much of it is due to experience. The learning opportunities afforded children and adults account for the sophistication of their perceptual modalities. Similarly, only through experience will the infant be able to acquire many of these capabilities. The infant's perceptual development is basic to later functioning and, as we will see, is intricately intertwined with the motor system.

METHODS OF STUDYING INFANT PERCEPTION

In the study of infant perceptual abilities, a number of techniques are used to determine the baby's response to various stimuli. Because of the infant's inability to verbalize a response or to fill out a questionnaire, indirect techniques of naturalistic observation were, until recently, used as the primary means of determining what infants could see, hear, feel, and so forth. Each of these methods compares the infant's state prior to introduction of the stimulus with its state during or immediately following the stimulus. The difference between the two measures provides the researcher with an indication of the level and duration of the infant's response to the stimulus. For example, if a uniformly moving pattern of some sort is passed across a neonate's visual field, repetitive following movements of the eyes occur. (Atkinson and Braddick, 1982). The occurrence of these eye movements provides evidence that the moving pattern is perceived at some level by the newborn. Similarly, changes in the infant's general level of motor activity (turning the head, blinking the eyes, crying, and so forth) have all been used over the years by researchers as visual indicators of the infant's perceptual abilities. Such techniques, however, have limitations. First, the observation may be unreliable in that two or more observers may not agree that the particular response actually occurred, or to what degree it occurred. Second, responses are difficult to quantify. Often the rapid and diffuse movements of the infant make it difficult to get an accurate record of the number of responses. The third, and most potent, limitation is that it is impossible to be certain that the infant's response was due to the stimulus presented or simply a change from no stimulus to a stimulus. The infant may be responding to aspects of the stimulus that are different from those identified by the investigator. Therefore, when using observational assessment as a technique for studying infant perceptual abilities, care must be taken neither to over-generalize from the data, nor to rely on one or two studies as conclusive evidence of a particular perceptual ability of the infant.

Observational assessment techniques have become much more sophisticated in recent years, thus reducing the limitations presented above. Film analysis of the infant's responses, heart and respiration rate monitors, and nonnutritive sucking devices are all used as effective tools in understanding infant perception. Film analysis permits researchers to study the infant's responses repeatedly and in slow motion. Precise measurements can be made of the infant's length and frequency of attention between two stimuli. Heart and respiration rate monitors provide the investigator with the number of heart beats or breaths taken when a new stimuli is presented. Numerical increases are used as a quantifiable indicator of increased attention to the new stimulus. Increases in *nonnutritive sucking* were first used as an assessment measure by Siqueland and Delucia (1969). They devised an apparatus which connected a baby's pacifier to a counting device. As stimuli were presented, changes in the infant's sucking behavior were recorded. Increases in the number of sucks was used as an indicator of the infant's attention to, or preference for, a given visual display.

Two additional techniques for studying infant perception have come into vogue in recent years: habituation-dishabituation and evoked potentials. The *habituation-dishabituation* technique is a method in which a single stimulus is presented repeatedly to the infant until there is a measurable decline (habituation) in whatever attending behavior is being observed. At that point a new stimulus is presented and any recovery (dishabituation) in responsiveness produced by it is recorded. If the infant fails to dishabituate and continues to show habituation, it is assumed that the baby is unable to perceive the new stimulus as different. The habituation-dishabituation paradigm has been used most extensively with studies of infants' auditory and olfactory perception.

Evoked potentials are electrical brain responses that may be determined to be related to a particular stimulus due to their proximal relationship to that stimulus. Electrodes are attached to the infant's scalp. Changes in the electrical pattern of the brain indicate that the stimulus is getting through to the infant's central nervous system and eliciting some form of response.

Each of the techniques discussed above provides the researcher with evidence that the infant can detect or discriminate between stimuli. Care must be taken, however, to remember that these measures are only indirect indicators of the infant's perceptual abilities. Rigid adherence to a chronological age classification of these abilities is unwise. But we do know, through sophisticated observational assessment and electrophysiological measures, that the neonate of only a few days is far more perceptually capable than previously thought to be.

VISUAL PERCEPTION

At birth, the infant's eyes have all of the parts necessary for sight and are completely formed with the exception of the fovea, which is incompletely developed. There is also an immaturity of the ocular muscles. These two factors result in poor fixation and focusing and lack of eye movement coordination. The blinking and lacrimal apparatuses are poorly developed at birth, and the neonate is unable to shed tears until one to seven weeks after birth. Visual acuity, accommodation, peripheral vision, binocularity, fixation, tracking, color vision, and form perception develop rapidly during the early weeks and months of life. Table 9.1 presents a list of the major developmental aspects of infant visual perception, along with the approximate age at which these abilities begin to emerge.

Contrast Sensitivity

The visual apparatus is anatomically complete at birth, although it may be functionally immature. Vision is first used by the newborn in responding to various light intensities. At birth the newborn exhibits a consensual pupillary reflex in which the pupils dilate or constrict in response to the intensity of a localized light source. Hershenson (1964) found that 2- to 4-day-old infants looked at medium intensity lights longer than at dim or high intensity lights. Peeples and Teller (1975) found that 2-month-old infants could discriminate between bars of light against a black background almost as well as adults. The babies were able to detect differences in brightness of as little as 5 percent, whereas adults were able to make 1 percent discriminations. McCandless (1967) noted that newborns tighten their eyelids when asleep in a brightly lit room and tend to be more active in dim light than in bright light. Perhaps this helps

Table 9.1 Developmental Aspects of Selected Infant Visual Perceptual Abilities

Visual Quality	Selected Abilities	Approximate Age of Onset
Sensitivity to Light (McCandless, 1967; Hershenson, 1964; Peoples & Teller, 1975)	Consensual pupillary reflex (contraction and dilation of the pupils)	Birth 2 to 3 hours
The visual apparatus is complete in the newborn and is first put to use by adjusting to varying intensities of the light source.	Strabismus	Birth to 14 days
	Turns head toward light source	Birth
	Closes eyes if light is bright	Birth
	Tightens eyelids when asleep	Birth
	More active in dim light than in bright light	Birth to 1 year
Visual Acuity (Cohen et al. 1979; Aslin & Dumais, 1980)	Organically complete visual apparatus	Birth
The length of focus increases daily as the eye matures.	Length of focus 4 to 10 in.	Birth to 1 week
	Length of focus about 36 in.	3 months
	Length of focus about 100 ft.	1 year
Accommodation (Hayes et al. 1965; Banks 1980)	Poor	Birth to 2 months
	Near adultlike	2 to 4 months
Accommodation is dependent upon functional maturity of the lens.		
Peripheral Vision (Tronick, 1972; Aslin, & Salapatak; 1975; Cohen, 1979)	15 degrees from center	Birth to 2 weeks
	30 degrees from center	1 to 2 months
Peripheral vision improves rapidly in a horizontal direction	40 degrees from center	5 months
Fixation (Atkinson & Braddick, 1982; Bower, 1966; Jeffrey, 1966, Zubek, 1954)	Fixates one eye on bright objects	Birth
	Fixates both eyes on bright objects	2 to 3 days
Fixation is monocular and essentially reflexive during the first weeks of life.	Turns head from one stationary bright surface to another	11 days
	Follows an object in motion, keeping the head stationary	23 days
	Directs eyes toward an object	10 weeks

Table 9.1 (continued)

Visual Quality	Selected Abilities	Approximate Age of Onset
Tracking (Dayton & Jones, 1964; Aslin, 1981; Field, 1976; Haith, 1966; Pratt, begin by 1954) Tracking is first saccadic and gradually smooths out. Develops far sooner than the motor component.	Horizontal Vertical Diagonal Circular	Saccadic pursuit begins at birth Smooth pursuits begin by 2 months Sequence is fixed
Depth Perception (Gibson & Walk, 1960; Walk, 1978; Von Hofsten, 1977; 79; 82; 86) Monocular vision at birth soon gives way to binocular vision and perception of depth.	Monocular vision Binocular vision Depth perception	Birth 2 months 2 to 6 months
Color Discrimination and Preference (Spear, 1964; Hershenson, 1964; Oster, 1975; Bornstein, 1976; Schaller, 1975) Inconsistent evidence. Color vision may be present at birth depending on the amount of rhodopsin present.	Color vision Color perception Prefers shape to color Color discrimination	Birth? 10 weeks 15 days 3 months
Form, Perception (Bower, 1977; Haith, 1980; Fantz, 1963; Salapatek, 1975; Hershenson, 1964, Cohen, 1979) Discrimination begins early and develops rapidly in complexity. The human face is the favorite object.	Prefers patterned objects to plain Imitates facial gestures Prefers human face Size and shape constancy Discriminates between two- and three-dimensional figures	Neonate Neonate Neonate 2 months 3 months 6 months

explain why the infant is frequently more active at night than during the daylight hours.

Visual Acuity, Accommodation, and Peripheral Vision

The eye grows and develops rapidly during the first two years of life. In the infant, the cornea is thinner and more spherical than in the adult.

As a result it is more refractive and the infant tends to be slightly myopic at birth. Normal *visual acuity* is gradually achieved as the cornea rounds out and the lens flattens (Wieczorek and Natapoff, 1981). The newborn has a focal distance of about 4 to 10 inches with the length of focus increasing almost daily and being within the range of normal adult acuity by 6 months to 1 year of age (Cohen et al., 1979; Aslin and Dumais, 1980)

Accommodation, the ability of the lens of each eye to vary their curvature in order to bring the retinal image into sharp focus, improves with age. The study by Hayes et al. (1965) demonstrated that adult-like accommodation does not occur until about the fourth month of age. Banks (1980), in a replication of the Hayes study, found partial accommodation at 1 month and near adult-like focusing around the second month. These studies demonstrate that, until at least 2 months of age, infants are not able to bring objects into sharp focus.

With regard to *peripheral vision*, Tronick's (1972) work suggests that the visual field of the 2-week-old is quite narrow (about 15 degrees from center) but expands during the first few months of postnatal life to about 40 degrees from center by the fifth month. In line with Tronick, Aslin and Salapatek (1975) found that 1- and 2-month-old infants had a visual field of about 30 degrees from center.

Cohen et al. (1979), p. 404) reported that "by 6 months of age both the infant's central and peripheral systems are quite mature." It appears, therefore, that visual acuity, accommodation, and peripheral vision improve dramatically as the eyes mature during early infancy. The interaction between these three developing systems is, at present, unknown.

Binocularity, Fixation, and Tracking

The topics of infant binocularity, fixation, and tracking have interested researchers for years. Prerequisite to efficient fixation and tracking behaviors is binocular vision. Binocularity requires that the eyes work together in visually attending to a stationary object (*fixation*) or to a moving object (*tracking*).

Binocular vision, according to the theoretical framework originally presented by Worth in 1915 as discussed by Aslin and Dumais (1980), occurs at three levels: bifoveal fixation, fusion, and stereopsis. In order for *bifoveal fixation* to occur, the foveas of the two eyes must be aligned and directed at the same instant toward the object of visual regard. If bifoveal fixation is absent, then, according to Aslin and Dumais (1980), fusion and stereopsis cannot occur.

Fusion is the second level of binocular vision. Fusion is a process in which the images on the two retinas are combined into a single visual percept. When looking at an object, each eye sends information to the retina and on to the brain from a different orientation. The two eyes are about 6 cm apart, therefore, a direct line from each eye to the object is quite different. Kreig (1978) noted that the interocular distance between the two eyes increases by about 50 percent from birth to adulthood. Limited data suggests that infants have fusion by the fourth to sixth month of postnatal life (Aslin, 1977). Fusion is required for stereopsis to occur.

Stereopsis is the third level of binocularity and enables one to detect depth. Stereopsis is based on the extent of retinal disparity or mismatch between the two eyes and has been demonstrated in infants 3 months and older (Fox et al. 1980). Aslin and Dumais (1980, p. 60) stated that "the presence of bifoveal fixation in infants does not guarantee that fusion and stereopsis are present." Therefore, although it is possible that these three levels of binocularity are hierarchical, it is also possible that they exist as three parallel functions interdependent upon one another. The primary developmental determiners of binocular vision, which makes fixation and tracking possible, are visual acuity, contrast sensitivity, accommodation and the distance between the eyes (Aslin and Dumais, 1980).

Visual fixation is monocular at birth. This is probably due to the infant's poor visual acuity and contrast sensitivity. Also, visual-motor control of the two eyes is immature. These conditions improve rapidly during the first 6 months, thus suggesting improvement in the infant's ability to binocularly fixate (Atkinson and Braddick, 1982).

Binocular tracking is the most basic aspect of visual-motor pursuit. Tracking involves directing the eyes from one line of sight to another. These eye movements are either of a high velocity (saccadic) or slow velocity (smooth pursuit). *Saccades* are quick movements of the eyes that involve a redirection of focus from one object of regard to another. Saccadic eye movements govern the object tracking of the very young infant. A series of saccadic movements are made as the infant tracks an object across the visual field. A variety of hypotheses are available for this yet-unexplained phenomena (See Aslin, 1984), but by the end of the second week of postnatal life the neonate is capable of making reliable saccadic tracking movements. Dayton and Jones (1964) were the first to demonstrate that the eye movements of the infant are totally saccadic until the end of the second month of life. However, Aslin (1981), using a very slow-moving target, found evidence of smooth pursuits beginning by the sixth week of age. Although the exact timing of the onset of smooth pursuits is debatable, the sequence is clear. Smooth pursuit tracking behaviors first occur in a horizontal direction, followed by vertical, then diagonal, and finally circular (Field, 1976; Haith, 1966; Pratt, 1954).

Depth Perception

Depth perception involves the ability to judge the distance of an object from oneself. Williams (1983) categorized depth perception into "static" and "dynamic" components. *Static depth perception* involves making depth or distance judgements with regard to stationary objects. *Dynamic depth perception* requires one to make distance judgements about moving objects.

Static depth perception has been extensively investigated in infants through the now-classic *visual-cliff* experiments by Gibson and Walk (1960). In their research paradigm, infants capable of self-produced locomotion, along with other animal species, were encouraged to crawl across a thick sheet of glass that contained a variety of depth cues. (Figure 9.1). The experiments concluded that mobile infants, even when coaxed, would not crawl across the "deep end" to their mothers.

More recently, Svejda and Schmid (1979) assessed the cardiac responses of pre-locomotor infants (mean age, 6.9 months) and locomotor infants (mean age 7.1 months) as they were lowered to either the shallow or to the deep side of the cliff. Pre-locomotor infants exhibited little or no difference in heart-rate levels when lowered to either side. Locomotor infants, however, showed significant increases in heart-rate responses to both sides but with a "more marked acceleration" on the deep side. The results of this experiment tend to confirm the Held and Hein (1963) and Walk (1978) hypotheses that the development of depth perception is at least, in part, a function of experience. It also indicates that sensorimotor feedback through early locomotor experience is sufficient to account for a developmental shift on the visual cliff between pre-locomotor and lo-

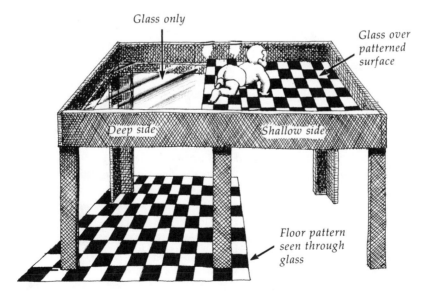

Figure 9.1. The visual cliff

comotor infants. Whether sensorimotor experiences are a necessary condition is still uncertain.

With regard to dynamic depth perception, a number of investigations have been conducted with infants in recent years. The reaching responses of young infants presented with a moving stimulus have been carefully studied by Von Hofsten (1979, 1982, 1986). The results of his investigations clearly demonstrated that infants as young as 5 days old make what appear to be purposeful, but poorly controlled, reaching movements toward moving objects. Dynamic depth perception appears to be present in a rather sophisticated form by the fourth month of postnatal life. Von Hofsten (1986, p. 174), states that:

> "Thus it seems without doubt that shortly before four months of age the infant starts to be able to use also the purely visual mode of control whereby the seen position of the hand is related to the seen position of the object"

It must be remembered that, at this point, the motor system lags behind the perceptual system. Movements toward an object, though purposeful, are crude, thus demonstrating poor integration between the visual and motor systems. Adult-like reaching behaviors do not appear until around the sixth month when differentiation of muscle groups and integration with sensory systems begin to be conjoined.

Color Perception

A large number of studies have been conducted over the years to determine if infants perceive color and are able to distinguish between different colors. Much of the experimentation prior to the 1960s yielded confusing and often conflicting information. Out of this research, however, came the realization that the infant responds to the brightness (i.e., *chromatic intensity*) of the colors presented prior to responding to hue. Hershenson (1964) was the first to demonstrate this in infants, leading to a new wave of studies that attempted to control for the brightness factor. As cited by Cohen et al. (1979), Oster (1975) found that by 10 weeks of age infants perceive colors over a large portion of the visible color spectrum. Schaller (1975) also found similar results with 11- to 12-week-old infants. These two experiments clearly demonstrate that infants as young as 10 weeks of age have the ability to perceive color. We do not know, however, whether infants younger than 10 weeks perceive color. The amount of *rhodopsin* present in the rods and cones may be insufficient for color vision. Similarly, we do not know categorically if the color perception of the infant is identical to that of adults, although limited evidence favors this notion.

Bornstein et al. (1976) demonstrated that 4-month-old infants were capable of discriminating between blue, green, yellow, and red. Another experiment by Bornstein (1976) with 3-month-olds yielded similar results. It appears, therefore, that infants as young as 3 months of age do have the ability to make adult-like color discriminations. The question concerning the favorite color of infants is open to further speculation and study. Spears (1964) notes that it is clear that babies as young as 15 days prefer colors to noncolors (i.e., unpatterned whites and grays), and that they prefer shape to color.

Form Perception

A number of investigators have examined form perception in infants. *Form perception* is the ability to distinguish between shapes and to discriminate among a variety of patterns. With regard to the neonate, Haith (1980) found that newborns placed in a darkened room would look for subtle shadows and edges. Moreover, Kessen et al. (1972), in a similar experiment, reported that newborns responded only to vertical high-contrast edges. Haith, however, found that they could also respond to horizontal lines. Fantz et al. (1975) reported that newborns were able to perceive form and preferred curved lines over straight lines. Salapatek (1975) reported that other researchers examining neonatal responses to squares, circles, and triangles found that the infants tend to fixate on a single line or edge at one month of age but spent much more time scanning the figures at 2 months of age. Salapatek (1975, p. 226) drew three important conclusions from the abundance of research on form perception in the newborn:

> "First, before 2 months of age, visual attention appears to be captured by a single or limited number of features of a figure or pattern. Second, before approximately 1 to 2 months of age, there is little evidence that the arrangement or pattern of figural elements plays any role in visual selection or memory. Third, before 1 to 2 months, there is little evidence that the line of sight is attracted by anything more than the greatest number of size of visible contour elements per unit area, regardless of type or arrangement of elements"

Infants over three months of age appear to exhibit a variety of sophisticated abilities with regard to form perception. Cohen et al. (1979) reported that several investigators have determined that infants can discriminate one pattern from another even when the pattern is placed in a variety of arrangements. Furthermore, he states, "the evidence is reasonably convincing that, at some point within the first 6 months of life, infants can perceive multiple forms and can respond to and prefer, a change in pattern arrangement" (Cohen et al. 1979, p. 412). Fantz (1963) found that 2-month-old infants prefer looking at the human face over all other simple stimuli. Cohen (1979) reported that by 6-month-old infants can distinguish between two-dimensional photographs of different human faces. Clearly, the ability of the infant to discriminate between shapes and patterns develops rapidly during this period and has reached rather sophisticated levels by the end of the first 6 months of postnatal life.

AUDITORY, OLFACTORY, AND GUSTATORY PERCEPTION

Available research data concerning the development of auditory, olfactory, and gustatory perception in the human infant are much less complete than for the visual modality. In the area of auditory perception we find that, as with vision, the development of auditory abilities does not unfold exclusively without the influences of the environment. Environmental conditions influence the extent of development of audition. The ear is structurally complete at birth, and the infant is capable of hearing just as soon as the amniotic fluid drains (usually within a day or two after birth). The fetus responds to sound before birth (Bernard & Sontag, 1947). These responses, however, may be in response to tactile sensations created by the vibrations produced (Aslin et al. 1983). At present, we do not know if the fetus is capable of hearing sound.

With regard to the neonate, research indicates that the newborn is less sensitive to sound than adults. (Aslin et al. 1983) reported that the difference is at least 10 decibels. Sensitivity to sound improves with age, and infants as young as 6 months old are more sensitive to high frequency sounds than their neonatal counterparts. (Trehub et al. 1980). Infant auditory perception may be adultlike by two years of age (Schneider et al. 1980). The infant can localize sounds at birth and reacts primarily to loudness and duration (Wertheiner, 1961). Crude pitch discriminations have been demonstrated by Leventhal and Lipsett (1964) as early as the first four days of postnatal life. Definite responses to tonal differences are seen around the third month, and the infant reacts with obvious pleasure to a parent's voice by the fifth month (Leventhal and Lipsett, 1964).

The research on olfactory and gustatory perception is much more sparse than on hearing. It is difficult to separate the developmental sequence of smell and taste simply because the nose and mouth are closely connected and stimuli applied to one are likely to affect the other. The newborn does, however, appear to react to certain odors, although this may be due more to pain caused by the pungent odors used than to smell. Lipsett et al. (1963) demonstrated that newborns less than 24 hours old made definite responses when exposed to a highly offensive odor. Engen and Lipsett (1965) showed that infants as young as 32 hours were able to discriminate between two different odors. McFarlane (1975), in studying 2- to 7-day-old infants, found that they could discriminate between their mother's breast pad and a clean pad, with a clear preference for their mother's pad. The same infants, however, failed to discriminate between their mother's breast pad and that of another. It may not be until the second week that recognition of mother's smell is developed. Newborns react to taste, preferring sweet tastes to sour ones and sour tastes to bitter ones. Table 9.2 presents a summary of the major developmental aspects of infant auditory, gustatory, and olfactory perception.

Table 9.2 Developmental Aspect of Selected Infant Auditory, Olfactory, and Gustatory Abilities

Perceptual Quality	Selected Abilities	Approximate Age of Onset
Auditory Perception (Bernard & Sontag, 1947; Levanthal and Lipsett, 1964; Wertheimer, 1961) The ear is structurally complete at birth, and the newborn can respond to sound.	Responds to loud, sharp sounds	Prenatal
	Ability to localize sounds	Birth
	Reacts primarily to loudness and duration	Birth
	Crude pitch discrimination	1 to 4 days
	Responds to tonal differences	3 to 6 months
	Reacts with pleasure to parent's voice	5 to 6 months
	Adultlike	24 months
Olfactory Perception (Bower, 1977; Lipsett et al. 1963; Engen & Lipsett, 1965; McFarlane, 1975) The olfactory mechanism is structurally complete at birth, and the newborn responds crudely to various odors.	Responds to odors	Birth
	Reduced sensitivity upon repeated application of the stimuli (habituation)	Neonate
	Distinguishes between pleasant and unpleasant odors.	2-3 days
	Shows preference to mother's odor	2 weeks
	Discrimination abilities improve with practice	Infancy
Gustatory Perception (Pratt, 1954; Bower, 1977) The newborn reacts to variation in sweet, sour, and bitter tastes. Little research data are available on this modality.	Shows preference in tastes (prefers sweet to sour, sour to bitter)	Neonate

SUMMARY

The study of infant perception has intrigued researchers for years. We now know that the newborn, neonate, and young infant is much more perceptually aware and capable than previously thought possible. Newer techniques for observing and recording infant responses to various stimuli have been responsible for a shift in our assumptions about the perceptual capabilities of the very young.

Observational assessment techniques that utilize film analysis, heart and respiration monitors, nonnutritive sucking devices, and electrical brain impulse recorders are making new inroads into our understanding of the perceptual world of the infant.

The visual world of the infant has been the most extensively studied perceptual modality. The newborn's eyes are structurally complete but functionally immature. Rapid progress is seen in the acqusition of a vast array of visual perceptual abilities. Although the age of onset of these abilities is difficult, if not impossible, to pinpoint, and generalizations to all infants is unwise, it is possible to chart the sequence of acquisition of many visual perceptual abilities. The motor developmentalist is especially interested in the visual modality because of its close, often essential, link to voluntary movement. Much of what we do as moving beings is governed by our perceptions. Although the visual perceptual world of the infant develops rapidly, the motor system tends to lag behind. It is not until later infancy that the motor cycle begins to catch up and a matching of perceptual and motor data occurs.

The other perceptual modalities (auditory, gustatory, olfactory), although important, are less clearly understood in the infant. Furthermore, their link to the motor system is less crucial than vision. Therefore, the visual-motor matching of perceptual and motor data in the infant and young child will probably continue to be a topic of keen interest to researchers and educators alike.

CHAPTER CONCEPTS

9.1 Development of the infant's motor system lags behind the perceptual system.

9.2 Infant perceptual abilities become refined as a function of both maturation and experience.

9.3 Indirect methods for assessing infant perceptual development must be used.

9.4 Observational assessment techniques for studying infant perception are limited in their ability to generalize.

9.5 The eye is structurally complete at birth but fuctionally immature.

9.6 Infant visual perceptual abilities develop rapidly during the first 6 months of postnatal life.

9.7 The newborn is myopic at birth, has a short focal distance and limited peripheral vision but responds to various light intensities.

9.8 Binocular vision occurs at three levels: bifoveal fixation, fusion, and stereopsis.

9.9 Saccadic eye movements govern the visual tracking of the young infant.

9.10 Smooth pursuit eye movements follow a predictable sequence but vary in their rate of appearance.

9.11 The perception of depth is a function of experience as well as maturation.

9.12 Infants tend to respond more to the chromatic intensity of colors rather than the actual hue itself.

9.13 Complexity governs the infants attending behaviors, in that the infant prefers shape to color, and prefers complex shapes to less complex ones.

TERMS TO REMEMBER

Perception
Sensation
Consensual Pupillary Reflex
Nonnutritive Sucking
Habituation
Dishabituation
Evoked Potentials
Contrast Sensitivity
Visual Acuity
Accommodation
Peripheral Vision
Binocular Vision
Fixation
Tracking
Bifoveal Fixation

Fusion Stereopsis
Visual Fixation
Binocular Tracking
Saccades
Depth Perception
Static Depth Perception
Visual Cliff
Dynamic Depth Perception
Color Perception
Chromatic Intensity
Rhodopsin
Form Perception
Auditory Perception
Olfactory Perception
Gustatory Perception

CRITICAL READINGS

Aslin, R. N. (1984). "Motor Aspects of Visual Development in Infancy." In Salapatek, P. and Cohen, L. B. (eds.) *Handbook of Infant Perception*. New York: Academic Press.

Cratty, B. J. (1986) *Perceptual and Motor Development in Infants and Children*. Englewood Cliffs, NJ: Prentice-Hall, (Chapter 11).

Wade, M. G. and Whiting, H. T. A. (1986). *Motor Development in Children: Aspects of Coordination and Control*. Dordrecht, The Netherlands: Martinus Nijhoff Publishers. (Section 4: Perception and Action).

Williams, H. G. (1983). *Perceptual and Motor Development*. Englewood Cliffs, NJ: Prentice-Hall (Chapter 4).

SECTION III
CHILDHOOD

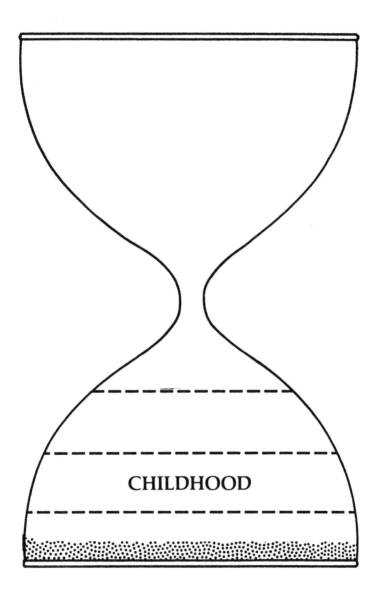

CHILDHOOD

10
Childhood Growth and Development

CHAPTER COMPETENCIES

Upon Completion of This Chapter You Should Be Able To:

* *Describe and interpret the normal curve and displacement and velocity graphs during childhood.*

* *Discuss secular trends in physical size and biological maturation.*

• *Discuss the influence of nutritional status on childhood growth processes.*

• *Distinguish between the terms "malnutrition" and "undernutrition" and discuss the causes and implications of each.*

• *Describe the relative influences of both exercise and injury on the childhood growth process.*

• *List and describe several factors associated with influencing the childhood growth process.*

• *List cognitive, affective, and motor development characteristics of the young child (2 to 6) and discuss implications for the developmental physical education program.*

• *List cognitive, affective, and motor development characteristics of the older child (6 to 10) and discuss implications for the developmental physical education program.*

The period of childhood marks a steady increase in height, weight, and muscle mass. Growth is not as rapid during this period as during infancy, and it shows a gradual deceleration throughout childhood until the adolescent growth spurt. Childhood is divided here into the early period from 2 to 6 years of age and the later period from about 6 to 10 years of age. Figures 10.1 through 10.4 present height and weight growth charts for males and females.

GROWTH IN EARLY CHILDHOOD (AGES 2-5)

During the early childhood years, growth in terms of height and weight is not as rapid as during infancy. The growth rate decelerates slowly. By 4 years of age, the child has doubled his or her birth length, which represents only about one-half the gain experienced during the first two years of life. The total amount of weight gain from 2 through 5 years of age is less than the amount gained during the first year of life. The growth process slows down after the first two years but maintains a constant rate until puberty. The annual height gain from the early childhood period to puberty is about 2 inches per year. Weight gains average 5 pounds per year. This, therefore, represents an ideal time during which the child can develop and refine a wide variety of movement tasks ranging from the fundamental movements of early childhood to the sport skills of middle childhood.

Gender differences may be seen between boys and girls in terms of height and weight, but they are minimal. The physiques of male and female preschoolers are remarkably similar when viewed from a posterior position, with boys being slightly taller and heavier. Boys have more muscle and bone mass than girls and both show a gradual decrease in fatty tissue as they progress through the early childhood period. The proportion of muscle tissue remains fairly constant (at about 25 percent of total body weight) throughout early childhood (Eckert, 1987).

Body proportions change markedly during early childhood because of the various growth rates of the body. The chest gradually becomes larger than the abdomen, and the stomach gradually protrudes less. By the time preschoolers reach the first grade, their body proportions more closely resemble those of older children in elementary school.

Bone growth during early childhood is dynamic, and the skeletal system is particularly vulnerable to malnutrition, fatigue, and illness (Brain and Moslay, 1968). The bones ossify at a rapid rate during early childhood and have been shown to be retarded by as much as three years in growth in deprived children (Scrimshaw, 1967).

Smart and Smart (1973a) report that the brain is about 75 percent of its adult weight by age 3, and almost 90 percent by age 6. The midbrain is almost fully developed at birth, but it is not until age 4 that the cerebral cortex is completely developed.

The development of myelin around the neurons (*myelination*) permits

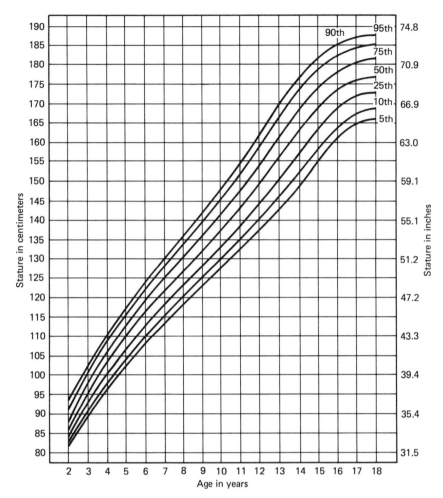

Figure 10.1. Male stature by age percentiles: ages 2 to 18 years (*Source*: National Center for Health Statistics)

the transmission of nerve impulses and is not complete at birth. Many nerves lack myelin at birth, but with advancing age greater amounts of myelin are laid down along nerve fibers. Myelination is largely complete by the end of the early childhood period, thus allowing for the complete transference of nerve impulses throughout the nervous system. It is interesting to note that increased complexity in the child's movement patterns are possible following myelination of the cerebellum. Also, Eckert (1987, p. 129) states that "myelination of the corpus callosum, which joins the two hemispheres of the brain, is a precursor to the development

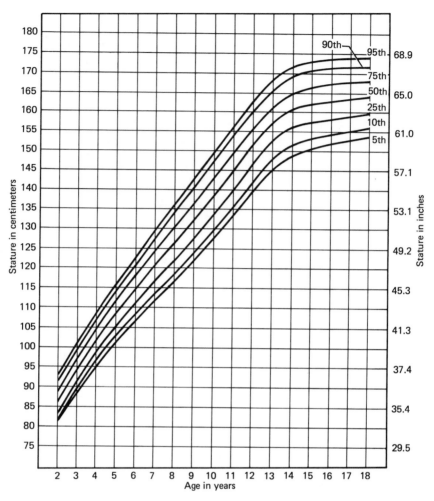

Figure 10.2. Female stature by age percentiles: ages 2 to 18 years (*Source*: National Center for Health Statistics)

of optimal alternate arm-leg action in such things as the throw and the kick." Therefore, as the cortex matures and becomes progressively organized, the child is able to perform at higher levels both motorically and cognitively.

The sensory apparatus is still developing during the preschool years. The eyeball does not reach its full size until about 12 years of age. the *macula* of the retina is not completely developed until about the sixth year, and the young child is generally *farsighted*. Preschool children have more taste buds than adults. They are generously distributed throughout the

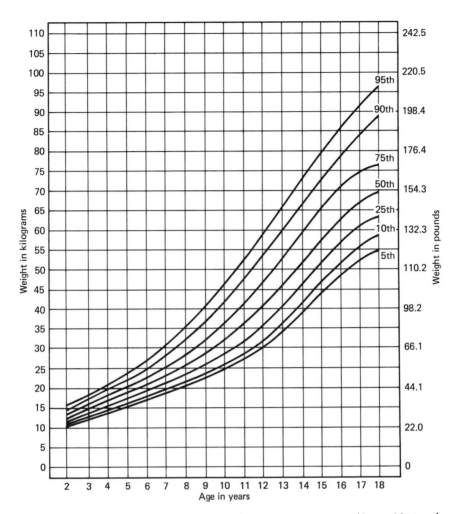

Figure 10.3. Male weight by age percentiles: ages 2 to 18 years (*Source*: National Center for Health Statistics)

insides of the throat and cheeks as well as on the tongue, causing greater sensitivity to taste. Because of the shorter *eustachian tube* connecting the midde ear with the throat, the child is also more sensitive to infections of the ear.

DEVELOPMENT IN EARLY CHILDHOOD (AGES 2-5)

Play is what young children do when they are not eating, sleeping, or complying with the wishes of adults. Play occupies most of their waking

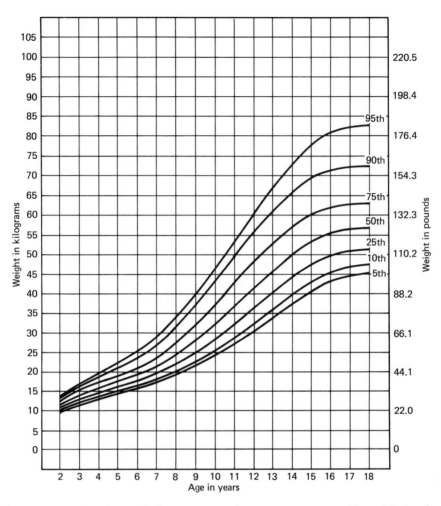

Figure 10.4. Female weight by age percentiles: ages 2 to 18 years (*Source*: National Center for Health Statistics)

hours, and it may be viewed as the child's equivalent of work as performed by adults. Children's play serves as the primary mode by which they learn about the body and its movement capabilities. It also serves as an important facilitator of cognitive and affective development in the young child, as well as an important means of developing both fine and gross motor skills.

Young children are actively involved in enhancing their cognitive abilities in a variety of ways. These early years are a period of important cognitive development and have been termed the "preoperational thought phase" by Piaget. During this time children develop cognitive functions that eventually result in logical thinking and concept formulation. Young children are incapable of thinking from any point of view other than their own. They are extremely egocentric and view almost everything in terms of themselves. Preschoolers' perceptions dominate their thinking, and what is experienced at a given moment in time has great influence on them. During this preconceptual phase of cognitive development, seeing is, literally, believing. In the thinking of preschool children, their conclusions need no justification and if they did, the children would be unable to reconstruct their thoughts to show others how they arrived at their conclusions. Play serves as a vital means by which higher cognitive structures are gradually developed. It provides a multitude of settings and variables for promoting cognitive growth.

Affective development is also dramatic during the early childhood years. During this period children are involved in the crucial social-emotional task of developing a sense of autonomy and a sense of initiative. Autonomy is expressed through a growing sense of independence, which may be seen in a child's delight in using the word "no" in response to almost any question. A child who wants to play outside may answer "No" when asked "Do you want to play outside?" not so much to express disobedience as to express a sense of independence and to exert control over environmental factors. Such a response can be avoided by replacing questions with positive suggestions like "Let's go play outdoors." In this way, the child is not confronted with a direct yes-or-no choice. Care must be taken, however, to give children abundant opportunities for reasonable and proper expression of their autonomy.

Young children's expanding sense of initiative is reflected in their curious exploring, and active behavior. Children engage in new experiences such as climbing, jumping, running, and throwing objects for their own sake and for the sheer joy of sensing and knowing their own capabilities. Failure to develop a sense of initiative and autonomy leads to feelings of shame, worthlessness, and guilt. Because it has an effect on both cognitive and psychomotor functions, the establishment of stable self-concept is crucial to proper affective development in young children.

Through the medium of play, young children develop a wide variety of fundamental locomotor, manipulative, and stability abilities. If they have a stable and positive self-concept, the gain in control over their musculature is a smooth one. The timid, cautious, and measured movements of the 2- to 3-year-old gradually gives way to the confident, eager, and often reckless abandon of the 4- and 5-year-old. Vivid imaginations make possible fantastic feats: jumps from "great heights," "high mountain" climbs, and leaps over "raging rivers."

Preschool-age children rapidly expand their horizons in complex and wondrous ways. They assert their individuality, develop their abilities, and test their limits as well as the limits of their family and others around them. Care must be taken, however, to understand their developmental characteristics, limitations, and potentials so we may effectively structure developmental experiences that reflect children's needs and interests and that are within their levels of ability.

The following developmental characteristics represent a synthesis of findings from a wide variety of sources and are presented to provide a complete view of the total child during the early childhood years.

Motor Development Characteristics

1. Boys and girls range from about 33 to 47 inches in height and 25 to 53 pounds.
2. Perceptual-motor abilities are rapidly developing, but confusion often exists in body, directional, temporal, and spatial awareness.
3. Good bladder and bowel control are generally established by the end of this period, but accidents may still occur.
4. Children during this period are rapidly developing fundamental movement abilities in a variety of motor skills. Bilateral movements such as skipping, however, often present more difficulty than unilateral movements.
5. Children are active and energetic and would often rather run than walk, but they still need frequent short rest periods.
6. Motor abilities are developed to the point where children are beginning to learn how to dress themselves, although they may need help straightening and fastening articles of clothing.
7. The body functions and processes become well regulated. A state of physiological homeostasis (stability) becomes well established.
8. The bodies of both boys and girls are remarkably similar. A back view of boys and girls reveals no readily observable structural differences.
9. Fine motor control is not fully established, although gross motor control is developing rapidly.
10. The eyes are not generally ready for extended periods of close work due to farsightedness.

Cognitive Development Characteristics

1. There is constantly-increasing ability to express thoughts and ideas verbally.
2. A fantastic imagination enables imitation of both actions and

symbols with little concern for accuracy or the proper sequencing of events.
3. There is continuous investigation and discovery of new symbols that have a primarily personal reference.
4. The "how" and "why" of the child's actions are learned through almost constant play.
5. This is a preoperational thought phase of development, resulting in a period of transition from self-satisfying behavior to fundamental socialized behaviors.

Affective Development Characteristics

1. During this phase children are egocentric and assume that everyone thinks the way they do. As a result, they often seem to be quarrelsome and exhibit difficulty in sharing and getting along with others.
2. They are often fearful of new situations, shy, self-conscious, and unwilling to leave the security of that which is familiar.
3. They are learning to distinguish right from wrong and are beginning to develop a conscience.
4. Two- and 4-year-old children often appear unusual and irregular in their behavior, while those who are 3 and 5 are often viewed as stable and conforming in their behavior.
5. Self-concept is rapidly developing. Wise guidance, success-oriented experiences, and positive reinforcement are especially important during these years.

Implications for the Developmental Movement Program

1. Plenty of opportunity for gross motor play must be offered in both undirected and directed settings.
2. The movement experiences should stress movement exploration and problem-solving activities to maximize the child's creativity and desire to explore.
3. The movement education program should include plenty of positive reinforcement in order to encourage the establishment of a positive self-concept and to reduce the fear of failure.
4. Stress should be placed on developing a variety of fundamental locomotor, manipulative, and stability abilities, progressing from the simple to the complex as the child becomes "ready" for them.
5. Interests and abilities of boys and girls are similar, with no need for separate activities during this period.
6. Plenty of activities designed specifically to enhance perceptual-motor functioning are necessary.

7. Advantage should be taken of the child's great imagination through the use of a variety of activities, including drama and imagery.
8. In consideration of their often awkward and inefficient movements, movement experiences should be geared to their maturity level.
9. Provide a wide variety of activities that require object handling and eye-hand coordination.
10. Begin to incorporate bilateral activities such as skipping, galloping, and hopping after unilateral movements have been fairly well established.
11. Encourage children to take an active part in the movement education program by showing and telling others what they can do to overcome tendencies to be shy and self-conscious.
12. Activities should stress arm, shoulder, and upper body involvement.
13. Mechanically-correct execution in a wide variety of fundamental movements is the primary goal, without emphasis on standards of performance.
14. Do not stress coordination in conjunction with speed and agility.
15. Poor postural habits are beginning. Reinforce good posture with positive statements.
16. Provide convenient access to toilet facilities and encourage the children to accept this responsibility on their own.
17. Allow individual differences and allow children to progress at their own rates.
18. Establish standards for acceptable behavior and abide by them. Provide wise guidance in the establishment of a sense of doing what is right and proper instead of what is wrong and unacceptable.
19. The motor development program should be prescriptive and based on each individual's readiness level.
20. A multisensory approach should be utilized, one in which a wide variety of experiences are incorporated using several sensory modalities.

GROWTH IN LATER CHILDHOOD (AGES 6-10)

The period of childhood from the sixth through the tenth years of life is typified by a slow but steady increase in height and weight and by progress toward greater organization of the sensory and motor systems. Changes in body build are slight during these years. Childhood is more a time of lengthening out and filling out prior to the prepubertal growth spurt that occurs around the eleventh year for girls and the thirteenth year for boys. Although these years are characterized by slow, steady growth, the child makes rapid gains in learning and functions at increasingly mature levels in the performance of games and sports. This period of slow growth in height and weight gives the child time to get used to his or her body and is an important factor in the typically dramatic improvement seen in coordination and motor control during the childhood years. The gradual change in size and the close relationship maintained between bone and tissue development may be an important factor in increased levels of functioning.

Differences between the growth patterns of boys and girls are minimal during the middle years. Both have greater limb growth than trunk growth, but boys tend to have longer legs, arms, and standing height during childhood. Likewise, girls tend to have greater hip width and thigh size during this period. There is relatively little difference in physique or weight exhibited until the onset of the preadolescent period (Figures 10.5 and 10.6). Therefore, in most cases, girls and boys should be able to participate together in activities.

During childhood there is very slow growth in brain size. The size of the skull remains nearly the same although there is a broadening and a lengthening of the head toward the end of childhood.

Perceptual abilities during childhood are becoming increasingly refined. The sensorimotor apparatus is working in greater harmony so that by the end of this period the child can perform numerous sophisticated skills. Striking of a pitched ball, for example, improves with age and practice due to improved visual acuity, tracking abilities, reaction and movement time, and sensorimotor integration. A key to maximum development of more mature growth patterns in the child is utilization. In other words, if the child has, through the normal process of maturation, improved perceptual abilities, they must be experimented with and integrated more completely with the motor structures through practice. Failure to have the opportunity for practice, instruction, and encouragement during this period will prevent many individuals from acquiring the perceptual and motor information needed to perform skillful movement activities.

DEVELOPMENT IN LATER CHILDHOOD (AGES 6-10)

Children in the elementary school years are generally happy, stable, eager, and able to assume responsibilities. They are able to cope with new situations and are anxious to learn more about themselves and their expanding world. Primary grade children take the first big step into their expanding world when they enter first grade. For many, first grade rep-

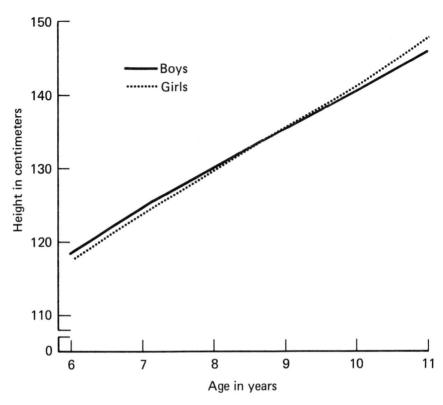

Figure 10.5. Mean height of U.S. children by age and gender (*Source*: U.S. Department of Health, Education and Welfare, DHEW Publication No.—HSM-73-1605, January 1973)

resents the first separation from the home for a regularly scheduled, extended block of time. It is the first step out of the secure play environment of the home and into the world of adults. Entering a school represents a major shift from the secure environment of the home and into the world of adults. Entering a school represents the first time that many children are placed in a group situation in which they are not the center of attention. It is a time when sharing, concern for others, and respect for the rights of and responsibilities of others are established. Kindergarten is a readiness time in which to begin making the gradual transition from an egocentric, home-centered play world to the group-oriented world of adult concepts and logic. In the first grade, the first formal demands for cognitive understanding are made. The major milestone of the first and second grader is learning how to read at a reasonable level. The 6-year-old is generally developmentally ready for the important task of "breaking the code" and learns to read. The child is also

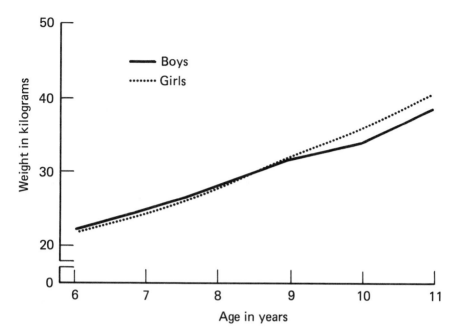

Figure 10.6. Mean weight of U.S. children by age and gender (*Source*: U.S. Department of Health, Education and Welfare, DHEW Publication No.—HSM-73-1605, January 1973)

involved in developing the first real understanding of time and money and numerous other cognitive concepts. By the second grade, children should be well on their way to meeting and surmounting the ever-broadening array of cognitive, affective, and psychomotor tasks that are placed before them.

The following is a listing of the general developmental characteristics of the child from ages 6 to 10. It is presented here to provide a more complete view of the total child and represents a synthesis of current findings.

Motor Development Characteristics

1. Boys and girls range from about 44 to 60 inches in height and from 44 to 90 pounds.
2. Growth is slow, especially from age 8 to the end of this period. There is a slow but steady pace of increments, unlike the more rapid gains in height and weight that occur during the preschool years.
3. The body begins to lengthen with an annual gain of only 2 to 3 inches and an annual weight gain of only 3 to 6 pounds.

4. The cephalocaudal (head to toe) and proximodistal (center to periphery) principles of development are now quite evident, in which the large muscles of the body are considerably better developed than the small muscles.
5. Girls are generally about a year ahead of boys in physiological development, and separate interests begin to develop toward the end of this period.
6. Hand preference is firmly established with about 85 percent preferring the right hand and about 15 percent preferring the left.
7. Reaction time is slow, causing difficulty with eye-hand and eye-foot coordination at the beginning of this period. By the end they are generally well established.
8. Both boys and girls are full of energy but often possess low endurance levels and tire easily. Responsiveness to training, however, is great.
9. The visual perceptual mechanisms are fully established by the end of this period.
10. Children are often farsighted during this period and are not ready for extended periods of close work.
11. Most fundamental movement abilities have the potential to be well defined by the beginning of this period.
12. Basic skills necessary for successful play become well developed.
13. Activities involving the eyes and limbs develop slowly. Such activities as volleying or striking a pitched ball and throwing require considerable practice for mastery to occur.
14. This period marks a transition from refining fundamental movement abilities to the establishment of transitional movement skills in lead-up games and athletic skills.

Cognitive Development Characteristics

1. Attention span is generally short at the beginning of this period but gradually lengthens. Boys and girls of this age, however, will often spend hours on activities that are of great interest to them.
2. They are eager to learn and to please adults but need assistance and guidance in decision-making.
3. Children have good imaginations and display extremely creative minds; but self-consciousness seems to become a factor toward the end of this period.
4. They are often interested in television, computers, video games, and reading.
5. They are incapable of abstract thinking and deal best with concrete examples and situations during the beginning of this pe-

riod. More abstract cognitive abilities are evident by the end of this period.

6. Children are intellectually curious and anxious to know "why."

Affective Development Characteristics

1. Interests of boys and girls are similar at the beginning of this period but soon begin to diverge.
2. The child is self-centered and plays poorly in large groups for extended periods of time during the primary years, although small group situations are handled well.
3. The child is often aggressive, boastful, self-critical, overreactive, and accepts defeat and winning poorly.
4. There is an inconsistent level of maturity; the child is often less mature at home than in school.
5. The child is responsive to authority, "fair" punishment, discipline, and reinforcement.
6. Children are adventurous and eager to be involved with a friend or a group of friends in "dangerous" or "secret" activities.
7. The child's self-concept becomes firmly established.

Implications for the Developmental Movement Program

1. There should be opportunities for children to refine fundamental movement abilities in the areas of locomotion, manipulation, and stability to a point where they are fluid and efficient.
2. Children need to be helped in making the transition from the fundamental movement phase to the specialized movement phase.
3. The assurance of being accepted and valued as a human being is important to children so they can know there is a stable and secure place in their school environment as well as in the home.
4. Abundant opportunities for encouragement and positive reinforcement from adults are necessary to promote continued development of a positive self-concept.
5. Opportunities and encouragement to explore and experiment through movement with their bodies and with objects in their environment enhances perceptual-motor efficiency.
6. There should be exposure to experiences in which progressively greater amounts of responsibility are introduced to help promote self-reliance.
7. Adjustment to the rougher ways of the playground and neighborhood without being rough or crude themselves is an important social skill to be learned.

8. Opportunities for gradual introduction to group and team activities should be provided at the proper time.
9. Storyplays and imaginary and mimetic activities may be effectively incorporated into the program during the primary years because of the child's still vivid imagination.
10. Activities that incorporate the use of music and rhythmics are enjoyable at this level and are valuable in enhancing fundamental movement abilities, creativity, and a basic understanding of the components of music and rhythm.
11. Children at this level learn best through active participation. Integration of academic concepts with movement activities provides an effective avenue for reinforcing academic concepts in science, mathematics, social studies, and the language arts.
12. Activities that involve climbing and hanging are beneficial to development of the upper torso and should be included in the program.
13. Discussion of play situations involving such topics as taking turns, fair play, cheating, and sportsmanship are valuable means of establishing a more complete sense of right or wrong.
14. Stress on accuracy, form, and skill in the performance of movement skills is important.
15. Children should be encouraged to "think" before engaging in an activity and helped to recognize potential hazards as a means of reducing their often reckless behavior.
16. Encouragement of small-group activities followed by larger-group activities and team sport experience is important.
17. Posture is important. Activities should stress proper body alignment.
18. Use of rhythmic activities to refine coordination is desirable.
19. Specialized movement skills begin to be developed and refined toward the end of this period. Plenty of opportunity for practice, encouragement, and selective instruction is important.
20. Opportunities should be provided for participation in youth sport activities that are developmentally appropriate and geared to the needs and interests of children.

FACTORS AFFECTING CHILD GROWTH AND DEVELOPMENT

Growth is not an independent process. Although heredity sets the limits of growth, environmental factors play an important role in the extent to which these limits are reached. The degree to which these factors affect motor development is unclear and needs further study. Nutrition, as well as exercise and physical activity, has been shown to be a major factor affecting growth.

Nutrition

The potentially harmful effects of poor nutrition during the prenatal period were highlighted earlier. Barness (1975, p. 345) noted that, among the factors influencing physical development during the prenatal period, nutrition "probably represents the most important single factor." Numerous investigations have also provided clear evidence that dietary deficiencies can have a very harmful effect on growth during infancy and childhood. The extent of growth retardation obviously depends on the severity, duration, and time of onset of undernourishment. For example, if severe chronic malnutrition occurs during the first four years of life, there is little hope of catching up to one's age-mates in terms of mental development, because the critical brain growth period has passed.

The physical growth process can be interrupted through malnutrition at any time between infancy and adolescence. Malnutrition may serve also as a mediating condition for certain diseases that affect physical growth. For example, lack of vitamin D in a diet can result in *rickets*, vitamin B-12 deficiencies may cause *pellagra*, and chronic lack of vitamin C results in *scurvy*. All are relatively rare in our modern society, but the effects of *kwashiorkor*, a debilitating disease, are seen in many parts of the world where there is a general lack of food and good nutrition. In the child with kwashiorkor, growth retardation can be expected as well as a large, puffed belly, sores on the body, and diarrhea.

Studies indicate that children suffering from *chronic malnutrition*, particularly during infancy and early childhood, never completely catch up to the growth norms for their age level and suffer from what is known as *growth retardation* (Behar, 1968; Eichenwald and Frye, 1969; Kallen, 1973). Evidence of this is shown in developing nations where adult height and weight norms are considerably lower than those in industrialized nations. Nutritional status is linked to income level. The results of the National Nutrition Survey as reported by Eichorn (1968, p. 266) indicate that in the United States "growth retardation was found in all ethnic groups and in all states, but the prevalence varied with sex, ethnic origin, and income level."

Popular opinion holds that children of low-income families most generally have a poor diet simply because food of low nutritional value is purchased. This is untrue. The results of the Preschool Nutrition Survey (Owen et al. 1974) indicated that the feeding style of low-income families is important. The quantity of food available to all members is less in low-income families, and there is a tendency toward greater permissiveness in the eating habits of children by low-income parents. The survey revealed that the quantity of food available increased with income level, and permissiveness about eating decreased.

Dietary excesses also represent nutritional factors affecting the growth of children. Among affluent countries, obesity is a major problem. Recent research (Oscai, 1974; Oscai et al. 1974; Eichorn, 1979) has proposed an interesting hypothesis linking obesity and its intractability to dietary habits during infancy and the preadolescent period. There is considerable concern among professionals over the high consumption of refined starches and sugars by children. The constant barrage of television commercials loudly extolling one junk food or another, the "fast food" addiction of millions, and the use of nonnutritive edibles as a reinforcer for good behavior all may have an effect on the nutritional status of children. What is not known, however, is where the critical point between adequate and inadequate nutrition lies. The individual nature of the child, with his or her own unique biochemical composition, makes it difficult to pinpoint where adequate nutrition ends and malnutrition begins. It seems, however, to be a critical question that needs further exploration. The welfare of a vast number of children hinges, in part, on the answer.

Exercise and Injury

One of the basic principles of physical activity is the concept of use and disuse. Basically, this principle revolves around the notion that a muscle that is used will *hypertrophy* (i.e., increase in size) and a muscle that is not used will *atrophy* (i.e., decrease in size). Anyone who has had a limb placed in a cast for several weeks knows about atrophy. In children, activity definitely promotes muscle development. Although the number of muscle fibers does not increase, the size of the fibers does increase. Muscles respond and adapt to increased amounts of stress. Maturation alone will not account for increases in muscle mass. An environment that promotes vigorous physical activity on the part of the child will do much to promote muscle development. Active children have less body fat in proportion to lean body mass. They do not have more muscle fibers; they simply have more muscle mass per fiber.

Although it is doubtful that permanent changes can be made in an individual's basic physique, it is certain that modifications within limits can be made. A popular method of classification of adult physique was developed by Sheldon et al. (1940), and later extended to children by Peterson (1967). This much-used system classifies individuals on the basis of fat, muscle, and bone length. An *endomorphic* physique is one that is soft and rounded in physical features (pear shape). The *mesomorphic* physique is well muscled, with broad shoulders, narrow waist, and thick chest (V shape). The *ectomorphic* physique is characterized by a tall, thin, lean look (angular shape). Within each classification a person is rated on a scale of 1 to 7, with 1 representing the least amount of a characteristic, 4 being average, and 7, the most of a characteristic. Therefore, the three-number sequence of 1-7-1 would represent a person very low on endomorphy, very high on mesomorphy, and very low on ectomorphy. A 2-3-6 would typify a person low on endomorphy, with some mesomorphic characteristics, and high on ectomorphy (perhaps a high jumper, or middle distance runner). Sheldon et al. (1954) found that males could typically be classified at the middle of the scale (i.e., 3-4-4 or 4-4-3) and females rated higher in endomorphy and lower in mesomorphy (i.e., 5-3-3).

Although physical activity generally has positive effects on the growth of children, it may have some negative effects if carried to the extreme. Seefeldt and Gould (1980) indicate that several studies have reported reduced growth rate in both height and weight of young athletes involved in moderate to intensive training programs, but that the controls in these investigations were weak at best. Clarke (1974) and Tipton and Tcheng (1970) did, however, report retarded growth in the height and weight of wrestlers. This was probably due to the unusually strenuous nature of training for this sport. Caine and Lindner (1984) raised the question of *growth plate injuries* to young long-distance runners. They reported that the literature is clear on the dangers of overusing a muscle. Overuse may result in epiphyseal injuries, and growth plate damage. Considerably more research needs to be conducted on the beneficial limits of strenuous physical activity during childhood. The critical point separating harmful and beneficial activity is not clear. The rapid rise of youth sport and the intensity of training that often accompanies it leave many unanswered questions. We can, however, assume that strenuous activity carried out over an extended period of time may result in injury to muscle and bone tissue of the child. "Swimmer's shoulder," "tennis elbow," "runner's knees" and stress fractures are but a few of the ailments plaguing children who exceed their developmental limits (Gilliam, 1981; Andrish, 1984). Care must be taken to supervise the exercise and activity programs of children. The potential benefits to the growth process are great, but the limits of the individual must be carefully considered.

Little evidence exists on the direct effects of regular exercise on stature (Malina, 1984, 1986). Bone growth is a hormonal process little affected by activity levels. Exercise does, however, increase bone width and promote *bone mineralization*, which makes for stronger, less brittle bones. Larson (1973) indicated that stress within the limits of the particular individual is beneficial to the bones. Chronic inactivity, on the other hand, has harmful effects on bone growth and may result in growth retardation (Krogman, 1980).

In summary, activity stimulates bone and muscle development and helps retard the depositing of fat. The vast majority of physical activity and athletic programs engaged in by children, other than the most strenuous forms of training such as marathon running, wrestling, and other heavy strength and endurance activities, have beneficial effects on growth. Injury, whether acute or chronic, may have negative effects depending on its severity and location. (Please refer to Chatper 11, Fitness Abilities of Children, for a further discussion of health-related fitness training).

Illness and Climate

A number of other factors have been associated with influencing the growth process. Such environmental factors as illness and disease, climate, emotions, and handicapping conditions have all been shown to influence the growth of the child (Krogman, 1972; Malina, 1980).

The standard childhood illnesses (chicken pox, colds, measles, and mumps) do not have a marked effect on the growth of the child. The extent to which illnesses and diseases may retard growth is dependent on their duration, severity, and timing. Krogman (1972, p. 144), reported that "there is some reason to use age three years as a cut-off point: before the age of three years the registry of health damage may be more marked and rebound may be slower." Often, the interaction of malnutrition and illnesses in the child makes it difficult to accurately determine the specific cause of growth retardation. But the combination of conditions puts the child at risk and greatly enhances the probability of measurable growth deficits.

A great deal of literature has reported the differences in height, weight, and onset of adolescence between individuals of varying climates (Krogman, 1972). The interacting effects of nutrition and health as well as possible genetic differences (e.g., when comparing black Africans with white Americans) make it impossible to demonstrate a direct causal relationship between climate and physical growth. The available data suggest that American children born and raised in the tropics have more linear physiques, but grow and mature at a slower rate than American children raised in more temperate climates. Malina (1980) reported that Eskimos show prolonged growth and are delayed in obtaining adult height. They also tend to have a more stocky physique and to mature earlier than individuals raised in the tropics.

Secular Trends

A *secular trend* is the tendency for children to be taller, heavier, and mature earlier, age for age, and to mature at an earlier age than children several generations ago. The trend for secular increases is not universal.

Increases in growth, maturation, and physical performance levels have been demonstrated in most developed countries. Developing nations throughout the world, however, have not demonstrated secular increases and in some cases have even shown decreases in stature (Gangirly, 1977). There may be many reasons for this, but it is largely a reflection of the little improvement in lifestyle and nutritional habits from one generation to another.

Malina (1978) reported that secular changes in length and weight are slight at birth but become progressively more pronounced until puberty, when there is again a lessening of differences. The largest differences in height and weight are found from ages 11 to 15 (the pubertal years) and are apparent across all socioeconomic classes and races in developed countries.

Children today mature more rapidly than they did 100 years ago. The age at menarche, for example, has decreased in European populations from an estimated range of 15.5 to 17.4 years to between 12.5 and 14 years (Eveleth and Tanner, 1976). Although secular trends in the maturation of boys are no doubt present, maturity data for them are lacking. It may be noted, however, that the average age at which the voice begins to change for members of boys' choirs today is considerably lower (about 13 years) than that estimated for boys performing in choirs more than 100 years ago (about 18 years) (Daw, 1974).

Malina (1978) reported that the secular trend in size and maturation in the United States and in many other developed nations has stopped. There has been little indication of secular trends in height, biological, and maturation in the past twenty years. This is probably due largely to the elimination of growth-inhibiting factors and a peaking of improved nutritional and health conditions. There is, however, clear evidence of a secular trend in weight during childhood (Ross and Pate, 1987). Comparison of National Children and Youth Fitness Study Scores (NCYFS, 1987) with data collected by the National Center for Health Statistics from 1963-1965 clearly indicates that today's children carry more body fat.

SUMMARY

Growth during childhood decelerates from the rapid pace characteristic of the first two years. This slow but steady increase in height and weight during childhood provides the child with an opportunity to coordinate perceptual and motor information. The child has time to lengthen, fill out, and gain control over his or her world. Numerous factors, however, can interrupt the normal developmental process. Nutritional deficiencies and excesses can severely affect growth and have a lasting negative impact on the child, depending on the severity and duration of poor nutrition. Severe and prolonged illness has also been shown to interrupt the growth process.

The effects of exercise both in acute and chronic forms as well as at low and high intensity levels is of great interest to researchers and youth sport coaches. Physical exercise has a positive influence on the growth process. Little evidence exists to support the claim that physical activity can be harmful to children, except in cases of extreme training requirements. The problem, however, lies in knowing when extremes have been reached for the individual child. Climatic factors also have been shown to accelerate or decelerate growth in children. North American children today are taller and heavier than their counterparts of 100 years ago. Definite secular trends can be seen in many but not all cultures. Differences in lifestyle and dietary circumstances play an important role in the presence or absence of secular trends.

CHAPTER CONCEPTS

10.1 Growth rates decelerate slowly during the early childhood period, with average annual gains in height and weight of 2 inches and 5 pounds, respectively.
10.2 Birth length is doubled by age 4.
10.3 Minimal gender differences are seen in children during the early childhood years, but boys tend to be taller, heavier, and have slightly more muscle mass.
10.4 Body proportions change markedly during early childhood.
10.5 The pace of growth is slow but steady during late childhood. It is a time of lengthening and filling out prior to puberty.
10.6 Boys and girls are similar in their growth patterns. Limb growth is greater than trunk growth.
10.7 Dietary deficiencies and excesses can have a serious impact on the growth patterns of children.
10.8 Body types have been classified as endomorphic, mesomorphic, and ectomorphic.
10.9 Physical activity generally has positive effects on growth except in cases of extreme exertion.
10.10 The critical line between beneficial and harmful levels of physical activity is not clear.
10.11 Exercise promotes bone mineralization and tends to increase bone width.
10.12 Illnesses may negatively affect growth, depending on the time of onset, duration, and severity.
10.13 Climatic conditions influence the growth process.
10.14 North American children are taller, heavier, and mature at an earlier age than their counterparts of past generations.
10.15 Secular changes are not universal and primarily reflect changes in lifestyle and nutritional habits.

TERMS TO REMEMBER

Myelination

Macula

Farsighted

Eustachian Tube

Rickets

Pellagra

Scurvy

Kwashiorkor

Growth Retardation

Chronic Malnutrition

Hypertrophy

Atrophy

Endomorphic

Mesomorphic

Ectomorphic

Growth Plate Injuries

Bone Mineralization

Secular Trend

CRITICAL READINGS

Bredekamp, S. (1987). *Developmentally Appropriate Practice in Early Childhood Programs Serving Children from Birth Through Age 8.* Washington, D.C.: National Association for the Education of Young Children.

Fishbein, H. D. (1976). *Evolution, Development, and Children's Learning.* Pacific Palisades, CA: Goodyear (Chapters 1 and 2).

Korgman, W. M. (1980) *Child Growth.* Ann Arbor: University of Michigan Press.

Malina, R. M. (1986). "Physical Growth and Maturation." In Seefeldt, V. (ed.) *Physical Activity and Well-Being.* Reston, VA: AAHPERD.

Morley, D. and Woodland, M. (1979). *See How They Grow—Monitoring Child Growth for Appropriate Health Care in Developing Countries.* New York: Oxford University Press, (Chapters 1, 8 and 9).

11

Fundamental Movement Abilities

CHAPTER COMPETENCIES

Upon Completion of This Chapter You Should Be Able To:

* *Compare and contrast intertask and intratask developmental sequences in selected fundamental movement skills.*

* *Categorize performer's movement into developmental stages.*

* *Demonstrate observational assessment skill in a variety of fundamental movement patterns.*

* *Discuss the uses of a developmental sequence checklist for assessing motor development.*

* *Distinguish between motor problems that students can assess and those they can't.*

* *Identify motor behavior characteristics or children who developmentally lag in motor skills.*

* *Discuss the concept of a developmental sequence of fundamental movement skill acquisition.*

* *Describe the meaning of the "initial," "elementary," and "mature" stages within the fundamental movement phase.*

* *Distinguish between "beween-child differences," "between-pattern differences," and "within-pattern differences" in movement skill acquisition.*

* *Devise a fundamental movement observational assessment checklist as an individual or group evaluative tool.*

* *Critically analyze the influences of opportunities for practice, encouragement, and instruction on the acquisition of fundamental movement abilities.*

As children approach their second birthday, a marked change can be observed in how they relate to their environment. By the end of the second year, they have mastered the rudimentary movement abilities that are developed during infancy. These movement abilities form the basis on which the child develops or refines the fundamental movement patterns of early childhood and the specialized movement skills of later childhood and adolescence. Children are no longer immobilized by their basic inability to move about freely or by the confines of their crib. They are now able to explore the movement potentials of their bodies as they move through space (locomotion). They no longer need to maintain a relentless struggle against the force of gravity but gain increased control over their musculature in opposition to gravity (stability). They no longer have to be content with the crude and ineffective reaching, grasping, and releasing of objects characteristic of infancy but rapidly develop the ability to make controlled and precise contact with objects in their environment (manipulation).

Young children are involved in the process of developing and refining fundamental movement abilities in a wide variety of stability, locomotor, and manipulative movements. This means that they should be involved in a series of coordinated and developmentally sound experiences designed to enhance knowledge of the body and its potential for movement. *Movement pattern* development is not so much concerned with developing high degrees of skill in a limited number of movement situations as it is with developing acceptable levels of proficiency and efficient body mechanics in a wide variety of movement situations. A *fundamental movement* involves the basic elements of that particular movement only. It does not include such things as the individual's style or personal peculiarities in performance. It does not emphasize the combining of a variety of fundamental movements into complex skills such as the lay-up shot in basketball or a floor exercise routine in gymnastics. Each movement pattern is first considered in relative isolation from all others and then linked with others into a variety of combinations. The locomotor movements of running, jumping, and leaping, or the manipulative movements of throwing, catching, kicking, and trapping are examples of fundamental movement abilities that are first dealt with separately by the child. They are then gradually combined in a variety of ways and elaborated upon to become sport skills. The basic elements of a fundamental movement should be the same for all children.

The development of fundamental movement abilities is basic to the motor development of children. A wide variety of movement experiences provide them with a wealth of information on which to base their perceptions of themselves and the world about them.

DEVELOPMENTAL SEQUENCE OF FUNDAMENTAL MOVEMENTS

With the renewed interest in the study of motor development that began in the 1960s, several scales appeared that illustrated a relationship between age and motor performance. Johnson (1962), using a large sample of boys and girls from grades 1 through 6, found that the mean scores on a variety of motor performance items showed a definite upward trend until the fifth grade. Cratty and Martin (1969) presented age-related sequences of acquisition for a variety of locomotor, manipulative, and perceptual abilities of 365 children ranging in age from 4 to 12 years. Williams' (1970) summary of the movement abilities of children between 3 and 6 years old revealed more advanced forms of movement with increases in age. Sinclair (1973) studied the motor development of 2- to 6-year-old children. The results of her longitudinal film analysis of 25 movement tasks at six-month intervals lent further support to the basic assumption that movement is a developing process during the early childhood years. Tables 11.1 through 11.3 provide a visual reference for appreciation of the sequence of emergence of selected locomotor, manipulative, and stability abilities, respectively.

These normative studies of motor development are interesting and informative about the quantity or outcome of movement in that they tell "how far," "how fast," and "how many." They fail, however, to provide information about *qualitative change* that occurs as the child progresses toward more mature form. As a result, a number of investigators, all using film and computer technqiues to analyze the intraskill aspects of a variety of fundamental movement patterns, began to collect data leading to a stage concept of movement skill acquisition during early childhood (Wild, 1938; Halverson, 1966; and Seefeldt, 1972). Seefeldt and Haubenstricker (1976), and several others conducted important investigations into the *intraskill sequences* of a variety of fundamental movement tasks. Out of these investigations have come three popular methods of charting the stage classification of children in actual observational settings. The systems devised by Roberton (1978c), McClenaghan and Gallahue (1978b), and Seefeldt and Haubenstricker (1976) have been used successfully in observational assessment with young children. The Roberton method expands the stage theory to an analysis of the separate components of movement within a given pattern, and is commonly referred to as the *segmental analysis* approach. The Seefeldt method assigns an overall stage classification score (Stage 1 through Stage 5), and is referred to as the *total body configuration* approach. The McClenaghan-Gallahue method provides opportunities for both, depending on the needs, interests, and abilities of

Table 11.1 Sequence of Emergence of Selected Locomotor Abilities

Movement Pattern	Selected Abilities	Approximate Age of Onset
Walking		
Walking involves placing one foot in front of the other while maintaining contact with the supporting surface	Rudimentary upright unaided gait	13 months
	Walks sideways	16 months
	Walks backward	17 months
	Walks upstairs with help	20 months
	Walks upstairs alone—follow step	24 months
	Walks downstairs alone—follow step	25 months
Running		
Running involves a brief period of no contact with the supporting surface	Hurried walk (maintains contact)	18 months
	First true run (nonsupport phase)	2–3 years
	Efficient and refined run	4–5 years
	Speed of run increases, mature run*	5 years
Jumping		
Jumping takes three forms: (1) jumping for distance; (2) jumping for height; and (3) jumping from a height. It involves a one- or two-foot takeoff with a landing on both feet	Steps down from low objects	18 months
	Jumps down from object with one foot lead	2 years
	Jumps off floor with both feet	28 months
	Jumps for distance (about 3 feet)	5 years
	Jumps for height (about 1 foot)	5 years
	Mature jumping pattern*	6 years
Hopping		
Hopping involves a one-foot takeoff with a landing on the same foot	Hops up to three times on preferred foot	3 years
	Hops from four to six times on same foot	4 years
	Hops from eight to ten times on same foot	5 years
	Hops distance of 50 feet in about 11 seconds	5 years
	Hops skillfully with rhythmical alteration, mature pattern*	6 years
Galloping		
The gallop combines a walk and a leap with the same foot leading throughout	Basic but inefficient gallop	4 years
	Gallops skillfully, mature pattern*	6 years
Skipping		
Skipping combines a step and a hop in rhythmic alteration	One-footed skip	4 years
	Skillful skipping (about 20 percent)	5 years
	Skillful skipping for most*	6 years

*The child has the developmental "potential" to be at the mature stage. Actual attainment will depend on environmental factors.

Table 11.2 Sequence of Emergence of Selected Manipulative Abilities

Movement Pattern	Selected Abilities	Approximate Age of Onset
Reach, Grasp, Release		
Reaching, grasping, and releasing involves making successful contact with an object, retaining it in one's grasp and releasing it at will	Primitive reaching behaviors	2-4 months
	Corralling of objects	2-4 months
	Palmar grasp	3-5 months
	Pincer grasp	8-10 months
	Controlled grasp	12-14 months
	Controlled releasing	14-18 months
Throwing		
Throwing involves inparting force to an object in the general direction of intent	Body faces target, feet remain stationary, ball, thrown with forearm extension only	2-3 years
	Same as above but with body rotation added	3.6-5 years
	Steps forward with leg on same side as the throwing arm	4-5 years
	Boys exhibit more mature pattern than girls	5 years and over
	Mature throwing pattern*	6 years
Catching		
Catching involves receiving force from an object with the hands, moving from large to progressively smaller balls	Chases ball; does not respond to aerial ball.	2 years
	Responds to aerial ball with delayed arm movements	2-3 years
	Needs to be told how to position arms	2-3 years
	Fear reaction (turns head away)	3-4 years
	Basket catch using the body	3 years
	Catches using the hands only with a small ball	5 years
	Mature catching pattern*	6 years
Kicking		
Kicking involves imparting force to an object with the foot	Pushes against ball. Does not actually kick it.	18 months
	Kicks with leg straight and little body movement (kicks *at* the ball)	2-3 years
	Flexes lower leg on backward lift.	3-4 years
	Greater backward and forward swing with definite arm opposition.	4-5 years
	Mature pattern (kicks *through* the ball)*	5-6 years
Striking		
Striking involves sudden contact to objects in an overarm, sidearm, or underhand pattern	Faces object and swings in a vertical plane	2-3 years
	Swings in a horizontal plane and stands to the side of the object.	4-5 years
	Rotates the trunk and hips and shifts body weight forward.	5 years
	Mature horizontal pattern with stationary ball	6-7 years

*The child has the developmental "potential" to be at the mature stage. Actual attainment will depend on environmental factors.

Table 11.3 Sequence of Emergence of Selected Stability Abilities

Movement Pattern	Selected Abilities	Approximate Age of Onset
Dynamic Balance		
Dynamic balance involves maintaining one's equilibrium as the center of gravity shifts	Walks 1-inch straight line	3 years
	Walks 1-inch circular line	4 years
	Stands on low balance beam	2 years
	Walks on 4-inch wide beam for a short distance	3 years
	Walks on same beam, alternating feet	3-4 years
	Walks on 2- or 3-inch beam	4 years
	Performs basic forward roll	3-4 years
	Performs mature forward roll*	6-7 years
Static Balance		
Static balance involves maintaining one's equilibrium while the center of gravity remains stationary	Pulls to a standing position	10 months
	Stands without handholds	11 months
	Stands alone	12 months
	Balances on one foot 3-5 seconds	5 years
	Supports body in basic three-point inverted positions	6 years
Axial Movements		
Axial movements are static postures that involve bending, stretching, twisting, turning, and the like	Axial movement abilities begin to develop early in infancy and are progressively refined to a point where they are included in the emerging manipulative patterns of throwing, catching, kicking, striking, trapping, and other activities	2 months– 6 years

*The child has the developmental "potential" to be at the mature stage. Actual attainment will depend on environmental factors.

the observer. Their method recognizes the differential rates of development within fundamental movement patterns as well as the need for an easy-to-apply tool for daily teaching situations.

In their book *Fundamental Movement: A Developmental and Remedial Approach*, McClenaghan and Gallahue (1978a) outlined three stages within the fundamental movement phase of development (Table 11.4).

Not all movement patterns fit precisely into an arbitrary three-stage progression. The developmental aspects of some movements may be more completely described in a four-, five-, or even an eight-stage sequence, depending on the specific pattern and the level of sophistication of the observer. The three-stage approach is used in the following sections because it accurately and adequately fits the developmental se-

Table 11.4 The Three Stages Within the Fundamental Movement Phase

Initial Stage:
Characterized by the child's first observable attempts at the movement pattern. Many of the components of a refined pattern, such as the preparatory action and follow-through, are missing.

Elementary Stage:
A transitional stage in the child's movement development. Coordination and performance improve, and the child gains more control over his movements. More components of the mature pattern are integrated into the movement, although they are performed incorrectly.

Mature Stage:
The integration of all the component movements into a well-coordinated, purposeful act. The movement resembles the motor pattern of a skilled adult [in terms of control and mechanics, but it is lacking in terms of movement performance as measured quantitatively*]. (p. 78).

*Author's Addition. From: McClenaghan, B. A., and Gallahue, D. L.(1978) *Fundamental Movement: A Developmental and Remedial Approach.* New York: Wiley. (p. 78)

---

quence of most fundamental movement patterns and provides the basis for a reliable, easy-to-use, observational assessment instrument.

MOVEMENT CONDITIONS

The fundamental movement phase of development has been extensively studied over the past several years. Most would agree that this phase follows a sequential progression that may be subdivided into stages. The cognitively and physically normal child progresses from one stage to another in a sequential manner that is influenced by both maturation and the environment. Children cannot rely solely on maturation to attain the mature stage in their fundamental movement abilities. Environmental conditions that include opportunities for practice, encouragement, and instruction are crucial to the development of mature patterns of fundamental movement. Miller (1978) investigated the facilitation of fundamental movement skill learning in children 3 to 5 years of age. She found that programs of instruction can increase fundamental movement patterns development beyond the level attained solely through maturation. She also found that an instructional program in skill development was more effective than a free-play program and that parents working under the direction of a trained specialist can be as effective as physical education teachers in developing fundamental movement skills. Luedke (1980) found similar results with fourth grade boys and girls by utilizing two different methods of instruction for the mature stage of throwing. Both instructional groups were more proficient in terms of form and performance than a noninstructed control group.

Care must be taken to remember that the mover's interaction with the environmental conditions and task goal may have a dramatic impact on the observed developmental maturity of a fundamental movement task (Figure 11.1).

Natural conditions within the environment such as temperature, lighting, surface area, and gravity may have an influence on the quantitative as well as the qualitative aspects of a movement task (Keogh and Sugden, 1985). Similarly, artificial conditions such as the size, shape, color, and texture of objects may dramatically influence performance (Payne and Isaacs, 1987). Furthermore, conditions such as ball velocity and trajectory may influence success in intercepting objects (Ridenour, 1974).

The goal of the task itself is another important influencer of the observed developmental status of a fundamental movement task. If, for example, the focus in a throwing task is on accuracy, such as with the game of darts, then it is reasonable to assume that the pattern of movement will be different than if the goal were distance. To this end Langendorfer (1988) observed two groups of subjects (children and adults) performing an overhand throwing pattern under two different goal conditions (force and accuracy). The results of his investigation indicated that "motor patterns are not absolutely robust to all environmental conditions, but some movers can accommodate their movements to shifting

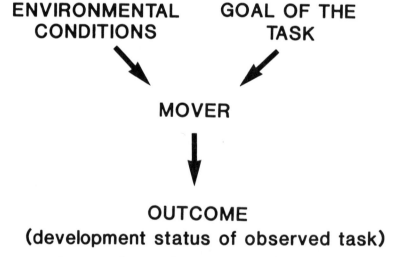

Figure 11.1. Interaction between the environment and the mover, and the task goal and the mover will impact on the apparent developmental maturity of a fundamental movement task.

environmental constraints." In other words, the degree to which a mover is able to make adjustments to an altered goal will be influenced by several factors within the mover as well as by the degree to which the task demands have changed. For example, the individual with limited ability to increase the velocity of a thrown ball (whether due to faulty body mechanics or lack of strength) will be limited in the adjustments he or she can make when switching from an accuracy throwing task to a distance throwing task.

The link between the mover, the conditions of the environment, and the demands of the task itself is not completely understood. It is interesting to note that many of the developmental descriptions of fundamental movement abilities that follow are laboratory-generated. That is, they are hypothesized, developmental sequences that are the product of research in an artificial setting—a setting quite unlike the real world in which children move. Little is known, as yet, about the changing ecology of the environment and its influence on the observed developmental status of children's movement. As we turn to methods of analyzing children's movement in more natural settings, we may find these hypothesized stages of development to be somewhat different. This point is echoed by Roberton (1987) who indicated that researchers have frequently been so concerned with describing changes in the movement characteristics of their subjects that they have failed to consider the powerful influence of the movement conditions (i.e., conditions of the environment and goal of the task) on the resulting observed developmental status of the fundamental movement pattern itself.

DEVELOPMENTAL DIFFERENCES

When observing and analyzing the fundamental movement abilities of children, it becomes apparent that there are various stages of development for each pattern of movement. It should also be obvious that differences in abilities exist between children, between patterns, and within patterns (McClenaghan and Gallahue, 1978a).

Between-child differences should remind us of the principle of individuality in all learning. The sequence of progression through the initial, elementary, and mature stages is the same for most children. The rate, however, will vary, depending on both environmental and hereditary factors. Whether or not a child reaches the mature stage depends primarily on instruction, encouragement, and opportunities for practice. When these are absent, normal differences between children will be magnified.

Between-pattern differences are seen in all children. A child may be at the initial stage in some, the elementary in others, and the mature in still others. Children do not progress at an even rate in the development of their fundamental movement abilities. Play and instructional experiences will greatly influence the rate of development of locomotor, manipulative, and stability abilities.

Within-pattern differences are an interesting and often curious phenomenon. Within a given pattern, a child may exhibit a combination of initial, elementary, and mature elements. In the throw, for example, the arm action may be at the elementary stage while the leg action is at the mature stage and the trunk action at the initial stage. Developmental differences within patterns are common and usually the result of: (1) incomplete modeling of the movements of others; (2) initial success with the inappropriate action; (3) failure to require an all-out effort; (4) inappropriate or restricted learning opportunities; or (5) incomplete sensorimotor integration. Children exhibiting within-pattern differences should be assessed utilizing the segmental analysis approach. This will permit the observer to accurately determine the stage of development of each body segment. With this knowledge, appropriate intervention strategies can be mapped out.

Creative, diagnostic teaching can do much to aid the child in the balanced development of his or her fundamental movement abilities. Observational assessment of the child's movement abilities will enable the teacher to plan experiences and instructional strategies that will help the child develop mature patterns of movement. Once movement control has been established, these mature patterns may be further refined in terms of force production and accuracy in the specialized movement phase. Failure to achieve proficiency in a wide variety of fundamental movement abilities is a barrier to the development of efficient and effective movement skills that may be applied to game, sport, and dance activities characteristic of one's culture.

FUNDAMENTAL LOCOMOTOR MOVEMENTS

Locomotion is a fundamental aspect of learning to move effectively and efficiently within one's environment. It involves projection of the body into external space by altering its location relative to fixed points on the surface. Activities such as walking, running, jumping, hopping, sliding, and skipping are considered fundamental locomotor movements. Performance of these movements must be sufficiently flexible so they can be altered as the requirements of the environment demand without deflecting attention from the purpose of the act. The child must be able to: (1) use any one of a number of types of movements to reach the goal; (2) shift from one type of movement to another when the situation demands; and (3) alter each movement as the conditions of the environment change. Throughout this process of alteration and modification, attention must not be diverted from the goal. For example, the locomotor pattern of walking may be used singularly or it may be used in conjunction with manipulative or stability movements. As a result, the pattern of walking is elaborated upon with the inclusion of object handling such as bouncing a ball while walking on a balance beam. Development and refinement of the following locomotor patterns in children is essential since it is through these movements that they explore the world about them.

Walking

Walking has often been defined as the process of continually losing and regaining balance while moving forward in an upright position. The walking pattern has been extensively studied in infants, children, and adults. The onset of walking behavior in the infant depends primarily on maturation but is also influenced by environmental factors such as the availability of handholds. Burnett and Johnson (1971) indicated that the average age for achieving independent walking is 12½ months, with a range of from 9 to 17 months. Once independent walking has been achieved, the child progresses rapidly to the elementary and mature stages. Several authors in describing the walking pattern have indicated that mature walking is achieved sometime between the fourth and the seventh year (Eckert, 1987; Grieve and Gaer, 1966; Guttridge, 1939; Saunders et al. 1953; Wickstrom, 1983; Williams, 1983). Many subtle changes continue to occur in the walking pattern but are unobservable through unaided visual assessment. Sophisticated film analysis and electromyography techniques must be used in order to detect progress in walking skill beyond this point (Wickstrom, 1983). Gad-Elmawla's 1980 dissertation is used as the basis for description of the following developmental sequence in the walking pattern (Table 11.5, Figure 11.2).

Running

Running is an exaggerated form of walking. It offers principally from the walk in that there is a brief flight phase during each step, in which the body is out of contact with the supporting surface. The flight phase is first seen around the second birthday. Prior to that, the run appears as a fast walk with one foot always in contact with the supporting surface. The initial stage of the running pattern does not depend on mature walking (Broer and Zernicke, 1979). Many young children begin to run prior to mastery of the mature walking pattern. The mature running pattern is fundamental to successful participation in a variety of sport-related activities. The running pattern has been extensively studied by a number of investigators (Seefeldt et al. 1972; Wickstrom, 1983; Robert-

Table 11.5 Developmental Sequence for Walking

I. Walking:
   A. Initial stage.
      1. Difficulty maintaining upright posture.
      2. Unpredictable loss of balance.
      3. Rigid, halting leg action.
      4. Short steps.
      5. Flat-footed contact.
      6. Toes turn outward.
      7. Wide base of support.
      8. Flexed knee at contact followed by quick leg extension.
   B. Elementary stage.
      1. Gradual smoothing out of pattern.
      2. Step length increased.
      3. Heel-toe contact.
      4. Arms down to sides with limited swing.
      5. Base of support within the lateral dimensions of trunk.
      6. Out-toeing reduced or eliminated.
      7. Increased pelvic tilt.
      8. Apparent vertical lift.
   C. Mature stage.
      1. Reflexive arm swing.
      2. Narrow base of support.
      3. Relaxed, elongated gait.
      4. Minimal vertical lift.
      5. Definite heel-toe contact.
II. Common Problems:
   A. Inhibited or exaggerated arm swing.
   B. Arms crossing midline of body.
   C. Improper foot placement.
   D. Exaggerated forward trunk lean.
   E. Arms flopping at sides or held out for balance.
   F. Twisting of trunk.
   G. Poor rhythmical action.
   H. Landing flat-footed.
   I. Flipping foot or lower leg in or out.

on & Halverson, 1984). The developmental sequence enumerated by McClenaghan (1976), based on film analysis, is used here (Table 11.6, Figure 11.3).

Horizontal Jumping

The jump for distance is an explosive movement requiring coordinated performance of all parts of the body. This is a complex movement

INITIAL

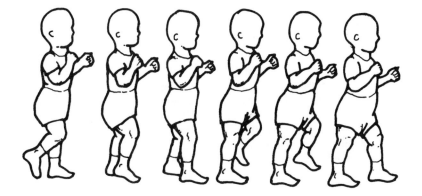

ELEMENTARY

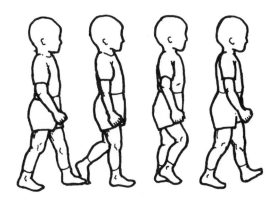

MATURE

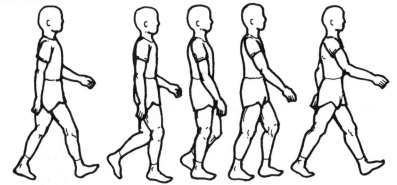

Figure 11.2. Stages of the walking pattern

Table 11.6 Developmental Sequence for Running

I. Running:
   A. Initial stage.
      1. Short, limited leg swing.
      2. Stiff, uneven stride.
      3. No observable flight phase.
      4. Incomplete extension of support leg.
      5. Stiff, short swing with varying degrees of elbow flexion.
      6. Arms tend to swing outward horizontally.
      7. Swinging leg rotates outward from hip.
      8. Swinging foot toes outward.
      9. Wide base of support.
   B. Elementary stage.
      1. Increase in length of stride, arm swing, and speed.
      2. Limited but observable flight phase.
      3. More complete extension of support leg at takeoff.
      4. Arm swing increases.
      5. Horizontal arm swing reduced on backswing.
      6. Swinging foot crosses midline at height of recovery to rear.
   C. Mature stage.
      1. Stride length at maximum; Stride speed fast.
      2. Definite flight phase.
      3. Complete extension of support leg.
      4. Recovery thigh parallel to ground.
      5. Arms swing vertically in opposition to legs.
      6. Arms bent at approximate right angles.
      7. Minimal rotary action of recovery leg and foot.
II. Common problems:
   A. Inhibited or exaggerated arm swing.
   B. Arms crossing the midline of the body.
   C. Improper foot placement.
   D. Exaggerated forward trunk lean.
   E. Arms flopping at the sides or held out for balance.
   F. Twisting of the trunk.
   G. Poor rhythmical action.
   H. Landing flat-footed.
   I. Flipping the foot or lower leg in or out.

pattern in which it is difficult to inhibit the tendency to step forward on one foot. Instead, the take-off and landing must be with both feet. The horizontal jumping pattern has been extensively studied (Wickstrom, 1983; Seefeldt et al., 1972; Roberton and Halverson, 1984; Clark & Phillips, 1985). The developmental sequence proposed by McClenaghan (1976), based on film analysis, is used here (Table 11.7, Figure 11.4).

INITIAL

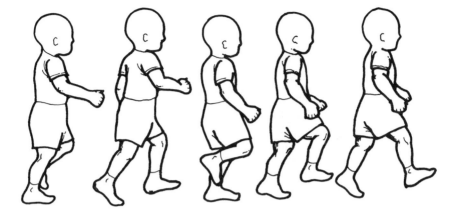

ELEMENTARY

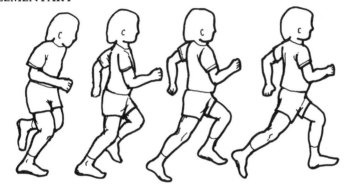

MATURE

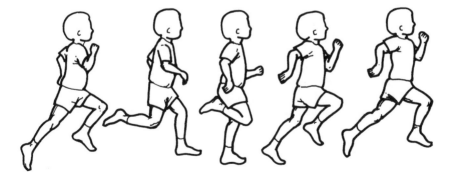

Figure 11.3. Stages of running pattern

Table 11.7 Developmental Sequence for Horizontal Jumping

I. Horizontal Jumping:
  A. Initial stage.
    1. Limited swing; arms do not initiate jumping action.
    2. During flight, arms move sideward-downward or rearward-upward to maintain balance.
    3. Trunk moves in vertical direction; little emphasis on length of jump.
    4. Preparatory crouch inconsistent in terms of leg flexion.
    5. Difficulty in using both feet.
    6. Limited extension of the ankles, knees, and hips at takeoff.
    7. Body weight falls backward at landing.
  B. Elementary stage.
    1. Arms initiate jumping action.
    2. Arms remain toward front of body during preparatory crouch.
    3. Arms move out to side to maintain balance during flight.
    4. Preparatory crouch deeper and more consistent.
    5. Knee and hip extension more complete at takeoff.
    6. Hips flexed during flight; thighs held in flexed position.
  C. Mature stage.
    1. Arms move high and to rear during preparatory crouch.
    2. During takeoff, arms swing forward with force and reach high.
    3. Arms held high throughout jumping action.
    4. Trunk propelled at approximately 45-degree angle.
    5. Major emphasis on horizontal distance.
    6. Preparatory crouch deep, consistent.
    7. Complete extension of ankles, knees, and hips at takeoff.
    8. Thighs held parallel to ground during flight; lower leg hangs vertically.
    9. Body weight forward at landing.
II. Common Problems:
  A. Improper use of arms (that is, failure to use arm opposite the propelling leg in a down-up-down swing as leg flexes, extends, and flexes again).
  B. Twisting or jerking of body.
  C. Inability to perform either a one-foot or a two-foot takeoff.
  D. Poor preliminary crouch.
  E. Restricted movements of arms or legs.
  F. Poor angle of takeoff.
  G. Failure to extend fully on takeoff.
  H. Failure to extend legs forward on landing.
  I. Falling backward on landing.

Vertical Jumping

Jumping for height, or vertical jump, has been studied by several investigators in recent years (Martin and Stull, 1969; Myers et al., 1977; Poe, 1976; Wickstrom, 1983; Williams, 1983). The jump for height involves projecting the body vertically into the air from a one- or two-foot

INITIAL

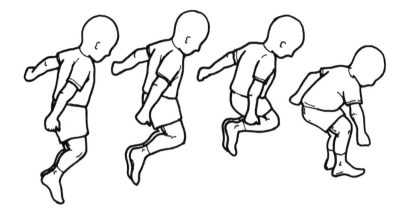

ELEMENTARY

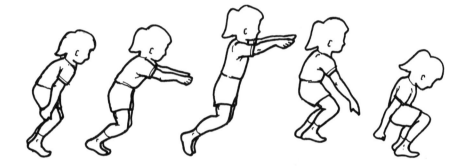

MATURE

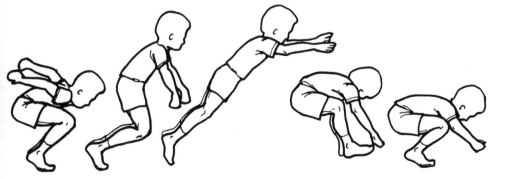

Figure 11.4. Stages of the horizontal jumping pattern

takeoff and landing on both feet. The developmental sequence proposed by Meyers et al. (1977), based on film analysis, is presented here (Table 11.8, Figure 11.5).

Jumping from a Height

The movements involved in jumping from a low height are somewhat similar to those found in the jump for distance and the jump for height, particularly at the initial stage. The jump from a low height has been studied by a few investigators (Bayley, 1935; McCaskill and Wellman, 1938) and has concentrated on the takeoff, flight phase, and landing aspects of the pattern. The description of stages that follows is based on this research and on my observation of numerous children. It is, therefore, subject to refinement and verification (Table 11.9, Figure 11.6).

Hopping

Hopping is similar to the jump for distance and the vertical jump, but both the takeoff and the landing are on the same foot. The hop has been studied by Seefeldt and Haubenstricker (1976); Roberton & Halverson (1984) and Halverson & Williams (1985). The four-stage developmental sequence proposed by Seefeldt & Haubenstricker (1976) is summarized here and condensed into three stages (Table 11.10, Figure 11.7).

Galloping and Sliding

Galloping and sliding involve the combination of two fundamental movements, the step and the hop, with the same foot always leading in the direction of movement. The movement is called a "gallop" when moving forward or backward, and a "slide" when progressing sideward. Sapp (1980) and Williams (1983) have described a developmental sequence for galloping that may also be applied for sliding (Table 11.11, Figure 11.8).

Leaping

The leap is similar to the run in that there is a transference of weight from one foot to the other, but the loss of contact with the surface is sustained, with greater elevation and distance covered than in the run. Leaping involves using greater amounts of force to produce more height and to cover a greater distance than that covered by a run. Biomechanic studies have been conducted on the hurdle event in track, but there is a dearth of information about the developmental aspects of the leaping pattern. The description of stages that follows is based on my observational assessment of numerous children and is subject to refinement and verification (Table 11.12, Figure 11.9).

Table 11.8 Developmental Sequence for Vertical Jumping

I. Vertical Jumping:
  A. Initial stage
    1. Inconsistent preparatory crouch.
    2. Difficulty in taking off with both feet.
    3. Poor body extension on takeoff.
    4. Little or no head lift.
    5. Arms not coordinated with the trunk and leg action.
    6. Little height achieved.
  B. Elementary stage.
    1. Knee flexion exceeds ninety degree angle on preparatory crouch.
    2. Exaggerated forward lean during crouch.
    3. Two-foot take off.
    4. Entire body does not fully extend during flight phase.
    5. Arms attempt to aid in flight (but often unequally) and balance.
    6. Noticeable horizontal displacement on landing.
  C. Mature stage.
    1. Preparatory crouch with knee flexion from 60 to ninety degrees.
    2. Forceful extension at hips, knees, and ankles.
    3. Simultaneous coordinated upward arm lift.
    4. Upward head tilt with eyes focused on target.
    5. Full body extension.
    6. Elevation of reaching arm by shoulder girdle tilt combined with downward thrust of nonreaching arm at peak of flight.
    7. Controlled landing very close to point of takeoff.
II. Common Problems:
  A. Failure to get airborn.
  B. Failure to take off with both feet simultaneously.
  C. Failure to crouch at about a ninety degree angle.
  D. Failure to extend body, legs, and arms forcefully.
  E. Poor coordination of leg and arm actions.
  F. Swinging of arms backward or to the side for balance.
  G. Failure to lead with eyes and head.
  H. One-foot landing.
  I. Inhibited or exaggerated flexion of hip and knee on landing.
  J. Marked horizontal displacement on landing.

Skipping

The skipping action puts two fundamental movement patterns, the step and the hop, into a combined pattern of movement. Seefeldt and Haubenstricker (1976) as well as Halverson and Roberton (1979) have studied the skipping pattern and report a three-stage developmental sequence which serves as the basis of the following description. The skip is a continuous flow of the step and hop involving rhythmical alteration of the leading foot (Table 11.13, Figure 11.10).

INITIAL

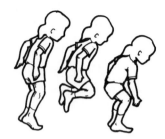

ELEMENTARY

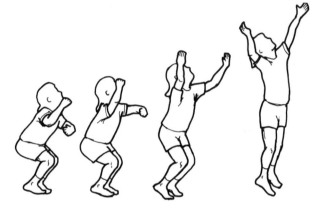

MATURE

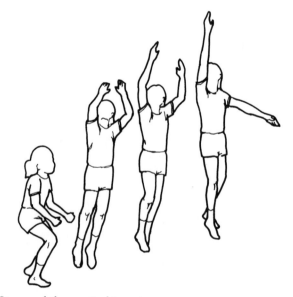

Figure 11.5. Stages of the vertical jumping pattern

Table 11.9 Developmental Sequence for Jumping from a Height

I. Jumping from a Height:
   A. Inital stage.
      1. One foot leads on takeoff.
      2. No flight phase.
      3. Lead foot contacts lower surface prior to trailing foot leaving upper surface.
      4. Exaggerated use of arms for balance.
   B. Elementary stage.
      1. Two-foot takeoff with one-foot lead.
      2. Flight phase, but lacks control.
      3. Arms used ineffectively for balance.
      4. One-foot landing followed by immediate landing of trailing foot.
      5. Inhibited or exaggerated flexion at knees and hip upon landing.
   C. Mature stage.
      1. Two-foot takeoff.
      2. Controlled flight phase.
      3. Both arms used efficiently out to sides to control balance as needed.
      4. Feet contact lower surface simultaneously with toes touching first.
      5. Feet land shoulder-width apart.
      6. Flexion at knees and hip congruent with height of jump.
II. Common Problems:
   A. Inability to take off with both feet.
   B. Twisting body to one side on takeoff.
   C. Exaggerated or inhibited body lean.
   D. Failure to coordinate use of both arms in the air.
   E. Tying one arm to side while using the other.
   F. Failure to land simultaneously on both feet.
   G. Landing flat-footed.
   H. Failure to flex knees sufficiently to absorb impact of landing.
   I. Landing out of control.

Climbing

Climbing is a fundamental movement similar to creeping. The primary difference between the two is that climbing requires the body weight to be pulled by the limbs in opposition to the force of gravity while creeping requires the body weight to be pushed by the limbs at right angles to the gravitational pull. Climbing may be performed with the legs alone, the arms alone, or with the legs and arms together. The terrain over which the child climbs or the object being climbed (e.g., rope, pole, ladder) dictates the exact form to be used. The following is a description of a vertical climbing pattern in which both the arms and the legs are used, as in climbing a ladder. It is based on my observations of children and is subject to verification and refinement (Table 11.14).

INITIAL

ELEMENTARY

MATURE

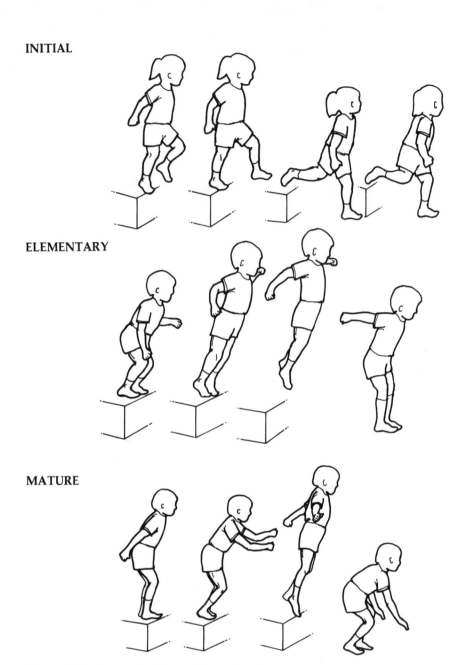

Figure 11.6. Stages of the jump from a height

Table 11.10 Developmental Sequence for Hopping

I. Hopping:
   A. Initial stage.
      1. Nonsupporting leg flexed 90 degrees or less.
      2. Nonsupporting thigh roughly parallel to contact surface.
      3. Body upright.
      4. Arms flexed at elbows and held slightly to side.
      5. Little height or distance generated in single hop.
      6. Balance lost easily.
      7. Limited to one or two hops.
   B. Elementary stage.
      1. Nonsupporting leg flexed.
      2. Nonsupporting thigh at 45-degree angle to contact surface.
      3. Slight forward lean, with trunk flexed at hip.
      4. Nonsupporting thigh flexed and extended at hip to produce greater force.
      5. Force absorbed on landing by flexing at hip and by supporting knee.
      6. Arms move up and down vigorously and bilaterally.
      7. Balance poorly controlled.
      8. Generally limited in number of consecutive hops that can be performed.
   C. Mature stage.
      1. Nonsupporting leg flexed at 90 degrees or less.
      2. Nonsupporting thigh lifts with vertical thrust of supporting foot.
      3. Greater body lean.
      4. Rhythmical action of nonsupporting leg (pendulum swing aiding in force production).
      5. Arms move together rhythmical lifting as the supporting foot leaves the contact surface.
      6. Arms not needed for balance but used for greater force production.
II. Common Problems:
   A. Hopping flat-footed.
   B. Exaggerated movements of arms.
   C. Exaggerated movement of nonsupporting leg.
   D. Exaggerated forward lean.
   E. Inability to maintain balance for five or more consecutive hops.
   F. Lack of rhythmical fluidity of movement.
   G. Inability to hop effectively on both left foot and right foot.
   H. Inability to alternate hopping feet in a smooth, continuous manner.
   I. Tying one arm to side of body.

INITIAL

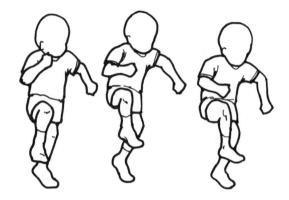

ELEMENTARY

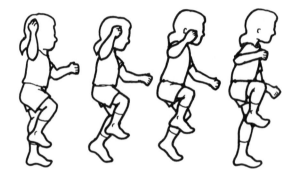

MATURE

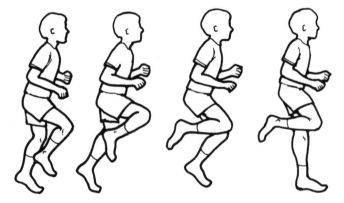

Figure 11.7. Stages of the hopping pattern

Table 11.11 Developmental Sequence for Galloping and Sliding

I. Galloping and Sliding:
    A. Initial stage.
        1. Arhythmical at fast pace.
        2. Trailing leg often fails to remain behind and often contacts surface in front of lead leg.
        3. 45-degree flexion of trailing leg during flight phase.
        4. Contact in a heel-toe combination.
        5. Arms of little use in balance or force production.
    B. Elementary stage.
        1. Moderate tempo.
        2. Appears choppy and stiff.
        3. Trailing leg may lead during flight but lands adjacent to or behind lead leg.
        4. Exaggerated vertical lift.
        5. Feet contact in a heel-toe, or toe-toe, combination.
        6. Arms slightly out to side to aid balance.
    C. Mature stage.
        1. Moderate tempo.
        2. Smooth, rhythmical action.
        3. Trailing leg lands adjacent to or behind lead leg.
        4. Both legs flexed at 45-degree angle during flight.
        5. Low flight pattern.
        6. Heel-toe contact combination.
        7. Arms not needed for balance; may be used for other purposes.
II. Common Problems:
    A. Choppy movements.
    B. Keeping legs too straight.
    C. Exaggerated forward trunk lean.
    D. Overstepping with trailing leg.
    E. Too much elevation on hop.
    F. Inability to perform both forward and backward.
    G. Inability to lead with nondominant foot.
    H. Inability to perform to both left and right.
    I. Undue concentration on task.

FUNDAMENTAL MANIPULATIVE MOVEMENTS

Gross motor *manipulation* involves the individual's relationship to objects and is characterized by giving force to objects and receiving force from them. Propulsive movements involve activities in which an object is moved away from the body. Fundamental movements such as throwing, kicking, striking, and rolling a ball are involved. Absorptive movements involve activities that are concerned with positioning the body or a body

INITIAL

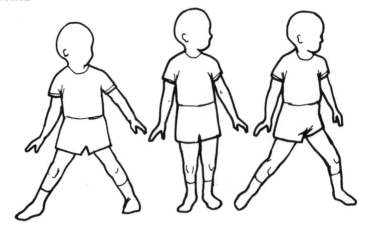

ELEMENTARY

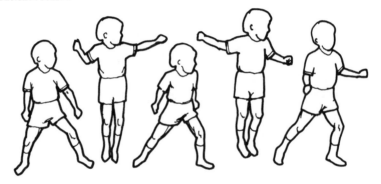

MATURE

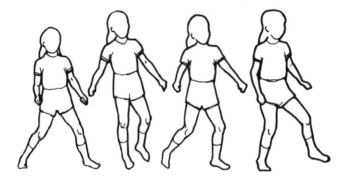

Figure 11.8. Stages of the sliding pattern

Table 11.12 Developmental Sequence for Leaping

I. Leaping:
  A. Initial stage.
    1. Child appears confused in attempts.
    2. Inability to push off and gain distance and elevation.
    3. Each attempt looks like another running step.
    4. Inconsistent use of takeoff leg.
    5. Arms ineffective.
  B. Elementary stage.
    1. Appears to be thinking through the action.
    2. Attempt looks like an elongated run.
    3. Little elevation above supporting surface.
    4. Little forward trunk lean.
    5. Stiff appearance in trunk.
    6. Incomplete extension of legs during flight.
    7. Arms used for balance, not as an aid in force production.
  C. Mature stage.
    1. Relaxed rhythmical action.
    2. Forceful extension of takeoff leg.
    3. Good summation of horizontal and vertical forces.
    4. Definite forward trunk lean.
    5. Definite arm opposition.
    6. Full extension of legs during flight.
II. Common Problems:
  A. Failure to use arms in opposition to legs.
  B. Inability to perform one-foot takeoff and land on opposite foot.
  C. Restricted movements of arms or legs.
  D. Lack of spring and elevation in push-off.
  E. Landing flat-footed.
  F. Exaggerated or inhibited body lean.
  G. Failure to stretch and reach with legs.

part in the path of a moving object for the purpose of stopping or deflecting that object. Fundamental movements such as catching and trapping are involved. The essence of manipulative movements is that they combine two or more movements and are generally used in conjunction with other forms of movement. For example, propulsive movements are generally a composite of stepping, turning, swinging, and stretching. Absorptive movements generally consist of bending and stepping.

It is through the manipulation of objects that children are able to explore the relationship of moving objects in space. These movements involve making estimates of the path, distance, rate of travel, accuracy, and mass of the moving object. At the point of contact, a check on previous estimates is possible. It is through such types of experimentation

INITIAL

ELEMENTARY

MATURE

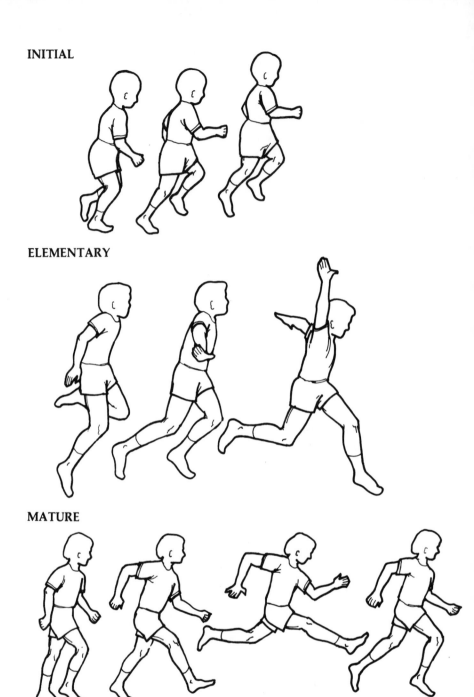

Figure 11.9. Stages of the leaping pattern

Table 11.13 Developmental Sequence for Skipping

I. Skipping:
   A. Initial stage.
      1. One-footed skip.
      2. Deliberate step-hop action.
      3. Double hop or step sometimes occurs.
      4. Exaggerated stepping action.
      5. Arms of little use.
      6. Action appears segmented.
   B. Elementary stage
      1. Step and hop coordinated effectively.
      2. Rhythmical use of arms to aid momentum.
      3. Exaggerated vertical lift on hop.
      4. Flat-footed landing.
   C. Mature stage.
      1. Rhythmical weight transfer throughout.
      2. Rhythmical use of arms (reduced during time of weight transfer).
      3. Low vertical lift on hop.
      4. Toe-first landing.
II. Common Problems:
   A. Segmented stepping and hopping action.
   B. Poor rhythmical alteration.
   C. Inability to use both sides of body.
   D. Exaggerated movements.
   E. Landing flat-footed.
   F. Exaggerated, inhibited, or unilateral arm movements.
   G. Inability to move in a straight line.
   H. Inability to skip backward and to side.

that children learn the nature and effect of the movement of objects. Because manipulative patterns commonly combine both locomotor and stabilizing movements, their efficient use should not be expected at the same time that locomotor and stability abilities are developing. Only after these patterns have been fairly well established do we begin to see the emergence of efficient manipulative movements. The following is a description of several manipulative patterns of movement.

Overhand Throwing

The overhand throw has been studied extensively over the past several years (Wild, 1938; Deach, 1951; Seefeldt et al. 1972; McClenaghan & Gallahue, 1978; Haubenstricker et al. 1983; Roberton, 1978 & 1984), with attention focused on form, accuracy, and distance. The components of the throw vary depending on which of these three factors the thrower is concentrating and on the starting position that is assumed. When view-

INITIAL

ELEMENTARY

MATURE

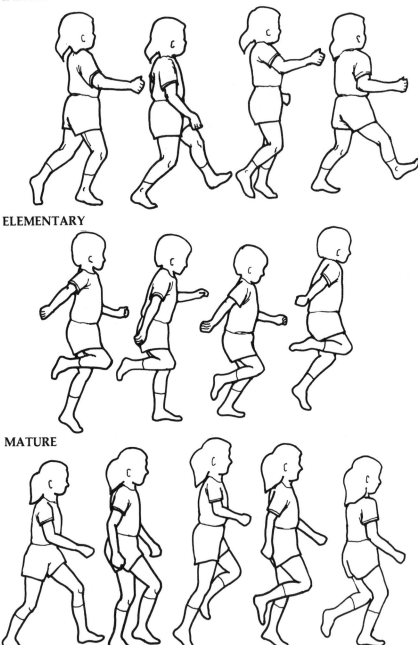

Figure 11.10. Stages of the skipping pattern

Table 11.14 Developmental Sequence for Climbing

I. Climbing:
   A. Initial stage.
      1. Leans body weight forward toward climbing surface to ensure balance.
      2. Begins action with feet.
      3. Uses a follow step and a follow grip.
   B. Elementary stage.
      1. Tends to lead with same foot and hand.
      2. Supports body weight with good balance.
      3. Begins action with preferred foot.
      4. Uses homolateral arm and leg action; appears in control.
   C. Mature stage.
      1. Good balance and body control.
      2. Can lead off with either hand or leg.
      3. Smooth, fluid, rapid motion.
      4. Uses a contralateral arm-leg action.
II. Common problems:
   A. Failure to wrap thumbs around grasping object.
   B. Improper sequencing of limb movements.
   C. Uneven or irregular use of two sides of the body.
   D. Inability to transfer basic elements to climbing other objects (e.g., rope, pole, ladder).
   E. Inability to use alternating hand and/or foot placement.

ing the overhand throw from the standpoint of the process or form, the developmental sequence depicted in Table 11.15 and Figure 11.11 is apparent.

Catching

The fundamental movement pattern of catching involves use of the hands to stop tossed objects. The elements of the underhand and overhand catch are essentially the same. The major difference is in the position of the hands upon impact with the object. The underhand catch is performed when the object to be caught is below the waist. The palms of the hands and the wrists are turned upward. When the object is above the waist, the palms face away from the individual in the direction of the object's flight.

Several researchers have investigated the development of catching abilities in children (Guttridge, 1939; Whiting, 1969; Pederson, 1973; McClenaghan & Gallahue, 1978; Haubenstricker et al. 1983, Roberton, 1984). The following developmental sequence of catching is based on these and McClenaghan's (1976) study (Table 11.16, Figure 11.12).

Table 11.15 Developmental Sequence for Overhand Throwing

I. Throwing:
  A. Initial stage.
    1. Action is mainly from elbow.
    2. Elbow of throwing arm remains in front of body; action resembles a push.
    3. Fingers spread at release.
    4. Follow-through is forward and downward.
    5. Trunk remains perpendicular to target.
    6. Little rotary action during throw.
    7. Body weight shifts slightly rearward to maintain balance.
    8. Feet remain stationary.
    9. There is often purposeless shifting of feet during preparation for throw.
  B. Elementary stage.
    1. In preparation, arm is swung upward, sideward, and backward to a position of elbow flexion.
    2. Ball is held behind head.
    3. Arm is swung forward, high over shoulder.
    4. Trunk rotates toward throwing side during preparatory action.
    5. Shoulders rotate toward throwing side.
    6. Trunk flexes forward with forward motion of arm.
    7. Definite forward shift of body weight.
    8. Steps forward with leg on same side as throwing arm.
  C. Mature stage.
    1. Arm is swung backward in preparation.
    2. Opposite elbow is raised for balance as a preparatory action in the throwing arm.
    3. Throwing elbow moves forward horizontally as it extends.
    4. Forearm rotates and thumb points downward.
    5. Trunk markedly rotates to throwing side during preparatory action.
    6. Throwing shoulder drops slightly.
    7. Definite rotation through hips, legs, spine, and shoulders during throw.
    8. Weight during preparatory movement is on rear foot.
    9. As weight is shifted, there is a step with opposite foot.
II. Common Problems:
  A. Forward movement of foot on same side as throwing arm.
  B. Inhibited backswing.
  C. Failure to rotate hips as throwing arm is brought forward.
  D. Failure to step out on leg opposite the throwing arm.
  E. Poor rhythmical coordination of arm movement with body movement.
  F. Inability to release ball at desired trajectory.
  G. Loss of balance while throwing.
  H. Upward rotation of arm.

INITIAL

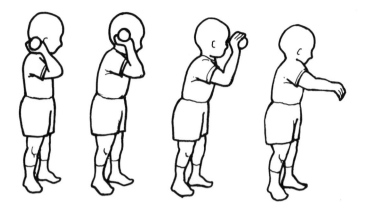

ELEMENTARY

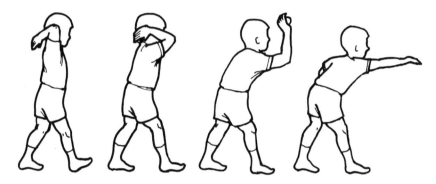

MATURE

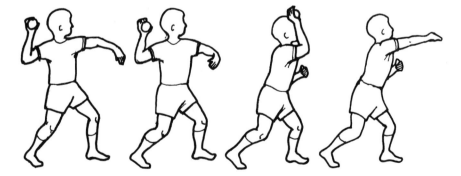

Figure 11.11. Stages of the overhand throwing pattern

Table 11.16 Developmental Sequence for Catching

I. Catching:
 A. Initial stage.
  1. There is often an avoidance reaction of turning the face away or protecting the face with arms (avoidance reaction is learned and therefore may not be present).
  2. Arms are extended and held in front of body.
  3. Body movement is limited until contact.
  4. Catch resembles a scooping action.
  5. Use of body to trap ball.
  6. Palms are held upward.
  7. Fingers are extended and held tense.
  8. Hands are not utilized in catching action.
 B. Elementary stage.
  1. Avoidance reaction is limited to eyes closing at contact with ball.
  2. Elbows are held at sides with an approximately 90-degree bend.
  3. Since initial attempt at contact with child's hands is often unsuccessful, arms trap the ball.
  4. Hands are held in opposition to each other; thumbs are held upward.
  5. At contact, the hands attempt to squeeze ball in a poorly-timed and uneven motion.
 C. Mature stage.
  1. No avoidance reaction.
  2. Eyes follow ball into hands.
  3. Arms are held relaxed at sides, and forearms are held in front of body.
  4. Arms give on contact to absorb force of the ball.
  5. Arms adjust to flight of ball.
  6. Thumbs are held in opposition to each other.
  7. Hands grasp ball in a well-timed, simultaneous motion.
  8. Fingers grasp more effectively.
II. Common Problems:
 A. Failure to maintain control of object.
 B. Failure to "give" with the catch.
 C. Keeping fingers rigid and straight in the direction of object.
 D. Failure to adjust hand position to the height and trajectory of object.
 E. Inability to vary the catching pattern for objects of different weight and force.
 F. Taking eyes off object.
 G. Closing the eyes.
 H. Inability to focus on, or track the ball.
 I. Improper stance, causing loss of balance when catching a fast-moving object.
 J. Closing hands either too early or too late.
 K. Failure to keep body in line with the ball.

INITIAL

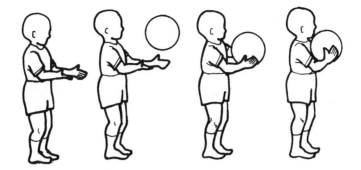

ELEMENTARY

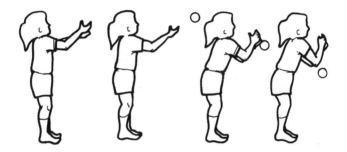

MATURE

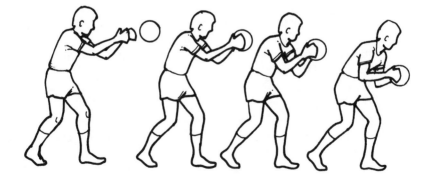

Figure 11.12. Stages of the catching pattern

Kicking

Kicking is a form of striking in which the foot is used to impart force to an object directed toward a goal. Precise variations of the kicking action may be accomplished by making adjustments with the kicking leg and by bringing the arms and trunk into play. The primary factors that influence the type of kick used are: (1) the desired trajectory of the ball, and (2) the height of the ball upon contact. The fundamental kicking pattern for a stationary ground ball is the only common striking movement that does not use the arms and hands directly. The developmental aspects of kicking a stationary ball have been studied extensively by Deach (1951) and Seefeldt and Haubenstricker (1981). The developmental sequence that follows (Table 11.17, Figure 11.13) is based on these studies and the work of McClenaghan (1976).

Striking

The first striking movements (other than kicking) appear in young children whenever they hit an object with an implement. Swinging at a ball in flight, on a batting tee, or on the ground is a familiar act to most children. Only a limited amount of scientific investigation has been conducted on the developmental aspects of striking in children (Deach, 1951; Roberton and Halverson, 1984; Seefeldt and Haubenstricker, 1976). The developmental sequence proposed by Seefeldt and Haubenstricker (1976) is summarized (Table 11.18, Figure 11.14).

Dribbling

Dribbling a ball with one hand is a fundamental movement pattern that has only recently received attention in the literature on children (Wickstrom, 1983; Williams, 1983; Payne and Isaacs, 1987). Dribbling is a complicated task requiring precise judgment of distance, force, and trajectory. Good figure, ground, and depth perception are also required for efficient dribbling. The following proposed developmental sequence is based on Wickstrom's work (1980) and on my observational assessment of numerous children and is subject to further refinement (Table 11.19, Figure 11.15).

Ball Rolling

Rolling an object is another fundamental movement pattern that has not been methodically studied. Ability in rolling a ball has most often been assessed by accuracy in knocking down bowling pins rather than from the standpoint of form. Numerous sport and recreational activities utilize the fundamental patterns found in rolling. Bowling, curling, shuffleboard, and the underhand pitch in softball utilize variations of the pattern found in mature rolling. The developmental sequence that follows is

Table 11.17 Developmental Sequence for Kicking

I. Kicking:
  A. Initial stage.
    1. Movements are restricted during kicking action.
    2. Trunk remains erect.
    3. Arms are used to maintain balance.
    4. Movement of kicking leg is limited in backswing.
    5. Forward swing is short: there is little follow-through.
    6. Child kicks "at" ball rather than kicking it squarely and following through.
    7. A pushing rather than a striking action is predominant.
  B. Elementary stage.
    1. Preparatory backswing is centered at the knee.
    2. Kicking leg tends to remain bent throughout the kick.
    3. Follow-through is limited to forward movement of the knee.
    4. One or more deliberate steps are taken toward the ball.
  C. Mature stage.
    1. Arms swing in opposition to each other during kicking action.
    2. Trunk bends at waist during follow-through.
    3. Movement of kicking leg is initiated at the hip.
    4. Support leg bends slightly on contact.
    5. Length of leg swing increases.
    6. Follow-through is high; support foot rises to toes or leaves surface entirely.
    7. Approach to the ball is from either a run or leap.
II. Common Problems:
  A. Restricted or absent backswing.
  B. Failure to step forward with nonkicking leg.
  C. Tendency to lose balance.
  D. Inability to kick with either foot.
  E. Inability to alter speed of kicked ball.
  F. Jabbing at ball without follow-through.
  G. Poor opposition of arms and legs.
  H. Failure to use a summation of forces by the body to contribute to force of the kick.
  I. Failure to contact ball squarely, or missing it completely (eyes not focused on ball).
  J. Failure to get adequate distance (lack of follow-through and force production).

based on my observational assessment of numerous children and is subject to verification and further refinement (Table 11.20, Figure 11.16).

Trapping

Trapping an object is actually a form of catching in which the feet or body is used to absorb the force of the ball instead of the hands and arms.

INITIAL

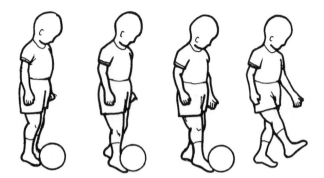

ELEMENTARY

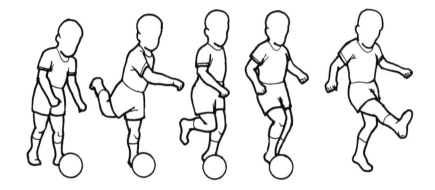

MATURE

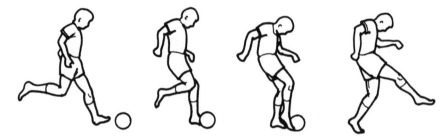

Figure 11.13. Stages of the kicking pattern

Table 11.18 Developmental Sequence for Striking

I. Striking:
    A. Initial stage.
        1. Motion is from back to front.
        2. Feet are stationary.
        3. Trunk faces direction of tossed ball.
        4. Elbow(s) fully flexed.
        5. No trunk rotation.
        6. Force comes from extension of flexed joints in a downward plane.
    B. Elementary stage.
        1. Trunk turned to side in anticipation of tossed ball.
        2. Weight shifts to forward foot prior to ball contact.
        3. Combined trunk and hip rotation.
        4. Elbow(s) flexed at less acute angle.
        5. Force comes from extension of flexed joints. Trunk rotation and forward movement are in an oblique plane.
    C. Mature stage.
        1. Trunk turns to side in anticipation of tossed ball.
        2. Weight shifts to back foot.
        3. Hips rotate.
        4. Transfer of weight is in a contralateral pattern.
        5. Weight shift to forward foot occurs while object is still moving backward.
        6. Striking occurs in a long, full arc in a horizontal pattern.
        7. Weight shifts to forward foot at contact.
II. Common Problems:
    A. Failure to focus on and track the ball.
    B. Improper grip.
    C. Failure to turn side of the body in direction of intended flight.
    D. Inability to sequence movements in rapid succession in a coordinated manner.
    E. Poor backswing.
    F. "Chopping" swing.

Trapping is a skill that must be highly refined in order to successfully play games such as soccer. With young children, however, trapping should be viewed very generally as the ability to stop a ball without use of the hands or arms. A developmental sequence for trapping in children follows. It is based on my observational assessment of numerous children and is subject to verification and further refinement (Table 11.21, Figure 11.17).

Volleying

Volleying is a form of striking in which an overhand pattern is used. It is a movement similar to the two-handed set shot once popular in bas-

INITIAL

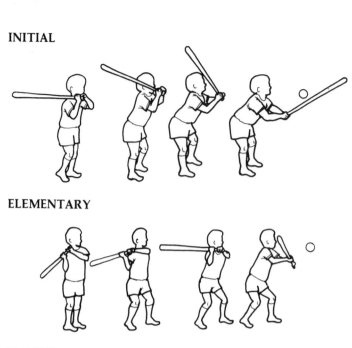

ELEMENTARY

MATURE

Figure 11.14. Stages of the striking pattern

ketball and is similar to the overhead set shot used in power volleyball. The developmental sequence that follows is based on my observation of children and is subject to verification and refinement (Table 11.22, Figure 11.18).

FUNDAMENTAL STABILITY MOVEMENTS

Stability is the most basic aspect of learning to move. It is through this dimension that children gain and maintain a point of origin for the explorations they make in space. *Stability* involves the ability to

Table 11.19 Developmental Sequence for Dribbling

I. Dribbling:
  A. Initial stage.
    1. Ball held with both hands.
    2. Hands placed on sides of ball, with palms facing each other.
    3. Downward thrusting action with both arms.
    4. Ball contacts surface close to body, may contact foot.
    5. Great variation in height of bounce.
    6. Repeated bounce and catch pattern.
  B. Elementary stage.
    1. Ball held with both hands, one on top and the other near the bottom.
    2. Slight forward lean, with ball brought to chest level to begin the action.
    3. Downward thrust with top hand and arm.
    4. Force of downward thrust inconsistent.
    5. Hand slaps at ball for subsequent bounces.
    6. Wrist flexes and extends and palm of hand contacts ball on each bounce.
    7. Visually monitors ball.
    8. Limited control of ball while dribbling.
  C. Mature stage.
    1. Feet placed in narrow stride position, with foot opposite dribbling hand forward.
    2. Slight forward trunk lean.
    3. Ball held waist high.
    4. Ball pushed toward ground, with follow-through of arm, wrist, and fingers.
    5. Controlled force of downward thrust.
    6. Repeated contact and pushing action initiated from fingertips.
    7. Visual monitoring unnecessary.
    8. Controlled directional dribbling.
II. Common Problems:
  A. Slapping at ball instead of pushing it downward.
  B. Inconsistent force applied to downward thrust.
  C. Failure to focus on and track ball efficiently.
  D. Inability to dribble with both hands.
  E. Inability to dribble without visually monitoring ball.
  F. Insufficient follow-through.
  G. Inability to move about under control while dribbling.

---

maintain one's relationship to the force of gravity. This is true even though the nature of the application of the force may be altered as the requirements of the situation change, causing the general relationship of the body parts to the center of gravity to be altered. Movement experiences designed to enhance children's stability abilities enable them to de-

INITIAL

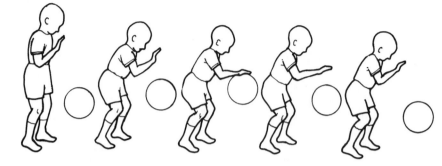

ELEMENTARY

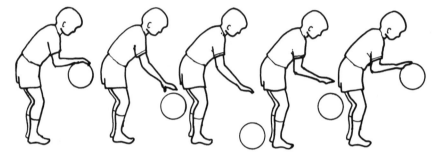

MATURE

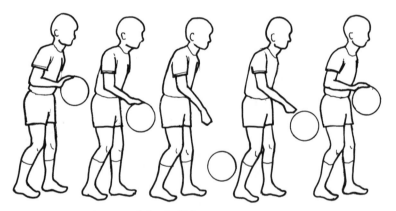

Figure 11.15. Stages of the dribbling pattern

Table 11.20 Developmental Sequence for Ball Rolling

I. Ball Rolling:
   A. Initial stage.
      1. Straddle stance.
      2. Ball is held with hands on the sides, with palms facing each other.
      3. Acute bend at waist, with backward pendulum motion of arms.
      4. Eyes monitor ball.
      5. Forward arm swing and trunk lift with release of ball.
   B. Elementary stage.
      1. Stride stance.
      2. Ball held with one hand on bottom and the other on top.
      3. Backward arm swing without weight transfer to the rear.
      4. Limited knee bend.
      5. Forward swing with limited follow-through.
      6. Ball released between knee and waist level.
      7. Eyes alternately monitor target and ball.
   C. Mature stage.
      1. Stride stance.
      2. Ball held in hand corresponding to trailing leg.
      3. Slight hip rotation and trunk lean forward.
      4. Pronounced knee bend.
      5. Forward swing with weight transference from rear to forward foot.
      6. Release at knee level or below.
      7. Eyes are on target throughout.
II. Common Problems:
   A. Failure to transfer body weight to rear foot during initial part of action.
   B. Failure to place controlling hand directly under ball.
   C. Releasing the ball above waist level.
   D. Failure to release ball from a virtual pendular motion, causing it to veer to one side.
   E. Lack of follow-through, resulting in a weak roll.
   F. Swinging the arms too far backward or out from the body.
   G. Failure to keep eyes on target.
   H. Failure to step forward with foot opposite hand that holds ball.
   I. Inability to bring ball to side of the body.

velop flexibility in postural adjustments as they move in a variety of different and often unusual ways relative to their center of gravity, line of gravity, and base of support.

The ability to sense a shift in the relationship of the body parts that alter one's balance is required for efficient stability. Also necessary is the ability to compensate rapidly and accurately for these changes with appropriate movements. These compensatory movements should ensure maintenance of balance, but they should not be overcompensating. They

INITIAL

ELEMENTARY

MATURE

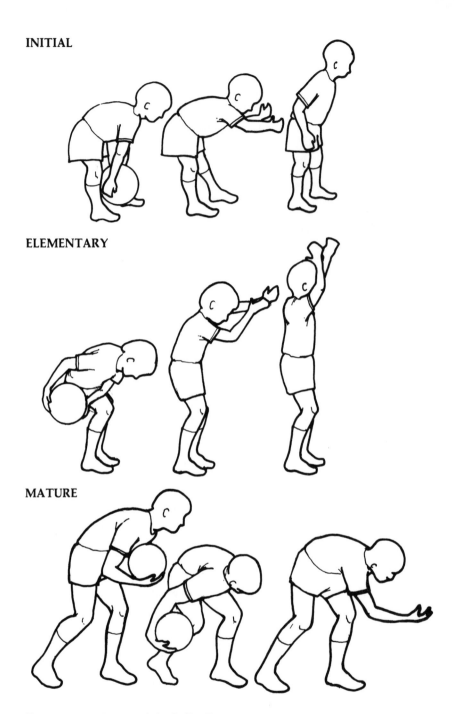

Figure 11.16. Stages of the ball rolling pattern

Table 11.21 Developmental Sequence for Trapping

I. Trapping:
   A. Initial stage.
      1. Trunk remains rigid.
      2. No "give" with ball as it makes contact.
      3. Inability to absorb force of the ball.
      4. Difficulty getting in line with object.
   B. Elementary stage.
      1. Poor visual tracking.
      2. "Gives" with the ball, but movements are poorly timed and sequenced.
      3. Can trap a rolled ball with relative ease but cannot trap a tossed ball.
      4. Appears uncertain of what body part to use.
      5. Movements lack fluidity.
   C. Mature stage.
      1. Tracks ball throughout.
      2. "Gives" with body upon contact.
      3. Can trap both rolled and tossed balls.
      4. Can trap balls approaching at a moderate velocity.
      5. Moves with ease to intercept ball.
II. Common Problems:
   A. Failure to position body directly in path of ball.
   B. Failure to keep eyes fixed on ball.
   C. Failure to "give" as ball contacts body part.
   D. Failure to angle an aerial ball downward toward feet.
   E. Causing body to meet ball instead of letting ball meet body.
   F. Inability to maintain body balance when trapping in unusual or awkward positions.

should be made only with those parts of the body required for compensation rather than readjusting the entire body to restore balance. Children's stability abilities should be flexible in order to make all kinds of movements under all sorts of conditions and still maintain their fundamental relationship to the force of gravity.

It should be noted here that the term "stability" as used in this text goes beyond the catch-all terms of "nonlocomotor" or "nonmanipulative" movements. The movement category of stability encompasses these terms but further implies maintenance of body control in movements that place a premium on maintaining balance. All movement involves an element of stability when viewed from the balance perspective. Therefore, strictly speaking, all locomotor and manipulative activities are, in part, stability movements. Certain fundamental movements may, however, be separated from all others that place a premium on the controlled maintenance of equilibrium.

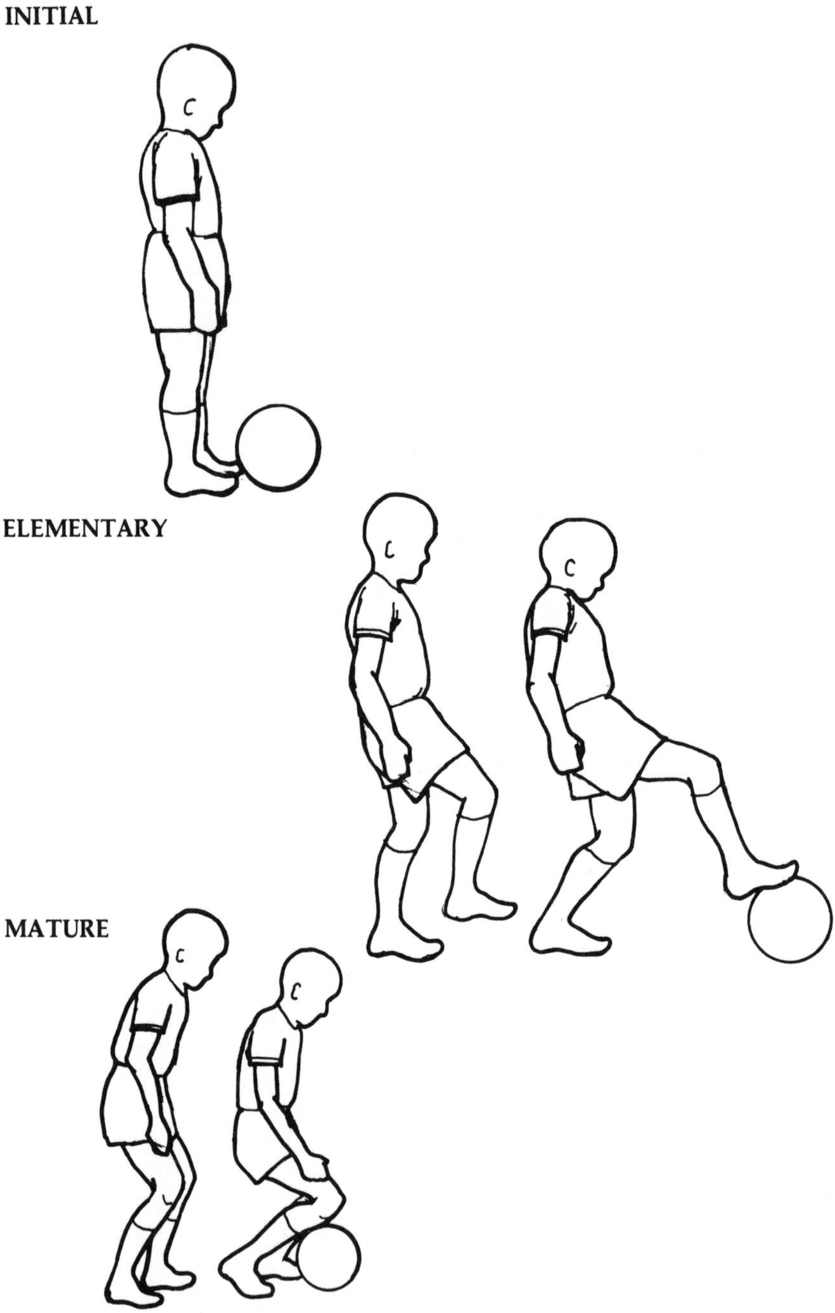

INITIAL

ELEMENTARY

MATURE

Figure 11.17. Stages of the trapping pattern

Table 11.22 Developmental Sequence for Volleying

I. Volleying:
    A. Initial stage.
        1. Inability to accurately judge path of ball or balloon.
        2. Inability to get under the ball.
        3. Inability to contact ball with both hands simultaneously.
        4. Slaps at the ball from behind.
    B. Elementary stage.
        1. Failure to visually track ball.
        2. Gets under the ball.
        3. Slaps at ball.
        4. Action mainly from hands and arms.
        5. Little lift or follow-through with legs.
        6. Unable to control direction or intended flight of ball.
        7. Wrists relax and ball often travels backward.
    C. Mature stage.
        1. Gets under the ball.
        2. Good contact with fingertips.
        3. Wrists remain stiff and arms follow through.
        4. Good summation of forces and utilization of arms and legs.
        5. Able to control direction and intended flight of ball.
II. Common Problems:
    A. Failure to keep eyes on ball.
    B. Inability to accurately judge flight of ball and to properly time movements of body.
    C. Failure to keep fingers and wrists stiff.
    D. Failure to extend all of the joints upon contacting ball (lack of follow-through).
    E. Inability to contact ball with both hands simultaneously.
    F. Slapping at ball.
    G. Poor positioning of body under ball.

Axial Movements

Axial movements are movements of the trunk or limbs that orient the body while it remains in a stationary position. Bending, stretching, twisting, turning, swinging, swaying, reaching, and lifting are axial movements. They are often combined with other movements to create more elaborate movement skills. Skilled performances in diving, gymnastics, figure skating, and modern dance typically incorporate a variety of axial movements along with various locomotor movements. Axial movements are included with a variety of manipulative skills in soccer, baseball, football, and track and field.

Little is known about the developmental sequence of axial movements. To date, no film analysis or observational studies have been con-

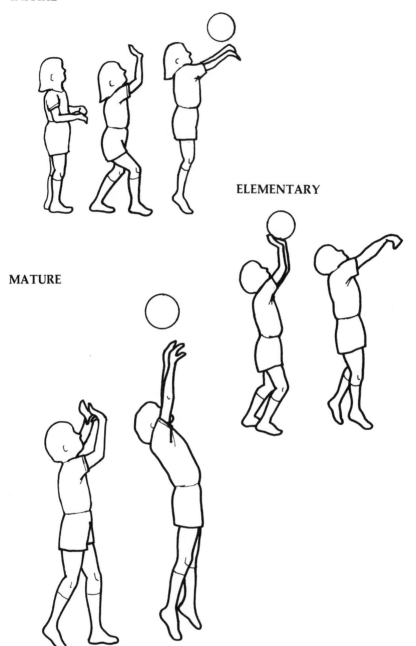

INITIAL

ELEMENTARY

MATURE

Figure 11.18. Stages of the volleying pattern

ducted with children. The following represents a proposed developmental sequence for axial movements in general. It is based on observation of numerous children and is subject to further verification and refinement (Table 11.23, Figure 11.19).

Postures

Postures are other body positions that place a premium on the maintenance of equilibrium while in a position of static or dynamic balance. Inverted supports, rolling, stopping, and dodging, as well as beam walking and one-foot balances, are dynamic or static balance postures.

Table 11.23 Developmental Sequence for Axial Movements

I. Axial Movements:
    A. Initial stage.
        1. Exaggerated base of support.
        2. Momentary loss of balance.
        3. Visual monitoring of body and model when possible.
        4. Combined movements appear jerky and segmented.
        5. Lack of fluid transition from one level or plane to another.
        6. Only one to two actions possible at a time.
    B. Elementary stage.
        1. Good balance.
        2. Appropriate base of support.
        3. Requires visual model.
        4. Does not have to monitor own body.
        5. Good coordination of similar movements.
        6. Poor transition in dissimilar movements.
        7. Can combine two to three actions into one fluid movement.
    C. Mature stage.
        1. Smooth, rhythmical flow.
        2. Sequences several movements with ease.
        3. Vision unimportant.
        4. Appears totally in control.
        5. Can combine four or more movements into one fluid movement.
II. Common Problems:
    A. Visually monitoring body.
    B. Visually mimicking a model.
    C. Poor rhythmical coordination.
    D. Segmented combination of movements.
    E. Loss of balance.
    F. Lack of smooth transition in flow of movement.
    G. Inability to perform at various tempos.
    H. Inability to perform at different levels.

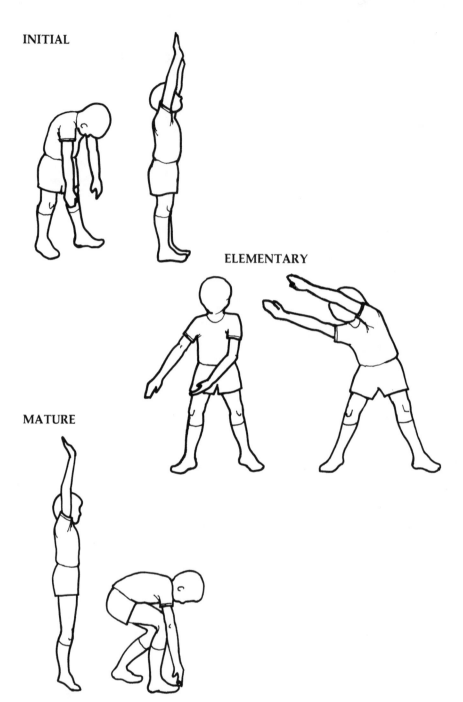

Figure 11.19. Stages of axial movement development

Inverted supports involve postures in which the body assumes an upside-down position for a number of seconds before the movement is discontinued. Stabilization of the center of gravity and maintenance of the line of gravity within the base of support apply to the inverted posture as well as to the erect standing posture. An inverted supporting posture, however, utilizes either the head, hands, forearms, or upper arms (or a combination) as the base of support. The shoulders are above the point of support. The tip-up, tripod, headstand, and handstand are examples of skills that incorporate the fundamental pattern of the inverted support. To date, no developmental studies have been conducted with inverted supports. The following represents a developmental sequence based on my observation of numerous children, and is subject to verification and refinement (Table 11.24, Figure 11.20).

Body rolling postures, although actually locomotor in nature, re-

Table 11.24 Developmental Sequence for Inverted Supports

I. Inverted Supports:
   A. Initial stage.
      1. Able to maintain triangular low level three-point balance positions.
      2. Able to assume inverted three-point postures for up to three seconds.
      3. Poor kinesthetic feel for unseen body parts.
      4. Minimal coordinated control of movements.
   B. Elementary stage.
      1. Can maintain controlled triangular three-point and low two-point contacts with surface.
      2. Able to hold balance for three seconds or longer with frequent brief addition of additional balance point.
      3. Gradual improvement in monitoring of unseen body parts.
   C. Mature stage.
      1. Good surface contact position.
      2. Good control of head and neck.
      3. Good kinesthetic feel for body part location.
      4. Appears to be in good control of body.
      5. Maintains inverted low and high level two- and three-point balance positions for three or more seconds.
      6. Comes out of static posture under control.
II. Common Problems:
   A. Inability to accurately sense location and position of body parts not visually monitored.
   B. Inability to keep line of gravity within base of support.
   C. Inadequate or exaggerated base of support.
   D. Overbalancing by shifting the body's weight too far forward.
   E. Inability to hold inverted balance position for three seconds or longer.

INITIAL

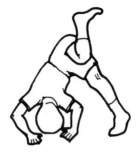

ELEMENTARY

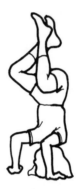

MATURE

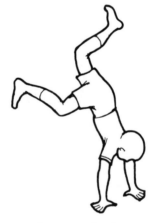

Figure 11.20. Stages of inverted support development

quire inordinate amounts of balance control. Considerable disturbance of the fluid in the semicircular canals results from rolling actions. Therefore, they are regarded as fundamental stability movements. Body rolling movements may involve rolling forward, sideways, or backward. In each, the body is momentarily inverted and must maintain positional control as it travels through space. The sport skills of the forward and backward somersault are elaborations of the fundamental forward and backward rolling patterns. Walkovers and handsprings are sophisticated combinations of rolling patterns combined with transitional inverted supports.

Developmental studies of body rolling are limited (Williams, 1980; Wickstrom, 1983; Roberton & Halverson, 1984). The following proposed sequence is based on these studies (Table 11.25, Figure 11.21).

Dodging is a fundamental stability pattern of movement that combines the locomotor movements of sliding with rapid changes in direction. Dodging involves rapid shifts in direction from side to side and requires good reaction time and movement speed. Extensive developmental studies of dodging have not been conducted with children. However, observational assessment of children and the work of Roberton and Halverson (1984) provides the basis for the following sequence (Table 11.26, Figure 11.22).

One-foot balancing is probably the most common measure of static balance ability. Several investigators have studied the one-foot balance with the eyes opened or closed and the arms at the sides, folded, or on the hips (Cratty, 1986; De Oreo, 1971, 1980; Eckert and Rarick, 1975). Performance trends for balancing on one foot are reported in a later chapter. The following appears to be the developmental sequence gleaned from these performance investigations, but it is subject to verification and refinement (Table 11.27, Figure 11.23).

Beam walking is the most frequently measured fundamental dynamic balance ability. A variety of investigations have been conducted, using walking boards that vary in length, width, and height from the supporting surface (De Oreo, 1971, 1980; Goetzinger, 1961; Seashore, 1949). Considerable information concerning the performance abilities of children from year to year is available, but little is known about the developmental sequence of the beam walking process itself. The following developmental sequence is based on my observational assessment of numerous children and is subject to refinement and verification (Table 11.28, Figure 11.24).

Table 11.25 Developmental Sequence for Body Rolling

I. Body Rolling:
   A. Initial stage.
      1. Head contacts surface.
      2. Body curled in loose "C" position.
      3. Inability to coordinate use of arms.
      4. Cannot get over backward or sideways.
      5. Uncurls to "L" position after rolling forward.
   B. Elementary stage.
      1. After rolling forward, actions appear segmented.
      2. Head leads action instead of inhibiting it.
      3. Top of head still touches surface.
      4. Body curled in tight "C" position at onset of roll.
      5. Uncurls at completion of roll to "L" position.
      6. Hands and arms aid rolling action somewhat but supply little push-off.
      7. Can perform only one roll at a time.
   C. Mature stage.
      1. Head leads action.
      2. Back of head touches surface very lightly.
      3. Body remains in tight "C" throughout.
      4. Arms aid in force production.
      5. Momentum returns child to starting position.
      6. Can perform consecutive rolls in control.
II. Common Problems:
   A. Head forcefully touching surface.
   B. Failure to curl body tightly.
   C. Inability to push off with arms.
   D. Pushing off with one arm.
   E. Failure to remain in tucked position.
   F. Inability to perform consecutive rolls.
   G. Feeling dizzy.
   H. Failure to roll in a straight line.
   I. Lack of sufficient momentum to complete one revolution.

INITIAL

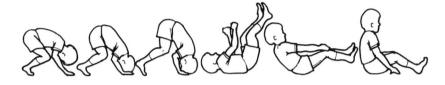

ELEMENTARY

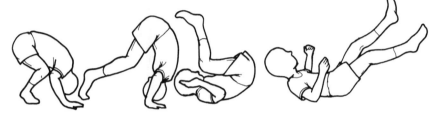

MATURE

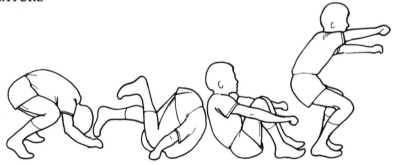

Figure 11.21. Stages of body rolling development

Table 11.26 Developmental Sequence for Dodging

I. Dodging:
   A. Initial stage.
      1. Segmented movements.
      2. Body appears stiff.
      3. Minimal knee bend.
      4. Weight is on one foot.
      5. Feet generally cross.
      6. No deception.
   B. Elementary stage.
      1. Movements coordinated but with little deception.
      2. Performs better to one side than to the other.
      3. Too much vertical lift.
      4. Feet occasionally cross.
      5. Little spring in movement.
      6. Sometimes outsmarts self and becomes confused.
   C. Mature stage.
      1. Knees bent, slight trunk lean forward (ready position).
      2. Fluid directional changes.
      3. Performs equally well in all directions.
      4. Head and shoulder fake.
      5. Good lateral movement.
II. Common Problems:
   A. Inability to shift body weight in a fluid manner in direction of dodge.
   B. Slow change of direction.
   C. Crossing feet.
   D. Hesitation.
   E. To much vertical lift.
   F. Total body lead.
   G. Inability to perform several dodging actions in rapid succession.
   H. Monitoring body.
   I. Rigid posture.

INITIAL

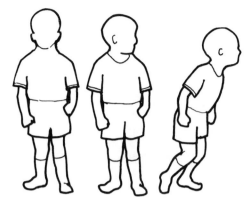

ELEMENTARY

MATURE

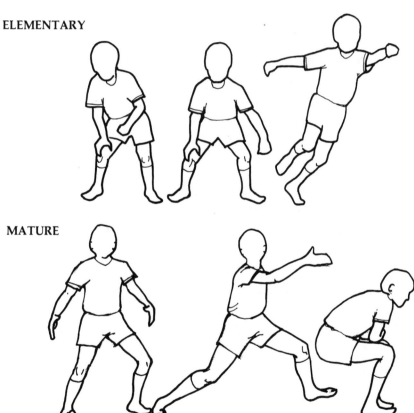

Figure 11.22. Stages of the dodging pattern

Table 11.27 Developmental Sequence for the One-Foot Balance

I. One-Foot Balance:
   A. Initial Stage.
      1. Raises nonsupporting leg several inches so that thigh is nearly parallel with contact surface.
      2. Either in or out of balance (no in-between).
      3. Overcompensates ("windmill" arms).
      4. Inconsistent leg preference.
      5. Balances with outside support.
      6. Only momentary balance without support.
      7. Eyes directed at feet.
   B. Elementary stage.
      1. May lift nonsupporting leg to a tied-in position on support leg.
      2. Cannot balance with eyes closed.
      3. Uses arms for balance but may tie one arm to side of body.
      4. Performs better on dominant leg.
   C. Mature stage.
      1. Can balance with eyes closed.
      2. Uses arms and trunk as needed to maintain balance.
      3. Lifts nonsupporting leg.
      4. Focuses on external object while balancing.
      5. Changes to nondominant leg without loss of balance.
II. Common Problems:
   A. Tying one arm to side.
   B. No compensating movements.
   C. Inappropriate compensation of arms.
   D. Inability to use either leg.
   E. Inability to vary body position with control.
   F. Inability to balance while holding objects.
   G. Visually monitoring support leg.
   H. Overdependence on outside support.

INITIAL

ELEMENTARY

MATURE

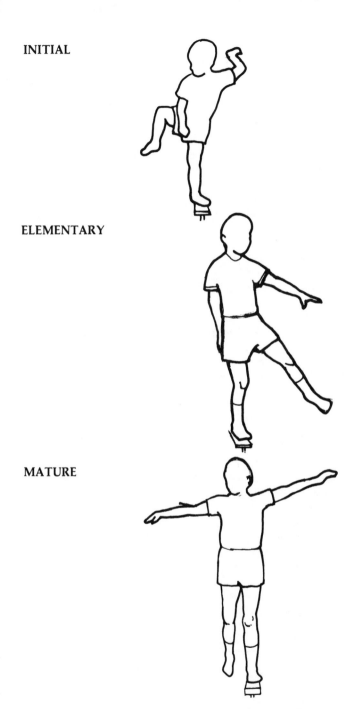

Figure 11.23. Stages of the one-foot balance

Table 11.28 Developmental Sequence for the Beam Walk

I. Beam Walk:
  A. Initial stage.
     1. Balances with support.
     2. Walks forward while holding on to a spotter for support.
     3. Uses follow-step with dominant foot lead.
     4. Eyes focus on feet.
     5. Body rigid.
     6. No compensating movements.
  B. Elementary stage.
     1. Can walk a 2-inch beam but not a 1-inch beam.
     2. Uses a follow-step with dominant foot leading.
     3. Eyes focus on beam.
     4. May press one arm to trunk while trying to balance with the other.
     5. Loses balance easily.
     6. Limited compensating movements.
     7. Can move forward, backward, and sideways but requires considerable concentration and effort.
  C. Mature stage.
     1. Can walk a 1-inch beam.
     2. Uses alternate stepping action.
     3. Eyes focus beyond beam.
     4. Both arms used at will to aid balance.
     5. Can move forward, backward, and sideways with assurance and ease.
     6. Movements are fluid, relaxed, and in control.
     7. May lose balance occasionally.
II. Common Problems:
  A. Overdependence on spotter.
  B. Visually monitors stepping leg.
  C. Tying one arm in.
  D. Rigid, hesitant movement.
  E. Failure to actually negotiate the problem of balance.
  F. Inability to perform without holding on to a spotter.
  G. Poor rhythmical coordination of both sides of body.
  H. Overcompensating for loss of balance.

INITIAL

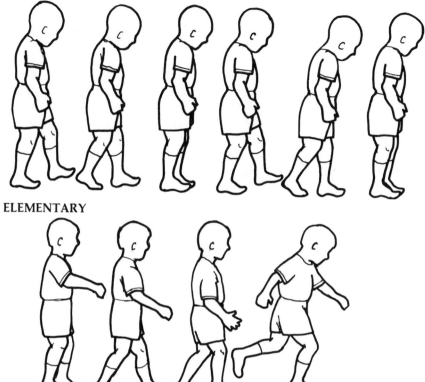

ELEMENTARY

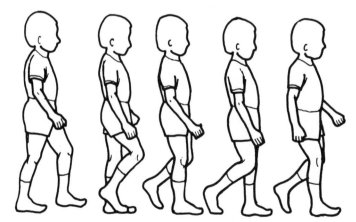

MATURE

Figure 11.24. Stages of the beam walk

SUMMARY

The fundamental movement pattern phase of development follows a sequential progression. The cognitively and physically normal child, under optimal circumstances, will progress through the initial, elementary, and mature stages in a sequential manner. Developmental sequences for several fundamental movements have been identified through biomechanical assessment of children at different age levels. Based on film, video tape, and observational assessment of numerous children developmental sequences have also been proposed. The fundamental movement phase of development is greatly influenced by the environment. Both conditions within the environment and task goals will create a variety of between-child, between-pattern and within-pattern differences. Developmental sequences have been proposed and are in the process of being validated. A thorough knowledge of these developmental sequences enables one to be more effective both in diagnosing movement problems and in programming meaningful movement experiences.

CHAPTER CONCEPTS

11.1 Classification of fundamental movements into "initial", "elementary", and "mature" stages is only one way of classifying basic movement.

11.2 Provided there is ample opportunity, instruction, and encouragement, children are capable of achieving the mature stage in most fundamental movements by age 6.

11.3 Fundamental movements should be sufficiently flexible so they can be altered as the requirements of the environment demand without deflecting attention from the movement purpose.

11.4 Fundamental movements may be dealt with in isolation or in combination with a variety of other movements.

11.5 Numerous differences can be observed between children, between patterns, and within patterns in the performance of fundamental movement abilities.

11.6 Locomotor movements involve activities in which the body is projected in a vertical, horizontal, or diagonal plane relative to a fixed point on the ground.

11.7 Manipulative movements involve activities in which force is either given to objects or received from objects.

11.8 Manipulative movements may be classified as either propulsive or absorptive.

11.9 The ability to impart force to objects and receive force from objects enables the individual to come into meaningful physical contact with the environment.

11.10 Effective manipulation of objects requires considerable coordination of both sensory and motor systems of the body.

11.11 Attention to form, accuracy, or precision in the performance of movements will alter the mechanics of the particular action.

11.12 Because all movement involves an element of stability, it is the most fundamental aspect of learning to move.

11.13 Axial movements involve movement of the limbs or trunk while the body remains in a static position.

11.14 Efficient performance of a variety of axial movements is basic to efficient performance of all movement.

11.15 Stability movements place a premium on the maintenance of equilibrium while the body is in either static or dynamic positions.

11.16 Static balance involves both upright and inverted body positions.

TERMS TO REMEMBER

Movement Pattern

Between-Pattern Differences

Fundamental Movement

Within-Pattern Differences

Qualitative Change

Locomotion

Intraskill Sequences

Manipulation

Segmental Analysis

Stability

Total Body Configuration

Axial Movement

Between-Child Differences

Postures

CRITICAL READINGS

Adrian, M. J., and Cooper, J. M. (1989). *Biomechanics of Human Movement*. Indianapolis: Benchmark Press. (Chapter 9, "Developmental Biomechanics").

Haubenstricker, J., and Seefeldt, V. (1986). "Acquisition of Motor Skills During Childhood." In Seefeldt V. (ed.) *Physical Activity and Well-Being*. Reston, VA: AAHPERD.

Roberton, M. A. and Halverson, L. E. (1984). *Developing Children-Their Changing Movement*. Philadelphia: Lea and Febiger.

Wickstrom, R. L. (1983). *Fundamental Motor Patterns*. Philadelphia: Lea and Febiger.

12

Physical Abilities of Children

CHAPTER COMPETENCIES

Upon Completion of This Chapter You Should Be Able To:

* Demonstrate knowledge of data available on performance scores and motor pattern changes during childhood.

* Describe gender differences and similarities in motor development.

* Discuss changes in movement dimensions such as balance, timing, or force production/control.

* Demonstrate knowledge of major changes in body composition and physiological functioning in males and females.

* Discuss the effect of exercise on body systems and body composition such as bone and muscle development and cardiorespiratory capacity.

• Draw conclusions concerning the merits and/or liabilities of strength and endurance training for prepubescent males and females.

• Distinguish between health-related and performance-related fitness during childhood.

• Interpret velocity curves on various parameters of children's fitness.

• Identify gender differences and similarities in motor performance.

The health-related fitness and motor fitness of children should be of great concern to all and not just the physical educator, coach, and physician. In the last several years the fitness level of boys and girls in North

America has become of great concern to many. This concern was originally highlighted by the results of a test of minimum muscular efficiency (Kraus-Weber Test) that was administered to several thousand American and European children during the 1950s. The results of this historic study indicated that the performance of American children was significantly poorer than that of their European counterparts. In fact, over 55 percent of the Americans failed the test, compared to less than 10 percent of the European youths. Although the comparison has been criticized for several reasons, it pointed out the important fact that American children are often in poor physical condition.

As a result of the Kraus-Hirschland study (1954), President Dwight D. Eisenhower established the President's Council on Youth Fitness in an effort to promote the upgrading of the physical fitness of our nation's children. Since that time, the President's Council and others concerned with the fitness level of our youth have made many important contributions toward that goal. The American Alliance for Health, Physical Education, Recreation, and Dance (AAHPERD) has developed the AAHPERD Youth Fitness Test (1976), and the AAHPERD Health Related Physical Fitness Tests (1980) that are among the most widely-used standardized physical fitness tests throughout the United States. The newest version of the health-related fitness test, "Physical Best" (1988), holds promise of being the preferred fitness test of the future because of its educational, motivational, and individualized approach to fitness testing.

The fact remains, however, that a great many of our children are still unfit. In fact, the National Children and Youth Fitness Study (Ross and Gilbert 1985) revealed that more than one-third of the children and youth tested (ages 10 to 18) were insufficiently active in their daily lives for aerobic benefit. A second survey, the National Children and Youth Fitness Study II (Ross, and Pate, 1987) of children 6 to 9 years old revealed that they are heavier and fatter than their counterparts of 20 years ago. Three factors seem to have contributed greatly to this state of affairs. First, the impact of the importance and need for enhancing fitness has centered on adults. Until recently, little attention has been focused on the fitness needs of children. As a result, our knowledge of the fitness of children and their capacity for work is limited. This has given rise to the second factor, namely, the child's "heart myth" and other basically false assumptions concerning the fitness of children.

According to the child's heart myth, there is a discrepancy in the development of the heart and blood vessels in children and, as a result, vigorous exercise should be avoided at the risk of straining the heart. This widely believed myth has since been disproven by Karpovich (1937), Astrand (1952), and others and is reflected in Corbin's (1980, p.20) statement that "a healthy child cannot physiologically injure the heart permanently through exercise unless the heart is already weakened." Recently, however, parents and educators have begun to realize that aerobic conditioning for children does not pose a health risk.

A third erroneous assumption is that children get enough vigorous physical activity by playing all day. The crowded conditions of apartment living and city dwelling for many, along with the ever-present television set and its fascination, has created a society of sedentary children (Groves, 1988). Children need regular, vigorous, physical activity every day, and the only way they will get it is through a drastic reorganization of their daily routines. Vigorous physical activity has been shown to be an important factor in the normal healthy growth of children.

HEALTH-RELATED FITNESS

Although there has been extensive study in the area of physical fitness over the past several years, comparatively little is known about the physical fitness of children. A review of the literature on fitness reveals a marked lack of information, particularly on children under 6 years of age. Most tests of physical fitness require the individual to go "all out" and perform at his or her maximum. Anyone familiar with young children will recognize the difficulty of this situation. The problems lie in: (1) being able to sufficiently motivate the youngster for maximal performance, (2) accurately determining whether a maximum effort has been achieved, and (3) overcoming the fears of anxious parents. Experts working with young children have in this situation a nearly untouched area for the study of physical fitness. The problems in conducting investigations of this nature are many, but carefully controlled, patient research will yield much valuable information.

Cardiovascular endurance, muscular strength, muscular endurance, joint flexibility and body composition are the components of health-related fitness. Each of these components is discussed briefly in the following paragraphs.

Aerobic Endurance

Aerobic endurance is an aspect of muscular endurance specific to the heart, lungs, and vascular system. It refers to the ability to perform numerous repetitions of a stressful activity requiring considerable use of the circulatory and respiratory system. *Maximal oxygen consumption* (VO_2 max) refers to the largest quantity of oxygen an individual can consume during physical work while breathing air at sea level. It is a measure of one's maximum ability to transmit oxygen to the tissues of the body. An increase in one's aerobic capacity is an excellent indicator of a higher energy output. Astrand (1952) indicated that improvement in VO_2 max is possible but by only about 20 percent. One's genetic inheritance plays a crucial role in the ability to consume oxygen. Maximal oxygen consumption tends to improve as a function of age until about ages 18 to 20. Improvement thereafter is primarily a function of training. Females possess about 75 percent of the capacity of males to consume oxygen. The differences between males and females prior to puberty are largely unexplored. The entire area of oxygen consumption in children has been investigated by relatively few researchers, and the results have often been conflicting. This is due largely to the questionable reliability and reproducibility of VO_2 max measures with children.

Maximal aerobic power as measured by maximal oxygen consumption is a universally accepted means of measuring status and change in cardiovascular fitness. It is not, however, universally understood how to express maximal aerobic ability in relation to body size. The literature concerning the aerobic capacity of children, particularly children under 6 years of age, is limited. Young children make difficult subjects, and the testing environment is limited to the extent of their interest in putting forth a maximal effort. Bar-Or (1983) has demonstrated that aerobic endurance can be assessed in preschool-age children on either a maximal or submaximal exercise test. In fact, an outgrowth of the Columbia University Study of Children's Activity and Nutrition has been a series of strategies and techniques for conducting treadmill tests on preschool children (Delozier et al., 1988).

Bailey et al. (1978, pp. 140-141) indicated that knowing how maximal aerobic power relates to body mass and body size is very important when dealing with children. "In fitness training studies on children there is a problem in determining if changes and maximal aerobic power are a result of training, growth, or both, since increasing size may result in changes similar to the training effect." Bailey and his colleagues studied 200 Canadian boys for 10 years beginning when the boys were 7 years old. The subjects received no special instruction or activity other than the performance of a yearly treadmill test of their aerobic capacity. The results of this study revealed yearly increases in their oxygen utilization. But, when the data were expressed in terms of the amount of oxygen utilized in proportion to body weight (i.e., liters-per-minute per kilogram of body weight), no consistent pattern with increasing age emerged. This finding indicates that the aerobic capacity of an individual is related in part to body weight and in part to age.

Anderson et al. (1978) conducted a 9-year longitudinal study of aerobic capacity with Norwegian boys and girls ranging in age from 8 to 12 years. The results of this investigation indicated that gains in aerobic power were greater than could be expected from growth in body size alone. Fitness expressed on the basis of body weight and on lean body mass increased as the children became older. The authors attributed this linear trend toward improved aerobic capacity over time (and without special training) and to informal environmental stimulation-not simply changes in body size.

Over the years several laboratory studies have been conducted with children to determine their VO_2 max values. Pate and Blair (1978), in their review of two decades of studies, concluded that values ranging from 45 to 55 had been consistently reported in the United States. Krahenbuhl et al. (1985), in a more recent review of 29 longitudinal studies, found similar mean values. They also noted that VO_2 max relative to weight remained stable for boys from year to year, but declined for girls as they advanced in years. It is interesting to note that a minimum VO_2 max threshold value of 42 has been recommended for adults (Cooper 1968) and, according to Simmons-Morton et al. (1987, p. 297) in their review of children and fitness, "it appears that most children are well above this level."

Heart rate responses to exercise are sometimes used as a crude measure of cardiovascular endurance in young children because of the difficulty in gathering accurate VO_2 max data. Mrzena and Macuek (1978) tested children 3 to 5 years old on the treadmill. Each subject was required to walk or run for 5 minutes at a level grade with the treadmill set at three different speeds (3, 4, and 5 km/h). The highest heart rates were recorded at 142 beats-per-minute. Another group performed the treadmill task at 4 kilometers per hour while the grade was increased from 5 to 10 to 15 inches. This group produced heart rates averaging 162 beats-per-minute. It was noted by the investigators that when the treadmill speed was increased to 6 kilometers per hour and the inclination to 20, "the children were not able to increase the step frequency and lost their balance" (p. 31). The maximum aerobic capacity of preschool children is certainly greater than the scores obtained in this experiment, but the maturity of movement as well as the psychological and emotional state of the young child will determine the degree of cooperation and effort put forth.

In an investigation by Parizkova (1977), heart rates of 160 beats-per-minute were recorded in a bench-stepping task with 3-year-old children. The children had considerable difficulty maintaining the cadence of 30 steps-per-minute on the low bench without the investigator holding one hand and stepping with the children. The children in this investigation also had difficulty maintaining the task even though normal play heart rates of young children often exceed 200 beats-per-minute. Cumming and Hnatiuk (1980) reported that normal maximal heart rates for children range from 180 to 234 beats-per-minute. This investigation again reminds us of the extreme difficulty in achieving a maximal effort for a sustained period of time with young children.

A study by Montoye (1970) used a 3-minute step test to evaluate an entire community. The results of Montoye's investigation indicate that resting, exercise, and recovery heart rates decrease with age between ages 10 and 20 and to a lesser degree between ages 20 and 35. Children are capable of working at much higher heart rates than previously expected.

Although it is now clear that children are capable of achieving maximal heart rates the same as or higher than those of their adult counterparts, it is doubtful that such levels are obtained during the daily routines of the vast majority of children. Gilliam and his colleagues (1981, p. 67) confirmed this hypothesis in an experiment in which they monitored the heart rate patterns of 6- and 7-year-olds during a 2- month summer period. The results of this investigation in which 22 boys and 18 girls wore a small heart monitoring device daily for 12 hours during their normal routine revealed:

> The voluntary activity patterns of the children studied may not be adequate in terms of duration and intensity to promote cardiovascular health . . . our data and others' show children . . . very seldom experience physical activity of high enough intensity to promote cardiovascular health. Furthermore, our data shows that boys are more active than girls.

The National Children and Youth Fitness Study II (Ross, and Pate, 1987) collected data on more than 4,500 children in grades one through four on five health-related fitness items. This study represents the most rigorously controlled national sampling to date of the fitness of children under 10 years of age. Data were collected by a small, highly trained traveling field staff. The data are thought to be highly reliable and representative of a broad cross section of the children of the United States (Errecart et al. 1987). Based on the results of these field tests, estimates of the various health-related components of fitness comparisons can be made by age and by gender. Figure 12.1 provides a graph of the mean scores for boys and girls ages 6 and 7 on the half-mile walk/run, and the mean scores for boys and girls ages 8 and 9 on the mile walk/run. Analysis of this graph reveals that boys are superior to girls in terms of mean times for both the half-mile and the mile walk/run at all ages. Furthermore, boys appear to maintain their margin of aerobic superiority at all ages.

Muscular Strength

Muscular strength is the ability of the body to exert force. In its purest sense, it is the ability to exert one maximum effort. Children engaged in daily active play are doing much to enhance their leg strength by

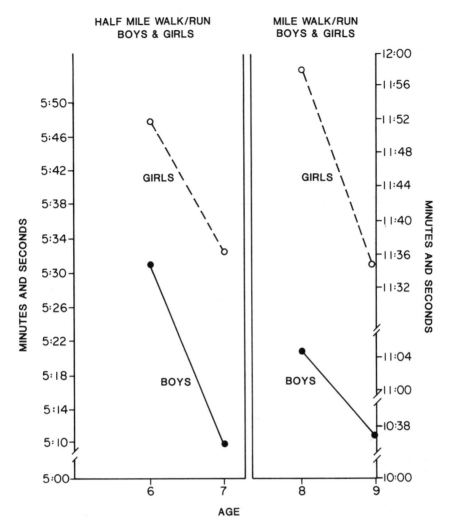

Figure 12.1 Half-mile walk/run (left) and one mile walk/run (right): mean scores for males and females 6-7 and 8-9, in minutes and seconds (*Source*: Ross, J. G., & Pate, R. R. [1987]. "The National Children and Youth Fitness Study II: A Summary of Findings." *Journal of Physical Education, Recreation and Dance*, 58, 9, 51-56)

running and bicycling. Their arm strength is developed through such activities as lifting, carrying objects, handling tools, and swinging on the monkey bars. Strength may be classified as isotonic, isometric or isokinetic. *Isometric strength* involves exerting force on an immovable object. The muscle contracts, but there is little change in its length. *Isotonic strength*, on the other hand, refers to the ability of a muscle to go through its full range of motion. The muscles involved contract, but they also shorten and lengthen during the activity. A barbell curl and a bench press are examples of isotonic strength activities. *Isokinetic strength* involves contracting a muscle and maintaining that contraction through its full range of motion. Isokinetic strength is measured by use of special machines that exert a constant resistance as the muscle works.

Static strength is commonly measured by using a dynamometer or tensiometer. These devices are highly reliable when utilized by trained personnel. *Dynamometers* are calibrated devices designed to measure grip strength, leg strength, and back strength. *Tensiometers* are more versatile than dynamometers in that they permit measurement of many different muscle groups. The classic longitudinal studies conducted by Clarke (1971) utilized 18 different cable tensiometer tests and revealed yearly strength increments in boys between 7 and 17 years. After age 12 or 13, girls tend to differ markedly from boys in their strength. According to Corbin (1980), girls without training tend to level off at this age, but boys continue to gain in strength. It seems probable that the strength levels of preschool and primary grade boys and girls are similar, with the edge being given to boys based on their tendency to be slightly taller and heavier than girls. Unfortunately, virtually nothing is known about the muscular strength of the young child.

Relatively few longitudinal investigations have been conducted into the development of strength in children at all ages. However, the information that is available indicates consistency in the development of strength in children over time. In fact, strength has been shown to increase more rapidly than muscle size during childhood (Armussen, 1973). This is probably due to the increasing skill and coordination with which a maximal contraction may be performed and indicates the interrelationship between strength, coordination, and motor performance in children.

Although strength is a relatively stable quality throughout childhood, the prediction of strength at later years from measures taken in childhood has met with little success. The strong child at age 8, for example, will not necessarily make the greatest gains in strength from childhood through adolescence. Neither will the weak child necessarily make the least gains in strength from childhood through adolescence. The rapid change in body size, which is positively correlated with strength, and the individual variability of growth patterns make prediction a precarious venture.

Muscular Endurance

Muscular endurance is the ability of a muscle or a group of muscles to perform work repeatedly against moderate resistance. Muscular endurance is similar to muscular strength in terms of the activities performed, but it differs in emphasis. Strength-building activities require overloading the muscles to a greater extent than endurance activities. Endurance-building activities require less of an overload on the muscle but more repetitions. Therefore, endurance may be thought of as the ability to continue in strength performance. Children performing sit-ups, push-ups, and pull-ups are actually engaged in endurance activities even though strength is required for any movement to begin. These three activities are among the most often used measures of muscular endurance and, according to Montoye (1970), are among the best tests available. There are, however, problems with pull-up measures because of the problem with body weight (Pate et al. 1987). The entire body weight must be lifted, and many children are unable to accomplish such a task. Therefore, a modified pull-up test is now frequently used.

The daily uninhibited play routines of young children, when viewed in toto, are excellent examples of endurance that most adults would find difficult to duplicate in terms of relative endurance. Relative endurance refers to the child's endurance level adjusted to body weight. It stands to reason that the adult's gross level of endurance and fitness is generally greater than that of the child but that when one's body weight is divided into the total fitness score, differences are less pronounced.

The results of the bent knee sit-up test and the flexed arm hang test administered as a part of both the AAHPERD Youth Fitness Test (1980) and the CAHPER Manitoba Physical Fitness Performance Test (1980) revealed developmental changes in muscular endurance. On both of these measures, boys and girls showed a tendency toward considerable improvement during childhood. The National Children and Youth Fitness Study II (1987) measured the strength/endurance of boys and girls ages 6 to 9. Abdominal strength/endurance was assessed by a 60-second bent-knee sit-up test (Figure 12.2). Upper body strength/endurance was tested through performance of a modified pull-up test (Figure 12.3). The results of the sit-up test (Figure 12.4) indicated that the mean scores for boys were slightly superior to those of girls at all ages. Both groups made steady improvements in terms of their abdominal strength/endurance from year to year.

In regard to upper body strength/endurance, boys were again slightly superior to girls in terms of the average number of completed modified pull-ups. Boys continued to improve with age while girls tended to level off in their average performance (Figure 12.5).

Flexibility

Joint Flexibility is the ability of the various joints of the body to move through their full range of motion. There are two types of flexibility: static and dynamic. *Static Flexibility* is the ability to flex the trunk of the body in different directions. *Dynamic flexibility* is the ability to perform

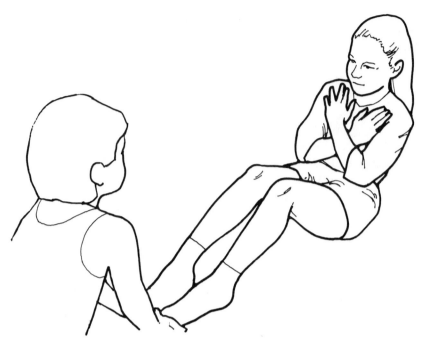

Figure 12.2 The bent-knee sit-up test

stretching muscular contractions of various limbs of the body. Flexibility is joint-specific and can be improved with practice. Hupperich and Sigerseth (1950) indicated, however, that dynamic flexibility in the shoulder, knee, and thigh joints decreases with age in children as evidenced by their investigation of girls 6, 9, and 12 years of age. Their investigation revealed also that static flexibility increased with age. Clarke (1975) reviewed the research on flexibility and concluded that flexibility begins to decline in boys around age 10 and in girls around age 12. This confirms Leighton's (1956) study of the flexibility of boys ages 10 to 18. His investigation revealed that the frequent assumption that boys have a high level of flexibility during childhood and adolescence is questionable. Boys showed no consistent pattern of increasing or maintaining flexibility with age but did show a definite tendency toward decreased flexibility with age. DiNucci (1976) reported that girls performed better than boys on five different measures of flexibility at all ages.

The National Children and Youth Fitness Study II (1987) tested thousands of children 6 to 9 years of age for flexibility. A sit-and-reach test (Figure 12.6) was used as a measure of joint flexibility in the lower back and hip area. Mean scores clearly favored the girls. They tended to be slightly more flexible than boys at all ages. Girls showed little im-

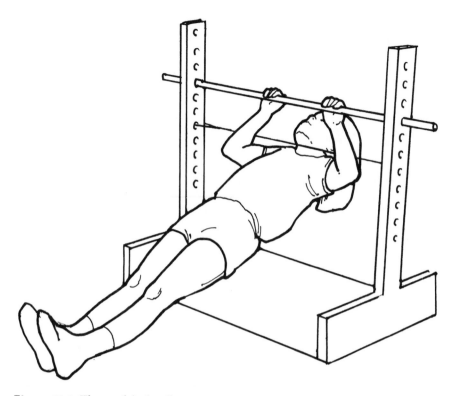

Figure 12.3 The modified pull-up test

provement with age, but neither did they regress. The boys were, however, on the average, slightly less flexible at age 9 than they were at age 6 (Figure 12.7).

Body Composition

Body composition is defined as the portion of lean body mass to fat body mass. Relative fatness can be determined through a variety of means. *Hydrostatic weighing* (under-water weighing) techniques, although the most accurate, are seldom used in studying the body composition of children. Instead, *skinfold calipers* are the preferred method of assessing children's body fatness, although the accuracy of measurement is sometimes questionable (Lohman, 1986). Measurement sites include the triceps, subscapular region, and the medial portion of the calf (Fig. 12.8). National surveys of body fatness have shown that children of all ages are fatter than they were 20 years ago (Gortmaker et al. 1987; Pate et al. 1985; Ross et al. 1987). This trend toward increased fatness of American

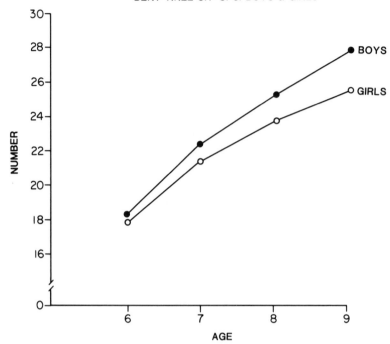

Figure 12.4 Bent-knee sit-ups: mean scores for males and females 6-9 years, number in 60 seconds (*Source*: Ross, J. G., & Pate, R. R. [1987]. "The National Children and Youth Fitness Study II: A Summary of Findings." *Journal of Physical Education, Recreation and Dance*, 58, 9, 51-56)

youth is probably reflective of changes in physical activity patterns and nutritional habits.

In regard to activity patterns, Parizkova (1972, 1973, 1977) demonstrated repeatedly that young athletes are less fat than their more sedentary age-mates. Conversely, it has been repeatedly documented that obese children are significantly less active than their lean peers (Parizkova, 1982; Bar-Or, 1983).

The reasons for adoption of a sedentary lifestyle among children are many, but the implications are clear: Lower activity levels result in increased body fat percentages, while higher activity levels tend to promote lower body fat levels. The activity habits of a lifetime are being formed during childhood. Parents, teachers, and other significant individuals in the child's environment can make a difference in activity levels both by example and by positive encouragement. Ward and Bar-Or (1986), after reviewing 13 school-based obesity intervention programs, reported that the success of these programs was dependent upon:

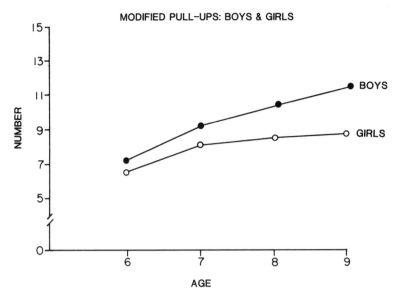

Figure 12.5 Modified pull-ups: mean scores for males and females 6-9, number completed (*Source*: Ross, J. G., & Pate, R. R. [1987]. "The National Children and Youth Fitness Study II: A Summary of Findings." *Journal of Physical Education, Recreation and Dance*, 58, 9, 51-56)

1. Multidisciplinary, integrating behavior modification, nutrition education, and physical activity.
2. Structured physical activity opportunities 4 to 5 times per week, with encouragement and incentives for after-school activities.
3. Team approach, with the participation of the school nurse guidance counselor, lunchroom supervisor, and PE teacher.
4. Parental involvement, in order to achieve continuity and to coordinate home support for the development of new behaviors (Bar-Or, 1987, p. 306).

Ward et al. (1987) found that a multicomponent intervention program with obese children could serve as a valuable means of reducing health risks associated with obesity. Parents, classroom teachers, health workers, and physical education teachers can all play an important role in reversing the trend toward increased body fatness in children. Working as a team, they stand the best chance of successfully intervening (Ross et al. 1987).

The National Children and Youth Fitness Study II (Ross, and Pate, 1987) represents the fourth large-scale, nationally representative sampling of 6 to 9-year-olds in terms of body composition. Skinfold measurements were made at three body landmarks (triceps, subscapular, and

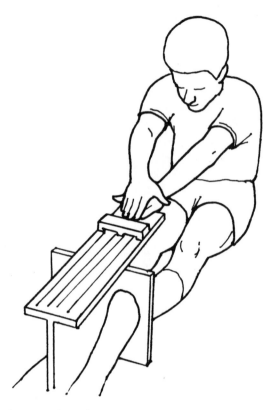

Figure 12.6 The sit-and-reach test

medial calf skinfolds) by use of a Lange skinfold caliper. When compared with the National Health Examination Survey and data from the National Center for Health Statistics, both the boys and the girls of the 1980s are fatter than their counterparts of the 1960s (Ross et al. 1987). Furthermore, there is a definite tendency for increased body fatness in both males and females as they advance in years from 6 to 9, with females leading males at all ages (Figure 12.9).

CHILDREN'S FITNESS TRAINING

During the last few years our knowledge base has expanded dramatically in the area of children's fitness training. Although we still have many unanswered questions, research is beginning to show that children are capable of much more in terms of aerobic conditioning, strength and endurance enhancement, and flexibility improvement than had previously been thought possible. Although we do not have adequate infor-

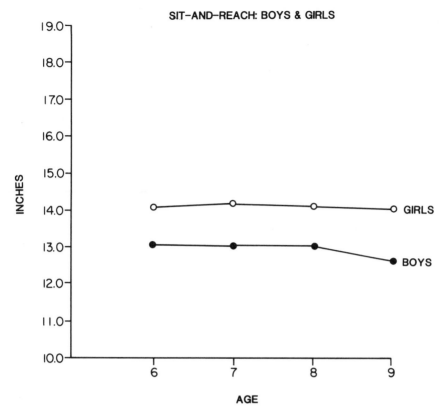

Figure 12.7 Sit-and-reach: mean scores for males and females 6-9 years, in inches (*Source*: Ross, J. G., & Pate, R. R. [1987]. "The National Children and Youth Fitness Study II: A Summary of Findings." *Journal of Physical Education, Recreation and Dance*, 58, 9, 51-56)

mation at this time to clearly deliniate what determines the physical activity patterns of children, we know that the active child can make significant health-related fitness gains.

Aerobic Training

The demonstrable effects of children's *aerobic training* programs are sometimes questionable. Some studies have reported increases in VO_2 max with training in children (Brown et al. 1972; Massicotte and Mac-Nab, 1974; Vrijens, 1978). Several studies, however, have failed to show a training effect with children (Cumming and Friesen, 1967; Cumming et al. 1969; Daniels and Oldridge, 1971; Ekbolm, 1969). This discrepancy in results is probably due to children not being predisposed to all-out physi-

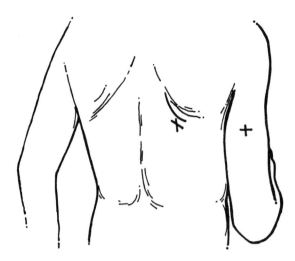

Figure 12.8 Triceps and subscapular skinfold caliper measurement sites

cal exertion. The use of scientific gadgets, the enduring of pain, and the length of time involved in data collection all make the results of any training study with children subject to further verification. Training effects have seldom been reported in elementary school physical education programs that focused on aerobic endurance. This, according to Simmons-Morton et al. (1987) may be due to a number of factors including: 1) naturally high levels of activity, 2) insufficient intensity in the training program, or 3) failure of all children to participate fully in the program. But, Pate and Blair (1978), Chausow et al. (1984) Krahenbuhl et al. (1985) and Savage et al. (1985) have all reported positive responses to training in laboratory settings where the frequency, intensity, and duration could be controlled and progress could be more carefully monitored. It appears, therefore, that prepubescent children can make positive adaptations to increased aerobic demands and that failure to do so is related to factors other than the child's inherent inability to adapt.

A second important consideration in aerobic training programs for children deals with aerobic activity carryover into adolescence and adulthood. Shepard (1984), Pate and Blair (1978), and others have hypothesized that active children will become active adults. Unfortunately, little data exists to support this claim. It seems, however, that vigorous activity during childhood alone is not the key to later activity patterns. Developing the movement skills necessary for participation in lifetime fitness activities in an atmosphere of fun, success, and enjoyment is essential if we expect to see real activity carry over from childhood into adulthood. The notion of "no pain, no gain" simply will not work with most children.

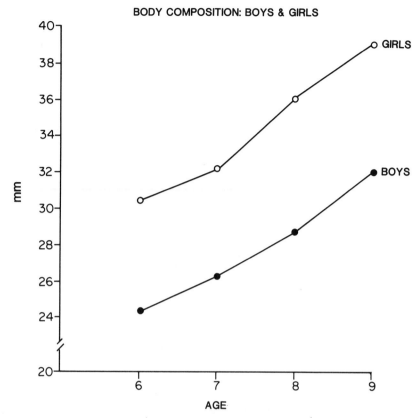

Figure 12.9 Sum of triceps, subscapular and medial calf skinfolds: mean scores for males and females 6-9, in millimeters (*Source*: Ross, J. G., & Pate, R. R. [1987]. "The National Children and Youth Fitness Study II: A Summary of Findings." *Journal of Physical Education, Recreation and Dance*, 58, 9, 51-56)

We must, therefore, strive to make children's aerobic training highly enjoyable and promote skill development so that aerobic conditioning becomes a natural outcome of a healthy lifestyle.

A third issue of importance to aerobic conditioning for children deals with knowing how much to promote the functional health of the child. Although we now know that the child is capable of infinitely more than previously thought possible, we do not know the optimal intensity frequency and duration of activity necessary to produce health benefits. In other words, although we can produce a training effect as measured by the ability of the cardiovascular system to adapt to increased stress, we do not know how much is required to produce positive health benefits. Recent studies with adults (Kannel and Sorlie, 1979; Paffenbarger et al.

1986) provide a convincing case for moderate activity levels of a regular nature over time as an essential promoter of positive health. Perhaps it is not the level of one's physical fitness, per se, that affects cardiovascular health but just that one takes part in moderate levels of physical activity as part of his daily activity pattern. At this juncture, we do not know if these results are applicable to children. Gilliam and Macconnie (1984, p. 183) stated that "programs and research efforts should be designed to study the long-range effect of physical activity and dietary intervention programs on CHD (coronary heart disease) risk in children." We do know, however, that overuse, injuries, burnout, and high attrition rates are common problems associated with children's programs that are too intense and which fail to stress skill and learning enjoyment (Andrish, 1984; Gould, 1987). Much needs to be done to determine optimal levels of activity and appropriate conditions for the maximal carry over of benefits into adulthood.

Cardiovascular endurance can be improved in children much as it can be in adults. Children need to be motivated to perform, to become familiar with pacing themselves, and to engage in intensive physical work over time.

The primary concern of the parent and teacher should not be how to improve maximum oxygen utilization but how to develop movement abilities and sufficiently motivate the child to the point that he or she improves as a function of a daily, self-programmed regimen of vigorous physical activity. The teacher of preschool and primary grade children needs to focus on developing and refining fundamental movement abilities. The intermediate and upper grade teacher needs to apply these movement abilities to a variety of game, sport, and dance activities that provide an avenue for enhancing maximum oxygen utilization and other fitness abilities.

Strength/Endurance Training

It has been widely assumed that prepubescent children will not benefit significantly from a monitored strength training program (Please refer to Table 12.1 for a description of common terms used in resistance training). Early negative findings resulted in the generally-held belief that, because of low levels of circulating androgens (male sex hormones) in prepubescent boys and in females of all ages, strength training programs were minimally effective (Vrijens, 1978; Legwold, 1982). In fact, a 1983 position paper by the American Academy of Pediatrics concluded that prepubescent strength training, although all right if properly supervised, was largely ineffective in terms of strength enhancement. Bar Or (1983), however, raised the question: if women, who have low levels of

Table 12.1 Terms Commonly Used in Strength/Endurance Training.[1]

RESISTANCE TRAINING: Any method used to overcome or bear force.

STRENGTH TRAINING: The use of resistance to increase the ability to overcome or bear force. Various devices, including machines, weights, or one's body may be used as a means of increasing strength.

WEIGHT TRAINING: The use of free weights (barbells, dumbbells), stationary weights, or machines to increase strength.

WEIGHT LIFTING: A competitive sport sometimes referred to as "power lifting" in which the participant attempts to lift the maximum weight possible in prescribed events (Olympic snatch and clean and jerk, or squat, bench press, and dead lift)

[1] Adapted from: National Strength and Conditioning Association (1985) "Position Paper on Prepubescent Strength Training." NSCA Journal, 7, 4, 27-31.

testosterone, are capable of making significant strength gains, why can't prepubescent children make similar gains? A number of recent studies clearly point out that children are, in fact, capable of making significant strength gains in properly conducted and supervised programs of sufficient duration and intensity (Sewell and Micheli, 1984; Cahill, 1986; Duda, 1986). It seems, therefore, that with proper supervision, strength training can be of benefit to prepubescent children in terms of strength enhancement (Micheli 1987), injury reduction (Hejna, 1982), and improved performance (Malina, 1986). It should be noted, however, that strength training is different from weight lifting. *Strength training* involves the use of progressive resistance techniques using the body, weights, or machines to improve one's ability to exert or resist a force. *Weight Lifting* is a sport in which one attempts to lift the maximum possible number of pounds. Weight lifting is not recommended for prepubescent children (Cahill, 1986; Micheli, 1987; National Strength Training Coaches Association, 1985).

Hormonal control of protein synthesis in muscle tissue involves the complex interaction of many *anabolic hormones* (muscle-enhancing) and *catabolic hormones* (muscle-destroying). One of the most important anabolic hormones is *growth hormone* (GH) which is found in prepubescent children. According to Bernuth et al. (1985, p. 100), "exercise has been found to be the most potent stimulus for GH release in children." It seems, therefore, that children have at least some of the hormones necessary for muscle hypertrophy.

Testosterone has been the primary sex hormone associated with the tremendous gains in muscular strength seen in adolescent males. Like growth hormone, it is an anabolic hormone, but it is unclear whether it enhances muscular development by a direct action on muscle tissue or by an indirect role through inhibition of the catabolic action of other hormones (Kuoppasalmi and Adlercrutz, 1985). It is, however, the combination of both testosterone and growth hormone that enhances protein synthesis and inhibits protein destruction in muscle tissue which contributes to increase in muscle size and strength (Tanner, 1978). So, although prepubescent males and females at all ages do not have high levels of circulating androgens, they do possess other anabolic hormones such as growth hormone that can facilitate protein synthesis and result in significant increases in strength under sufficiently enhanced levels of training.

Prepubescent children can increase their strength through resistance training and endurance training due to enhanced stimulation of the central nervous system beyond that which normally would occur with growth and maturation. The term *physiological adaptation* is used for the changes that are caused by training. In other words, when the body is subjected over time to significant amounts of anatomical or physiological stress, the natural reaction of the body is to adapt to the new conditions to which it is being subjected. Although children may differ biochemically and hormonally from adults, there is little to suggest that they do not undergo the same sort of physiological adaptation processes that adults do when involved in certain types of training programs. There are, however, special concerns of the preadolescent involved in a strength/endurance training program.

Specifically, there has been concern over the possibility that weight training and endurance training harms the still-growing *epiphyseal growth plates* in young bones. Indeed, these cartilaginous structures, by their soft and spongy nature, are susceptible to injury, especially those resulting from shearing forces and chronic stress (Micheli, 1983; Micheli and Melhonian, 1987). The potential vulnerability of the growth plates through overuse must not be minimized. In fact, a high correlation exists between damage to these areas and children involved in the sport of weight lifting (Gumbs et al. 1982; AAP, 1983). As a result, the National Strength and Conditioning Association (1985) recommends against the sport being engaged in by prepubescent athletes due to the inability of their bones to handle the shearing force common to this sport. Furthermore, it has been frequently reported that the repetitive nature of training resulting in chronic stress for some sports (i.e., distance running and swimming) can cause damage and premature closing of the growth plates resulting in shorter bones (Wilkerson, 1982).

Another prime cause of epiphyseal damage in children engaged in weight training and chronic stress activities is improper training techniques. Although much has been written, there is little support for the notion that weight training and endurance training is dangerous as long, as the proper mechanics are used in asserting particular movement, and as long as the muscles are not overused. Some weight training equipment, however, may be unsuitable with or without proper technique. Most machine-type resistance equipment is made to adult body proportions with little or no consideration given to youth proportions.

In summary, it appears that prepubescent strength training can, if properly supervised, result in significant gains in strength by both boys and girls. One must be careful, however, to use this information with care. Overuse injuries resulting in damage to the epiphyseal growth end plates of the long bones may occur if the young body is required to go beyond its physiological ability to adapt to increased resistance. As a result, carefully supervised weight-training programs that emphasize proper technique and actively discourage maximal lifts are recommended. Furthermore, programs that utilize equipment adapted to the child's size and that stress low resistance training are encouraged. In no case should prepubescent athletes be encouraged or permitted to engage in the sport of weight lifting (i.e., "max-out"). Care should be taken to recognize that endurance training programs, may, if carried to extremes, result in growth plate and other overuse injuries.

Flexibility Training

In addition to strength and endurance training, another key health-related fitness component considered essential to injury prevention is joint flexibility. Historically, it was believed that any type of weight training would decrease one's flexibility by not allowing the muscle to work through the full range of motion. The isokinetic weight training equipment of today is deigned to answer this problem. Through the principle of variable resistance throughout a joint range of motion, the inherent weak areas in that joint's range are compensated for through the use of an intricate system of cams and pulleys. Thus, flexibility can be maintained or even augmented with both proper technique and certain types of weight training equipment (Duda, 1986). Micheli and Michel's (1985) reported less flexibility in males and females during the prepubescent growth spurt. The reason for this is explained by bone growth preceding muscle and tendon growth. As a result, there is a tightening of musculotendonous units. Thus, it seems essential for the prepubescent athlete to be engaged in a good stretching program along with any form of strength or endurance training to help counter the tendency for reduced flexibility. Furthermore, overuse injuries such as "swimmers shoulder" have been shown to be related to a lack of flexibility. Care should be taken not to assume that endurance-type activities such as running and swimming promote flexibility. The young performer must be encouraged to engage in a proper stretching program prior to and after the endurance workout in order to help minimize the possibility of injury to the area around the joints.

HEALTH-RELATED FITNESS AND MOVEMENT ABILITIES

The interaction between the components of health-related fitness and physical activity is obvious. Performance of any movement task, whether it be at the rudimentary, fundamental, or sport skill level, requires varying degrees of cardiovascular fitness, muscular strength, muscular endurance, and joint flexibility. All movement involves overcoming inertia and, in order to overcome inertia, force must be exerted. In order to exert that force, one must possess some degree of strength. If a movement task is to be performed repeatedly, as with dribbling a ball, endurance is also required. If the action is to be repeated over an extended period of time at a rapid pace, as in dribbling a ball up and down a basketball court, both cardiovascular endurance and flexibility are required. The reciprocal nature of the components of physical fitness may also be viewed from the standpoint that performance of movement activities maintains and develops higher levels of physical fitness. The components of physical fitness are inseparable from movement activity. Rarely, if ever, is a movement activity performed that does not involve some aspect of strength, endurance, or flexibility.

It is impossible under normal conditions to isolate the basic components of skill performance. Tests have been devised that, by their very nature, require more of one fitness component than another. It is through this indirect means of measuring health-related fitness that we are able to determine estimates of one's functional health (Table 12.2).

MOTOR FITNESS

Considerable research has been conducted on the motor skill performance of the adolescent, adult, and skilled performer. The literature is replete with information dealing with their performance levels, biomechanics, and neurophysiological capabilities, but relatively little has been done with preschool and elementary school-children. The situation is much the same as with health-related fitness. Only recently have investigators begun to more closely analyze the motor fitness abilities of children. Studies on the specific factors that make up the child's *motor*

Table 12.2 Common Measures of the Components of Health-Related Fitness and a Synthesis of Findings

Health-Related Fitness Components	Common Tests	Specific Aspect Measured	Synthesis of Findings
Cardiovascular endurance	Step test	Physical work capacity	Max VO_2 estimates are tenuous with young children. Children can achieve maximum VO_2 values similar to adults when corrected for body weight. Maximal heart rates decrease with age. Trend for improved Max VO_2 values in both boys and girls with age. Girls level off after age 12 or so. Boys continue to improve.
	Distance run	Aerobic endurance	
	Treadmill stress test	Max VO_2	
	Bicycle Ergometer	Max VO_2	
Muscular strength	Hand dynamometer	Isometric grip strength	Annual increase for boys from age 7 on. Girls tend to level off after age 12. Boys slow prior to puberty, then gain rapidly throughout adolescence. Boys superior to girls at all ages.
	Back and leg dynamometer	Isometric back and leg strength	
	Cable tensiometer	Isometric joint strength	
Muscular endurance	Push-ups	Isotonic upper body endurance	Similar abilities throughout childhood slightly in favor of boys on most items. Lull in performance prior to age 12. Large increases in boys from 12 to 16, then a leveling off. Girls show no significant increases without special training after age 12.
	Sit-ups	Isotonic abdominal endurance	
	Flexed arm hang	Isometric upper body endurance	
	Pull-ups	Isotonic upper body endurance	
Flexibility	Bend and reach	Hip joint flexibility	Flexibility is joint specific. Girls tend to be more flexible than boys at all ages. Flexibility decreases with reduced activity levels.
	Sit and reach	Hip joint flexibility	
Body composition	Hydrostatic weighing	Percent body fat	Children at all ages are more fat than their age-mates of 20 years ago. Active children are leaner than obese children at all ages. Obese children are less active than nonobese children.
	Skinfold calipers	Estimate of percent body fat	
	Body mass index	Estimate of percent body fat	

fitness indicate that a well-defined structure is present during early childhood but that these factors may differ somewhat from those of older age groups (Peterson et al. 1974, Seefeldt, 1980). There is a factor structure of motor abilities in children generally consisting of four or five items depending on the age level investigated (Bergel, 1978; Peterson et al. 1974; Rarick and Dobbins, 1975). *Movement control factors* of balance (both static and dynamic balance) and coordination (both gross motor and eye-hand coordination), coupled with the *force production factors* of speed, agility, and power, tend to emerge as the components that most influence motor performance. The movement control factors (balance and coordination) are of particular importance during early childhood when the child is gaining control of his or her fundamental movement abilities. The force production factors (speed, agility, and power) begin to assume greater importance after the child has gained control of his or her fundamental movements and passes into the specialized movement phase of later childhood.

It should be remembered that, as with the components of health-related fitness, one's motor fitness abilities are intricately interrelated with movement-skill acquisition. One depends in large part on the other. Without adequate motor fitness abilities, the child's level of skill acquisition will be limited. Without adequate skill acquisition, the level of attainment of motor fitness components will be impeded. The components of motor fitness are discussed here and synthesized in Table 12.3.

Coordination

Coordination is the ability to integrate separate motor systems with varying sensory modalities into efficient patterns of movement. The more complicated the movement tasks, the greater the level of coordination necessary for efficient performance. Coordination is interrelated with balance, speed, and agility but not closely aligned with strength and endurance (Barrow and McGee, 1979). Coordinated behavior requires that the child perform specific movements in a series both quickly and accurately. Movement must be synchronous, rhythmical, and properly sequenced in order to be coordinated.

Eye-hand and eye-foot coordination are characterized by integrating visual information with limb action. Movements must be visually controlled and precise in order to project, make contact with, or receive an external object. Bouncing, catching, throwing, kicking, and trapping a ball all require considerable amounts of visual input integrated with motor output in order to result in efficient coordinated movement.

Gross body coordination in children involves moving the body rapidly while performing various fundamental movement skills. Peterson et

Table 12.3 Common Measures and the Components of Motor Fitness and a Synthesis of Findings

Motor Fitness Component	Common Tests	Specific Aspect Measured	Synthesis of Findings
Coordination	Cable jump	Gross body coordination	Year by year improvement with age in gross body coordination. Boys superior from age 6 on in eye-hand and eye-foot coordination.
	Hopping for accuracy	Gross body coordination	
	Skipping	Gross body coordination	
	Ball dribble	Eye-hand coordination	
	Foot dribble	Eye-foot coordination	
Balance	Beam walk	Dynamic balance	Year by year improvement with age. Girls often outperform boys, especially in dynamic balance activities until about age 8. Abilities similar thereafter.
	Stick balance	Static balance	
	One-foot stand	Static balance	
Speed	20-yd dash	Running speed	Year by year improvement with age. Boys and girls similar until age 6 or 7, at which time boys make more rapid improvements. Boys superior to girls at all ages.
	30-yd dash	Running speed	
Agility	Shuttle run	Running agility	Year by year improvement with age. Girls begin to level off after age 13. Boys continue to make improvements.
	Side straddle	Lateral agility	
Power	Vertical jump	Leg strength and speed	Year by year improvement with age. Boys outperform girls at all age levels.
	Standing long jump	Leg strength and speed	
	Distance throw	Upper arm strength and speed	
	Velocity throw	Upper arm strength and speed	

al. (1974) have indicated that measures such as the shuffle run, 30-yard dash, various hopping and skipping tests, and the standing long jump load high with the factor of gross body coordination. Gross body coordination and eye-hand and eye-foot coordination appear to improve with age in a roughly linear fashion. Also, the performance of boys tends to be superior to that of girls throughout childhood (Frederick, 1977; Van Slooten, 1973).

Balance

Balance is the ability to maintain the equilibrium of one's body when it is placed in various positions. Balance is basic to all movement and is influenced by a variety of factors. Maintenance of balance is influenced by visual, tactile-kinesthetic, and vestibular stimulation.

Vision plays an important role in balance with young children. Cratty and Martin (1969) found that boys and girls age 6 and under could not balance on one foot with their eyes closed. But by age 7 they were able to maintain balance with their eyes closed, and balancing ability continued to improve with age. Use of the eyes enables the child to focus on a reference point in order to maintain balance. The eyes also enable the young child to visually monitor the body during a static or dynamic balance task.

Tactile and kinesthetic abilities play an important role in balance. The famous rod-and-frame experiments conducted by Wapner and Werner (1957) emphasize the importance of the tactile and kinesthetic senses. Verticality of a luminous rod in a frame was predicted by subjects seated in a darkened room and tilted to one side. The hypothesis was that children do not have control of their kinesthetic abilities to the point of being able to compensate for changes in body tilt and, therefore, must rely on visual information for accurate prediction of verticality. The experiment by Comalli et al. (1959) confirmed this hypothesis and revealed that in subjects from 6 to 16 years of age the rod appeared to be vertical when it was actually tilted in the same direction as the individual. Older subjects (age 16 to age 50) were able to more accurately locate the apparent vertical plane but often overcompensated and predicted verticality of the rod in the direction opposite their own tilt. In other words, tactile and kinesthetic abilities tend to improve with age and contribute to balance more in adults than in children (Parker, 1980).

Balance is profoundly influenced by the vestibular apparatus. The fluid contained in the *semicircular canals* and in the *otolith* plays a key role in maintaining equilibrium. The receptors in the semicircular canal respond to changes in angular acceleration (dynamic and rotational balance). While the otolith receptors respond to linear accelerations (static balance), the movement of *macula* (hairs) in either the otolith or the semicircular canals triggers nerve impulses by changing the electrical potential of adjoining nerve cells (Parker, 1980). Movement of the body and gravity are sensed by these vestibular receptors and aid the individual in awareness of both static and dynamic postural changes as well as of changes in acceleration. The vestibular apparatus coordinates with the visual, tactile, and kinesthetic systems in governing balance. It appears that vestibular development in terms of balance occurs very early in life and that the vestibular apparatus is structurally complete at birth. The body musculature, however, and the other sensory modalities involved in maintaining balance must further mature and be integrated with vestibular clues to be of real use to the child in maintaining either static or dynamic balance.

Balance is often defined as static or dynamic. *Static balance* refers to the body's ability to maintain equilibrium in a stationary position. Balancing on one foot, standing on a balance board, and performing a stick balance are common means of assessing static balance abilities. Research on the static balance abilities of children shows a linear trend toward improved performance with age from ages 2 through 12 (De Oreo, 1971; Keogh, 1965; Van Slooten, 1973). Prior to age 2, children generally are not able to perform a one-foot static balance task, probably because of their still-developing abilities to maintain a controlled upright posture. De Oreo (1980) indicated that clear-cut boy-girl differences are not seen in static balance performance as with other motor performance tasks. In fact, girls tend to be more proficient that boys until about age 7 to 8, whereupon the boys catch up. Both sexes level off in performance around age 8, prior to a surge in abilities from ages 9 to 12.

Dynamic balance refers to the ability to maintain equilibrium when moving from point to point. Balance beam walking tests are used most often as measures of dynamic balance in children. The available literature on dynamic balance indicates a trend similar to static balance. Girls are often more proficient than boys until age 8 or 9, whereupon they perform at similar levels (De Oreo, 1971; Frederick, 1977). Both slow in their progress around age 9 prior to making rapid gains to age 12 (Goetzinger, 1961; Heath, 1949).

Speed

Speed is the ability to cover a short distance in as short a period of time as possible. Speed is influenced by *reaction time* (the amount of elapsed time from the signal "go" to the first movements of the body) as well as *movement time* (the time elapsed from the initial movement to completion of the activity). Reaction time depends on the speed with which the initial stimulus is processed through the efferent and afferent neural pathways and is integrated with the initial response pattern. Reaction time has been shown to decrease in children as they get older.

Cratty (1986) reported that the information available concerning simple reaction time indicates that it is about twice as long in 5-year-olds as it is in adults for an identical task and that there is rapid improvement from ages 3 to 5. These developmental differences are probably due to neurological maturation and differences in the information processing capabilities of children and adults.

Speed of movement in children is most generally measured through various tests of running speed. Frederick (1977), in testing the running speed of five groups of children 3 to 5 years of age on the 20-yard dash, found linear improvement with age but no gender differences. In a study of the running speed of elementary school children, Keogh (1965) found that boys and girls are similar in running speed at ages 6 to 7, but that boys were superior from ages 8 to 12. Both boys and girls improve with age at about 1 foot per second per year from ages 6 to 11 (Cratty, 1979). Keogh also found similar improvement and boy-girl differences in the 50-foot hop for speed, although girls tended to perform better than boys on hopping and jumping tasks that require greater precision and accuracy of movement.

Fifty-yard sprint run scores are recorded as part of the AAU Physical Fitness Program (1988). These data are viewed as highly representative of the running speed of children and adolescents because of the very large sample size, geographical distribution, and randomization techniques utilized. Both boys and girls are reported to make annual incremental improvements with males slightly outperforming females at all ages, except at age 9 years where they are identical (Figure 12.10). Similarity in performance on the sprint run does not appear to carry over into the adolescent years (see Figure 17.11). Males continue to make dramatic improvements throughout the teen years, while females tend to regress slightly after age 14. Both factors are more closely associated with sociocultural mores than with anatomical or physiological change.

Speed of movement generally improves until about age 13 in both boys and girls. After this, however, girls tend to level off and even regress in their performance, while boys tend to continue improving throughout the adolescent years. The movement speed of both boys and girls may be fostered during childhood and beyond through opportunities for vigorous physical activity that incorporate short bursts of speed.

Agility

Agility is the ability to change the direction of the body rapidly and accurately as it moves from one point to another as fast as possible. It is

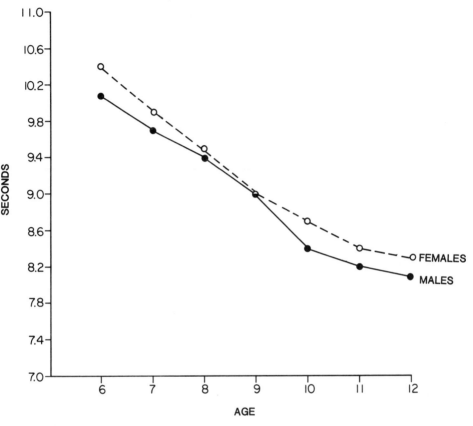

50 YARD SPRINT RUN: MALES & FEMALES

Figure 12.10 50 yd. sprint run, mean scores for males and females 6-12 years, in seconds (Data courtesy of: Chrysler—AAU Physical Fitness Program [1987] Indiana University, Bloomington, IN)

the ability to make quick and accurate shifts in body position during movement. A variety of agility runs have been used as indirect measures of agility. Unfortunately, the wide variety of ways in which these scores have been obtained makes it impossible to compare studies. Scores from the 30-foot shuttle run are typically used as a measure of running. Figure 12.11 depicts mean shuttle run scores for both boys and girls 6 to 10 years of age. Annual incremental improvements are seen throughout the period of childhood with a slight edge given to boys at all ages. Highly similar results were obtained from both the AAHPER Youth Fitness Test (1976) and the Manitoba Physical Fitness Performance Test (CAHPER, 1980).

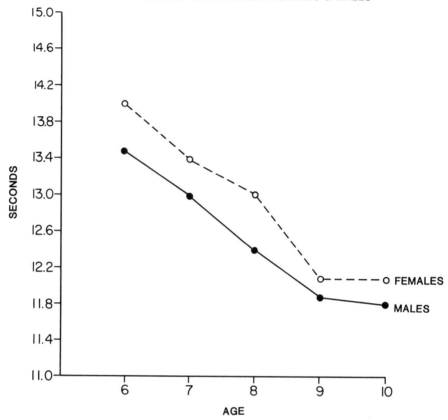

Figure 12.11 30 ft. shuttle run, mean scores for males and females 6-10 years, in seconds (Data courtesy of: Chrysler—AAU Physical Fitness Program [1987] Indiana University, Bloomington, IN)

Power

Power is the ability to perform a maximum effort in as short a period as possible. Power is sometimes referred to as "explosive strength" and represents the product of strength-times-speed. This combination of strength and speed is exhibited in children's activities that require jumping, striking, throwing for distance, and other explosive, all-out efforts. The speed of contraction of the muscles involved, as well as the strength and coordinated use of these muscles, determines the degree of power of the individual.

Because power involves a combination of motor abilities, it is difficult, if not impossible, to obtain a pure measure of this component. The often-used throwing and jumping measures can only give us an indirect indication of power because of the obvious requirements for skill involved in both of these tasks. Frederick (1977) did, however, find significant yearly increments in vertical jump, standing long jump, and distance throwing tasks for children ages 3 through 5. Also, the boys outperformed the girls on all measures at all age levels. The same results were found by Keogh (1965) for boys and girls from 6 to 12 years of age and by Van Slooten (1973) for children 6 to 9 years of age on the throw for distance but with gender differences magnified beyond age 7. Luedke's (1980) excellent review of the literature on throwing supports these studies.

Figure 12.12 represents mean standing long jump scores for boys and girls 6 to 10 years of age. This figure is based on a national sampling

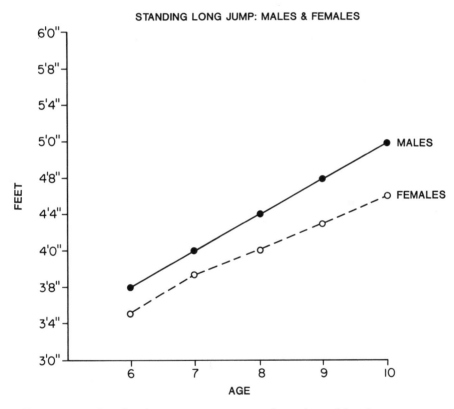

Figure 12.12 Standing long jump, mean scores for males and females 6-10 years, in feet (Data courtesy of: Chrysler—AAU Physical Fitness Program [1987] Indiana University, Bloomington, IN)

of thousands of children taking the AAU Physical Fitness Program (AAU, 1988). These data are considered to be highly representative of standing long jump abilities because of the sample size and randomization techniques used. Boys outperform girls at all ages. The gap that begins to widen at age 10 increases in magnitude throughout adolescence (see Figure 17.13).

Similar linear improvements and differences between boys and girls have been demonstrated in the standing long jump from age 3 through age 5 (Frederick, 1977), 6 through 12 (Keogh, 1965), and 10 through 17 (AAHPERD, 1976). Differences in throwing velocity based on age and sex have also been shown in samples of children from ages 6 to 14 (Glassow and Kruse, 1960; Luedke, 1980). But, differences from age to age and between sexes are closely related to yearly strength and speed of movement increments as well as to the varying sociocultural influences on boys and girls.

SUMMARY

Although specific questions remain unanswered, there is general agreement regarding the advisability of vigorous physical activity in children. The growth patterns of almost all the internal organs are in proportion to the remainder of the body. Hence the lungs, heart, and so forth, are able to cope with the demands placed on them. Proportional to their mass, young children can transport and utilize oxygen volumes comparable to adults. There seems to be no appreciable difference in the fatigability patterns between children and high-school youth and adults. The general consensus among researchers is that a sound heart cannot be injured by vigorous physical activity. Precautionary measures need to be taken, of course, in the case of a child with a suspected or known cardiac and/or pulmonary dysfunction.

Muscular strength, muscular endurance, and flexibility are also components of health-related fitness. They are related to one's positive state of health in much the same way as aerobic endurance. Good levels of fitness tend to reduce the likelihood of suffering from numerous physical ailments. The components of health-related fitness improve with age but not in a linear fashion. There is a strong tendency to make small gains during early and later childhood followed by a lull during the preadolescent period. During adolescence, boys often make rapid gains in all measures of fitness, while girls tend to level off and sometimes decline in their performance scores after age 15.

The motor fitness components of coordination and balance are closely aligned with the development of movement control during early childhood. Once good control has been established, the child is able to focus on improvement in the force components of motor fitness. Speed, agility, and power improve dramatically during later childhood as balance and coordination improve during early childhood. There is a linear trend for improvement in all measures of motor fitness. The motor abilities of both boys and girls improve with age and effort, with boys outperforming girls at all levels except during the prepubescent period.

CHAPTER CONCEPTS

12.1 There has been a growing realization of the importance of and necessity for vigorous physical activity for children and youth as well as adolescents and adults.

12.2 The normal daily routine of millions of North American children tends to exclude regular vigorous physical activity.

12.3 Accurately determining the fitness levels of young children is difficult and time-consuming. Therefore, information concerning children under 6 years of age is limited.

12.4 The components of health-related fitness are considered to be aerobic endurance, muscular strength, muscular endurance, joint flexibility, and body composition.

12.5 Aerobic endurance is meaured by determining the volume of oxygen consumed per kilogram of body weight (VO_2 max).

12.6 Children can achieve VO_2 max values similar to adult values when corrected for body weight.

12.7 The sedentary child will not develop the same degree of aerobic fitness as his or her active counterparts.

12.8 Muscular strength may be classified as isotonic, isometric, or isokinetic and involves one maximum exertion.

12.9 Predicting strength scores in later years on the basis of strength scores achieved during childhood is imprecise.

12.10 Boys tend to be stronger than girls at all ages even when body weight corrections are made.

12.11 Endurance levels of children approach and often exceed those of adults when adjusted for body weight.

12.12 Differences in endurance levels between genders and within gender may be partially accounted for by differences in achievement motivation levels.

12.13 Flexibility is joint-specific and as such has often revealed conflicting results in research measures of this fitness component.

12.14 Age is a poor predictor of flexibility. Activity levels offer a better guide.

12.15 Today's children tend to be more fat than their counterparts of 20 or 30 years ago.

12.16 Health-realted fitness abilities, motor fitness abilities, and movement abilities are interrelated. One affects the other, and none operates in isolation of the others except in controlled reserach settings.

12.17 Factor analytic studies with young children tend to indicate that the components of motor fitness may be grouped into a movement control factor and a movement force factor.

12.18 Balance and coordination are considered to be movement control factors, while speed, agility, and power are regarded as movement force factors.

12.19 Coordinated movement requires integration of sensory and motor systems into a congruent and harmonious action pattern.

12.20 Balance is critical to all movement behavior and is influenced by a variety of sensory mechanisms. Disturbance of any of these systems will have negative results on both static and dynamic balance behavior.

12.21 Speed, agility, and power are all influenced by both reaction time and movement time and improve up to about age 13 in most males and females. Improvement beyond this time requires special training.

TERMS TO REMEMBER

Health-Related Fitness
Aerobic Endurance
Maximal Oxygen Consumption
Heart Rate Response
Muscular Strength
Isotonic Strength
Isometric Strength
Isokinetic Strength
Dynamic Strength
Dynamometer
Tensiometer
Muscular Endurance
Joint Flexibility
Static Flexibility
Dynamic Flexibility
Body Composition
Hydrostatic Weighing
Skinfold Calipers
Aerobic Training
Strength Training
Weight Lifting

Anabolic Hormones
Catabolic Hormones
Growth Hormone
Testosterone
Physiological Adaptation
Epiphyseal Growth Plates
Motor Fitness
Coordination
Balance
Semicircular Canals
Otolith
Macula
Movement Control Factors
Force Production Factors
Static Balance
Dynamic Balance
Speed
Reaction Time
Movement Time
Agility
Power

CRITICAL READINGS

Bar-Or, O. (Ed.) (1989). *Advances in Pediatric Sport Science (Volume 3: Biological Issues)*. Champaign, IL: Human Kinetics.

Bar-Or O. (1983). *Pediatric Sports Medicine for the Practitioner*. New York: Springer-Verlag, (Chapter 1).

NSCA *Journal* (1985). "National Strength and Conditioning Association Position Paper on Prepubescent Strength Training," 7, 27-31.

Research Quarterly for Exercise and Sport. (1987). "Review and Commentary: Children and Fitness," 58, 295-333.

Ross, J. G., and Pate, R. R. (1987). "The National Children and Youth Fitness Study II." *Journal of Physical Education Recreation and Dance*, 58, 49-96.

13

Childhood Perception and Perceptual-Motor Development

CHAPTER COMPETENCIES

Upon Completion of This Chapter You Should Be Able To:

* *Discuss changes in perceptual functioning during childhood.*

* *Analyze the relationship and interaction between perceptual and motor development.*

* *Identify motor behavioral characteristics of children who developmentally lag in motor skills.*

* *Analyze the effect of cognitive processing differences within and across age groups on motor skill development and performance.*

* *Evaluate cognitive processing demands on motor skill performance.*

• *Discuss the developmental aspects of visual acuity, figure-ground perception, depth perception and visual motor coordination, and their interaction with motor performance.*

• *Demonstrate an understanding of perceptual training and its impact on the skill learning process.*

• *Define the term "perceptual-motor" and diagram the perceptual-motor process.*

• *Describe the perceptual-motor components and give examples of each.*

• *Distinguish between various forms of perceptual-motor training and provide a rationale for each.*

• *Draw conclusions from perceptual-motor research findings regarding what we know about its relationship to cognitive development and academic achievement.*

Study of the perceptual process and perceptual-motor development attempts to answer the age-old question of how we come to know our world. The nature of the perceptual process and its impact on movement and cognition have been topics of considerable interest to researchers and educators for years. From the moment of birth, children begin to learn how to interact with their environment. This interaction is a perceptual as well as a motor process. This chapter will focus on developmental aspects of visual perception and perceptual-motor behavior. The importance of developing perceptual and perceptual-motor abilities will be discussed along with factors that influence their development.

PERCEPTUAL DEVELOPMENT IN CHILDHOOD

By the time the child reaches 2 years of age, the ocular apparatus is mature. The eyeball is nearly adult size and weight. All anatomical and physiological aspects of the eye are complete, but the perceptual abilities of the young child are still incomplete. Although the child is able to fixate on objects, track them, and make accurate judgments of size and shape, numerous refinements still need to be made. The young child is unable to intercept a tossed ball with any degree of control (Payne, 1981). Difficulty with letter and number reversals is commonly experienced (Davidson, 1934; Rudel and Teuber, 1963). Children's perception of moving objects is poorly developed (Wapner, and Werner, 1957) and so are figure-ground perceptual abilities (Gallahue, 1968), and perception of distance (Smith and Smith, 1966).

The extent to which movement plays a role in visual perceptual development is speculative. Held and his colleagues (1961, 1963, 1964, 1965), Smith and Smith (1966), and Riesen and Aarons (1959) all speculated on the importance of movement in the development and refinement of visual perceptual abilities. They conducted investigations based on the hypothesis that self-produced movement is both a necessary condition and a sufficient condition for *visual-motor adjustment* to occur within a visually altered environment. They contended that without movement, visual perceptual adjustments will not occur and that the muscles and the motor aspect of the nervous system are intimately involved with perception and, in fact, that one is dependent on the other. The concept of a relationship between movement activity and perceptual development has also been indirectly supported by the decline in performance on both perceptual and motor deprivation experiments (Hebb, 1949; Riesen and Aarons, 1959) and experiments testing visual perceptual adjustment to an optically rearranged environment (Held and Blossom, 1961; Held and Mikaelian, 1964; Hoepner, 1967). This research has lead to what Payne and Isaacs (1987) termed the "movement hypothesis" which simply means that one must attend to objects that move in order to develop a normal visual-spatial reperitoire of skills.

The fact remains, however, that the results of each of these experiments are speculative at best when applied to the development of perceptual abilities in children. We still do not know the extent of the role that movement plays in perceptual development. It is probably safe to say that movement is a sufficient condition for encouraging the development of perceptual abilities. Whether it is, in fact, a necessary condition is doubtful (Gallahue, 1982).

There is little doubt that the developmental level of one's visual perceptual abilities will have an impact on the performance level of movement skills. It is important, therefore, that we become familiar with the child's developing perceptual abilities and their perceptual impact on skill development and refinement. Visual acuity, figure-ground perception, depth perception, and visual-motor coordination are all important visual perceptual qualities that are developmentally based and influence movement performance. Table 13.1 provides a summary of these qualities and a hypothesized developmental sequence.

Visual Acuity

Visual acuity is the ability to distinguish detail in objects. The finer the details that can be distinguished the better one's visual acuity, and vice versa. Visual acuity may be measured in both static and dynamic settings. *Static visual acuity* is the degree of detail distinguishable when both the individual and the object of visual regard are stationary. Static visual acuity is most commonly measured by use of a Snellen eye chart. A Snellen assessment is expressed in fractions. Therefore, a 20/20 rating indicates that one can distinguish objects at a distance of 20 feet in the same manner as others with normal vision at 20 feet. Similarly, a 20/200 rating indicates the ability to distinguish at 20 feet what others with normal vision could distinguish at 200 feet.

Dynamic visual acuity is the ability to distinguish detail in moving objects. It is less frequently assessed than static visual acuity but is of interest to anyone required to make precise judgements based on visually guided tracking. Therefore, the baseball player preparing to strike or catch a ball needs to have good dynamic visual acuity as does the volleyball player or skeet shooter. Dynamic visual acuity is measured by flashing on a screen checkerboard targets with varying levels of grid precision. These targets are made to travel horizontally at varying speeds and the individual is asked to indicate when the small checks can be seen in the moving object.

With regard to static visual acuity, Williams (1983) reported that it is mature by age 10 and, in general, is less developed in 5 and 6 year olds.

Table 13.1 Selected Developmental Aspects of Children's Visual Perception

Visual Quality	Selected Abilities	Approximate Age
VISUAL ACUITY The ability to distinguish detail in static and dynamic settings (Whiting, 1974; Williams, 1983)	Rapid Improvement	5-7
	Plateau	7-8
	Rapid Improvement	9-10
	Mature (Static)	10-11
	Plateau (Dynamic)	10-11
	Mature (Dynamic)	11-12
FIGURE-GROUND PERCEPTION The ability to separate an object from its surroundings (Frostig, 1966; Gallahue, 1968; Williams, 1983)	Slow Improvement	3-4
	Rapid Improvement	4-6
	Slight Spurt	7-8
	Mature	8-12
DEPTH PERCEPTION The ability to judge distance relative to oneself (Williams, 1983; Sage, 1984, Payne & Isaacs, 1987)	Frequent Judgement Errors	3-4
	Few Judgement Errors	5-6
	Rapid Improvement	7-11
	Mature	By age 12
VISUAL-MOTOR COORDINATION The ability to integrate use of eyes and hands in terms of object tracking and interruption (Dorfman, 1977; Jeannerod, 1986; Williams, 1983)	Rapid Improvement	3-7
	Slow Slight Improvement	7-9
	Mature	10-12

Rapid improvement occurs between 5 and 7 years of age, with little change seen from ages 7 to 9, followed by rapid improvement between ages 9 and 10. By age 12 static visual acuity is adultlike (Whiting, 1974).

Dynamic visual acuity appears to mature somewhat later than its static counterpart. Morris (1977) found improvement up to 20 years of age. Williams (1983) reported that dynamic visual acuity becomes increasingly refined during three separate time periods: 5-7 years, 9-10 years, and 11-12 years of age. Furthermore, boys display better visual acuity (both dynamic and static) than girls at all ages. This information may help us better understand why making adjustments in the skill requirement in a sport such as baseball is essential if we are to encourage the child to sustain efforts over time. Furthermore, the fact that females lag behind their male counterparts may explain why they often do less well on object-interception tasks and tend to drop out of these sports earlier. Recognition of these facts makes it essential that adult leaders modify the rules in order to enhance the potential for success and sustained participation.

Figure-Ground Perception

Figure-ground perception is the ability to separate an object of visual regard from its surroundings. Gallahue (1968) demonstrated that 6-year-old children were influenced in their ability to distinguish an object of visual regard from its surroundings by using various combinations of a blending and/or distracting background. Basically, he found that combinations which caused a maximum amount of blending and distraction were most disruptive in terms of distinguishing the figure from its background in the performance of a simple stepping test. Treatment conditions in which only color blending or visual distractors were present were less disruptive. With regard to the developmental nature of visual figure-ground perception, Williams (1983), interpreting Frostig's et al. (1966) data, reported stable figure-ground perception between 8-10 years. Prior to that slow improvement occurs between 3 and 4 years, with large improvement seen from ages 4 through 6. Smaller changes were reported from ages 6 to 7 followed by a slight spurt between 7 and 8 years of age. Williams (1973) further suggested that figure-ground perception becomes increasingly refined from 8 to 13 years and may even continue to improve to 17 or 18 years of age.

The significance of visual figure-ground perception is obvious. Along with good dynamic visual acuity, figure-ground perception enables the performer to not only clearly distinguish an object, but to separate it from its background. Such a highly refined skill is essential for batters or outfielders in baseball, for wide-receivers or quarterbacks in football, or for performers on the uneven bars in gymnastics. The ability to clearly extract the object of regard (figure) from its background (ground) is essential for success. With children it is important to recognize that this perceptual quality is still developing. Modifications of the task requirements or manipulation of the background against which certain movement tasks are performed may do much to enhance performance.

Depth Perception

Depth Perception is one of the most intriguing aspects of visual perception. It provides us with the ability to see three-dimensionally, an astonishing feat when you consider that separately our retinas function two-dimensionally but combined provide us with a visual image complete with minute depth cues. These cues to depth are both monocular and binocular.

Monocular depth cues are those that can be picked up by one eye. Such things as size, texture gradient, shading, convergence, overlap, proportanealty and linear perspective are common monocular cues to depth. Each of these are used by the artist to give the illusion of depth on canvas.

They are also used by us to give important three-dimensional visual cues to depth.

Binocular depth cues require both eyes working in concert. *Retinal Disparity*, an important component of depth perception, is the viewing of objects of visual regard from slightly different angles by each eye. Therefore, the image projected on each retina is slightly different and the information passed on to the visual area of the cortex results in binocular disparity. Hence the images that we receive have the impression of depth.

Little is known about the developmental aspects of depth perception. Williams (1983) however, reported that binocularity and depth perception continues to improve from 2 through 5 years of age. She also indicated that by age 7 children can accurately judge depth with monocular cues. Based on this and the extensive literature on infant depth perception, it is probably safe to conclude that depth perception begins developing in a very basic way during the first months of life but that it continues to improve throughout early childhood. It is doubtful whether depth perception in general can be improved through special training. It is possible, however, that depth perception in specific situations can be improved (Sage, 1984).

Teachers, parents, and coaches need to consider the visual perception of depth when teaching new ball skills. Ball size, color, and texture, as well as distance, trajectory, and speed all play an important role in providing depth cues for successful object interception (Isaacs, 1980; Payne, 1985; Payne, & Isaacs, 1987). One need only observe the child that exhibits a head-turning avoidance reaction to an approaching ball to see the importance of depth cues to successful catching. Turning the head to one side eliminates binocular vision and forces the child to depend on monocular cues. All too often these monocular cues are insufficient to make the accurate and refined adjustments required for mature catching. As a result, the child reverts to a less mature catching pattern, or the ball hits the face or chest before being dropped. Successful object interception requires making use of all the depth cues available, especially during the early stages of skill development.

Visual-Motor Coordination

Visual-motor coordination refers to the ability to track and make interception judgements with a moving object. The development of visual abilities begins early in infancy and continues to improve with age. Morris (1980) indicated that by age 5 or 6 children can accurately track moving objects in a horizontal plane, and that by age 8 or 9 they can track balls moving in an arc. Payne and Isaacs (1987, p. 191) noted that "as dynamic visual acuity improves, so does the ability to track fast-moving objects, because whenever an object is moving at an angular velocity at which smooth eye movements are no longer possible, the pursuit task becomes a function of dynamic visual acuity." Williams (1983) reported that accurate perception of movement continues to develop to about 10 to 12 years of age.

Object interception is the second aspect of visual-motor coordination. Object interception, or *coincidence-anticipation* as it is frequently referred to in the motor learning literature, involves the ability to make accurate estimates of an object's location in harmony with a specific motor response. For example, the batter in baseball must estimate where the ball will be at a certain time and simultaneously bring the motor system into play in an attempt to make contact with the bat at just the right moment. Object interception abilities improve greatly with age and with practice (Dorfman, 1977). Due to the vast number of confounding variables, it is difficult to propose a developmental model for object interception ability. But, observation of numerous children attempting to hit a pitched ball leads me to conclude that younger children and less experienced individuals make numerous judgement errors, but that older children and more experienced persons make fewer errors. Therefore, experience clearly appears to be an essential element in making accurate estimates of object interception. Whether experience alone, or maturation of the visual-motor apparatus in conjunction with experience, is responsible for improved judgments awaits further study.

Perceptual Training

That the visual perceptual sophistication of the individual is intricately related to success in the performance of numerous movement skills makes it essential for the teacher or coach to be aware of the developmental nature of children's visual abilities. The perceptual requirements of fundamental manipulative skills that involve imparting force to an object or receiving force from an object are especially great. Therefore, when working with young children we must make appropriate adjustments in the equipment used in order to take into account the developmental level of their perceptual abilities. The ball texture chosen, for example, (foam, fleece, plastic, or soft rubber) can have a dramtic influence on the level and success experienced. Making modification in the color and size of the object will also have an impact.

Modifying the rules of play to permit greater clarity and consistancy of perception, time to react, or ease of tracking is also recommended. In baseball, for example, use of a pitching machine set at a predetermined speed and trajectory will help children develop their tracking skills. Hitting a ball off a tee enables younger children to experience greater success and to focus on developing a level swing without compounding the complexity of the task with object-tracking.

A third consideration in perceptual training is recognition that the mechanics of the movement itself are influenced by the level of perception required for successful performance. If the visual requirements are great, the mechanics are more likely to be negatively influenced (a tennis serve), than if vision is less crucial (swimming, or skipping).

Finally, it is essential that those working with children recognize that perceptual development as well as motor development is crucial to successful movement performance. It is important that this point not be overlooked and that we adjust our level of expectations to the perceptual as well as to the physical maturity of the individual.

PERCEPTUAL-MOTOR DEVELOPMENT IN CHILDREN

The visual perceptual abilities of young children are not the same as in adults. Children's visual world is in the developmental stages and is, therefore, restricted. The development of perceptual abilities significantly inhibits or enhances children's movement performance. From the previous section we have seen that the converse of this may be true, that is, movement performance may significantly inhibit or enhance the development of children's perceptual abilities. The child restricted in perceptual development often encounters difficulties in performing perceptual-motor tasks.

The realization that the process of perception is not entirely innate enables one to hypothesize that the quality and quantity of movement experiences afforded young children are related to some extent to the development of their perceptual abilities. The initial responses of young children are motor responses, and all future perceptual and conceptual data are based, in part, on these initial responses. Young children must establish a broad base of motor experience for these higher learnings to develop properly. Meaningfulness is imposed on perceptual stimulation through movement. The matching of perceptual and motor data is thought by many to be necessary for the child to establish a stable spatial world (Barsch, 1965; Kephart, 1971). The more motor and perceptual learning experiences children have, the greater the opportunity to make this perceptual-motor match and to develop a plasticity of response to various movement situations.

Unfortunately, the complexity of our modern society often deters the development of many perceptual-motor abilities. The environment in which today's children are raised is so complicated and dangerous that they are constantly being warned not to touch and to stay away from situations that potentially offer great amounts of motor and perceptual information. Children who grow up in large cities, or in apartment buildings, seldom are given the opportunity to climb trees, walk fences, jump streams, or ride horses. They miss out on many of the experiences that children need as part of their daily life experiences that help to develop their movement abilities. The lack of these movement experiences and the adaptability of response that comes with practice and repetition often deter perceptual development.

Artificial means must be devised to provide additional experiences and practice in the perceptual-motor activities that modern society is unable to provide naturally. Providing children with substitute experiences for those they are unable to get or fully explore on their own may have a positive effect on the development of their visual perceptual abilities. This seems to support the essentiality of a physical education teacher in the child's educational curriculum. A sound physical education program will contribute to the development of a child's perceptual-motor skills and help develop many of the basic readiness skills prerequisite to success in school.

What is "Perceptual-Motor"

There are two reasons for the hyphen in the term *perceptual-motor*. First, it signifies the dependency of voluntary movement activity upon some forms of perceptual information. All voluntary movement involves an element of perceptual awareness resulting from some sort of sensory stimulation. Second, the hyphen indicates that the development of one's perceptual abilities is dependent, in part, on motor activity. Perceptual-motor abilities are learned abilities and, as such, use movement as an important medium for this learning process.

It has long been recognized that the quality of one's movement performance depends on the accuracy of perception and the ability to interpret these perceptions into a series of coordinated movement acts. The terms "eye-hand coordination" and "eye-foot coordination" have been used for years as a means of expressing the dependency of efficient movement on the accuracy of one's sensory information. The individual in the process of shooting a basketball free-throw has numerous forms of sensory input that must be sorted out and expressed in the final perceptual-motor act of shooting the ball. If the perceptions are accurate, and if they are put together into a coordinated sequence, the basket is made. If not, the shot misses. All voluntary movement involves the use of one or more sensory modalities to a greater or lesser degree, depending on the movement act to be performed. What has not been recognized until recently is the important contribution that movement experiences have on the development of the children's perceptual-motor abilities.

The term perception means "to know" or "to interpret information." Perception is the process of organizing incoming information with stored information which leads to a modified response pattern. Therefore, perceptual-motor development may be described as a process of attaining increased skill and ability to function. It involves:

1. *Sensory Input*: receiving various forms of stimulation by way of specialized sensory receptors (visual, auditory, tactile, and kinesthetic and transmitting this stimulation to the brain in the form of a pattern of neural energy.

2. *Sensory Integration*: organizing incoming sensory stimuli and integrating it with past or stored information (memory).

3. *Motor Interpretation*: making internal motor decisions (recalibration) based on the combination of sensory (present) and long-term memory (past) information.

4. *Movement Activation*: executing the actual movement (observable act) itself.

5. *Feedback*: evaluating the movement act by way of various sensory modalities (visual, auditory, tactile, and/or kinesthetic) which in turn feeds back information into the sensory input aspect of the process, thus beginning the cycle over again.

The Perceptual-Motor Components

Although the movement experiences found in the regular physical education program are by general definition perceptual-motor activities, there is a difference in emphasis in programs that focus on the perceptual-motor quality being reinforced rather than the gross motor quality. In remedial and readiness programs emphasis is placed on improving specific perceptual-motor components. Therefore, movement activities are grouped according to the perceptual-motor qualities they enhance, namely: body awareness, spatial awareness, directional awareness, and temporal awareness. Activities designed to enhance these abilities are used in the regular instructional physical education program, with a primary objective of movement skill acquisition rather than perceptual-motor acquisition.

The development and refinement both of children's *spatial world* and *temporal world* are two of the primary contributions of perceptual-motor training programs. The jargon used in programs across North America varies greatly. There does seem to be general agreement, however, that the following perceptual-motor qualities are among the most important to be developed and reinforced in children.

Body Awareness

The term *body awareness* is often used in conjunction with the terms body image and body schema. Each term refers to the developing capacity of children to accurately discriminate among their body parts. The ability to differentiate among one's body parts and to gain a greater understanding of the nature of the body occurs in three areas. The first of these is knowledge of the body parts. This means being able to accurately locate the numerous parts of the body on oneself and on others. Second is knowledge of what the body parts can do. This refers to the child's developing abilities to recognize the parts of a given act and the body's actual potential for performing it. Knowledge of how to make the parts move efficiently is the third component of body awareness. This refers to the ability to reorganize the body parts for a particular motor act and the actual performance of a movement task.

Spatial Awareness

Spatial awareness is a basic component of perceptual-motor development that may be divided into two subcategories: (1) knowledge of how much space the body occupies and (2) the ability to project the body effectively into external space. Knowledge of how much space the body occupies and its relationship to external objects may be developed through a variety of movement activities. With practice and experience, children progress from their egocentric world of locating everything in external space relative to themselves (*egocentric localization* to the development of an objective frame of reference (*objective localization*). For example, preschoolers tend to determine the location of an object relative to where they are standing. Older children, however, are able to locate an object relative to its proximity to other nearby objects without regard to the location of their body.

As adults, our spatial awareness is generally adequate, but we may still encounter difficulties in locating the relative position of various objects. For example, when reading a road map while traveling through unfamiliar territory, many people become uncertain of whether they are traveling north, south, east, or west. Decisions regarding which way to turn sometimes seem to necessitate literally placing oneself on the map in order to project a mental image of turning options. The absence of familiar landmarks and the impersonality of the road map make it difficult for many to objectively localize themselves in space relative to this particular task. Young children encounter much the same difficulty but on a broader scale. They must first learn to orient themselves subjectively in space and then proceed carefully to venture out into unfamiliar surroundings in which subjective clues are useless. Providing children with opportunities to develop spatial awareness is an important attribute of a good physical education program that recognizes the importance of perceptual-motor development.

Directional Awareness

An area of great concern to many classroom teachers is that of *directional awareness*. It is through directional awareness that children are able to give dimension to objects in external space. The concepts of left-right, up-down, top-bottom, in-out, and front-back are enhanced through movement activities that place emphasis on direction. Directional awareness is commonly divided into two subcategories: laterality and directionality.

Laterality refers to an internal awareness of the various dimensions of the body with regard to their location and direction. Children who have adequately developed the concept of laterality do not need to rely on external cues for determining direction. They do not need, for example, to have a ribbon tied to their wrist to remind them which is their left and which is their right hand. The concept of laterality seems so basic to most adults that it is difficult to conceive how anyone could possibly not develop it. Yet, we need only to look into our rear-view mirror to be confused by reversed directions. Backing up a trailer hitched to a car or truck is an experience that most of us prefer to avoid due to the difficulty encountered in deciding whether to turn the wheel to the left or right. The pilot, astronaut, and deep-sea diver must possess a high degree of laterality or "feel" for determining up from down and left from right.

Directionality is the external projection of laterality. It gives dimension to objects in space. True directionality depends on adequately established laterality. Directionality is important to parents and teachers because it is a basic component in learning how to read. Children who do not have fully established directionality will often encounter difficulties in discriminating between various letters of the alphabet. For example, the letters (*b, d, p,* and *q*) are all similar. The only difference lies in the direction of the "ball" and the "stick" that make up the letters. As a result, the child encounters considerable difficulty in discriminating between several letters of the alphabet. Entire words may even be reversed for the child with a directionality problem. The word "cat" may be read as "tac," or "bad" as "dab" due to the inability to project direction into external space. Some children encounter difficulty in the top-bottom dimension, which is more basic than the left-right dimension. They may write and see words upside-down and are totally confused when it comes to reading.

It should be pointed out that established directional awareness is a developmental process and relies on both maturation and experience. It is perfectly normal for the 4- and 5-year-old to experience confusion in direction. We should, however, be concerned for the 6- or 7-year-old child who is consistently experiencing these confusions; this is the time when most schools traditionally begin instruction in reading. Adequately developed directional awareness is one important readiness skill necessary for success in reading, and movement in one way in which this important perceptual-motor concept may be developed.

Temporal Awareness

The preceding discussion of the various aspects of perceptual-motor development dealt with the development of the child's spatial world. Body awareness, spatial awareness, and directional awareness are closely interrelated and combine to help children make sense out of their spatial world. *Temporal awareness*, on the other hand, is concerned with the development of an adequate time structure in children. It is developed and refined at the same time the child's spatial world is developing.

Temporal awareness is intricately related to the coordinated interaction of various muscular systems and sensory modalities. The terms "eye-hand coordination" and "eye-foot coordination" have been used for years to reflect the interrelationship of these processes. The individual with a well-developed time dimension is the one we refer to as coordinated. One who has not fully established this is often called clumsy or awkward.

Everything we do possesses an element of time. There is a beginning point and an end point, and no matter how minute, there is a measurable span of time between the two. It is important that children learn how to function efficiently in this time dimension as well as in the space dimension. Without one, the other cannot develop to its fullest potential.

Rhythm is the basic and most important aspect of developing a stable temporal world. The term has many meanings but is described here as the synchronous recurrence of events related in such a manner that they form recognizable patterns. Rhythmic movement involves the synchronous sequencing of events in time. Rhythm is crucial in the performance of any act in a coordinated manner. Cooper (1982) tape-recorded the sounds of the movement pattern of selected sport skills in outstanding performers. The sounds made by these performers were transcribed into musical notation illustrating that a recordable rhythmical element was present. The recorded rhythms of these outstanding athletes were beaten out on a drum in several teaching situations with beginners. The results were startling in that the beginners learned the movements of the champions more rapidly when this technique was used than in a standard teaching situation. Cooper and Andrews (1975, p. 66) concluded that "it appears that beginning performers can profit by listening to and emulating certain elements of the rhythmic pattern of the good performers. Teachers should take full advantage of this phenomenon." Surely this statement applies to children as well as to athletes. We must recognize the rhythmic element in all efficient movement and, in so doing, be sure that we emphasize the rhythmic component of all movement (Adrian and Cooper, 1989).

H. Smith (1970) indicated that children begin to make temporal discriminations through the auditory modality before the visual and that there is transfer from the auditory to the visual but not the reverse. Activities that require performing movement tasks to auditory rhythmic patterns should begin with young children and be a part of their daily lives. The activity possibilities are endless. Moving to various forms of musical accompaniment ranging from the beat of a drum to instrumental selections can be an important contributor to temporal awareness.

PERCEPTUAL-MOTOR TRAINING

During the 1960s and 1970s several *perceptual-motor training programs* were established throughout North America. These programs were given considerable exposure in the popular press. Based on their articles and the claims of some, many people formed the impression that perceptual-motor programs were panaceas for the development of cognitive and motor abilities. Considerable confusion and speculation developed over the values and purposes of perceptual-motor training programs. Programs adhering to one technique or another emerged almost overnight. All too often, people were inadequately trained, ill-informed, and frankly, uncertain of just what they were trying to accomplish. The smoke has now cleared, and concerned educators have taken a closer, more objective look at perceptual-motor training programs and their role in the total educational spectrum. Instead of claiming they are panaceas or adhering to one training technique or another, many are viewing perceptual-motor programs as important facilitators of *readiness development*. Perceptual-motor activities are being recognized as important contributors to the general readiness of children for learning. The contribution of perceptual-motor activities to specific perceptual readiness skills is being closely reexamined.

Readiness programs may be classified as concept developing, and concept reinforcing. *Concept development programs* are generally designed for children who, for a variety of reasons, have been limited or restricted in their experiential background (e.g., socioeconomic status, prolonged illness, ethnic background, television). Head Start programs and Frostig's (1969) developmental program are examples of concept developing programs in which a variety of multisensory experiences including perceptual-motor activities are used as a means of developing fundamental readiness skills.

Concept reinforcement programs are those in which movement is used in conjunction with traditional classroom techniques to develop basic cognitive understandings. In this type of program, movement is used as an aid or vehicle for reinforcing cognitive concepts dealt with in the nursery school or primary grade classroom. Cratty (1973), Humphrey (1974), Werner and Burton (1979), Blatt and Cunningham (1981), and others have outlined a variety of concept reinforcing activities for use by children.

Remedial training programs are the third and most controversial type of perceptual-motor training program. They have been established as a means of alleviating perceptual inadequacies and increasing academic achievement. Programs have been developed by Delacato (1959), Getman (1952), Kephart (1971), and others in attempts to aid cognitive development through perceptual-motor remediation techniques. The avowed purpose of these programs is to enhance academic achievement. There is, however, little solid support for this claim although abundant testimony and opinions are available. In fact, a recent meta-analysis of more than 180 research studies designed to measure the efficacy of perceptual-motor training on academic achievement and cognition clearly reveals that such programs make little or no direct contribution to these areas (Kavale, & Mattson, 1983). Figure 13.1 presents an overview of the various types of perceptual-motor training programs.

READINESS AND REMEDIATION

Research indicates that, as children pass through the normal development stages, their perceptual abilities become more acute and refined. This is due partly to the increasing complexity of the neuromuscular apparatus and sensory receptors and partly to children's increasing ability to explore and move throughout their environment (Williams, 1983). Piaget's (1954) work has traced the gradual development of perception from crude, meaningless sensations to the perception of a stable spatial world. His stages of development rely heavily on motor information as a primary information-gathering process. As the perceptual world of children develops, they try to construct it with as much stability as they can to reduce variability as far as possible. As a result, they learn to differentiate between those things that can be ignored, that are easily predictable, or that are wholly unforeseen and must be observed and examined in order to be understood, according to Piaget and others. Movement plays an important role in this process of developing perceptual readiness for cognitive tasks. Table 13.2 provides a comparison of Piaget's (1962) stages of development with those proposed by Kephart (1971), and by this author.

The majority of our perceptions (visual perceptions in particular) result from the elaboration and modification of these basic reactions by

Table 13.2 Comparison of Piaget's, Kephart's, and Gallahue's Phases and Stages of Development

Approximate Chronological Age	Piaget's Intellectual Evolution	Kephart's Developmental Sequences	Gallahue's Phases of Motor Development
0 to 6 months	**Sensorimotor Phase** Use of reflexes Primary circular reactions Coordination of prehension and vision, secondary circular reactions.	**Reflexive Stage**	**Reflexive Phase** Encoding stage Decoding stage
6 to 12 months	Secondary schemata Discovery of new means, tertiary circular reactions	**Motor Stage** Rudimentary motor pattern development Balance Receipt and propulsion Globular Form	**Rudimentary Phase** Reflex inhibition stage
1 to 2 years	Beginnings of insight and cause/effect relationships Egocentric organization Perceptive movement	**Motor-Perceptual Stage** Laterality Hand-eye coordination Gross motor pattern development Syncretic form Form recognition	Precontrol stage
2 to 4 years	**Preoperational Thought Phase** Perceptually oriented, period from self-satisfying behavior to rudimentary social behavior Awareness of a conceptual hierarchy, beginnings of cognition		**Fundamental Movement Phase** Initial stage Elementary stage

Age			
4 to 6 years	Beginning abstractions	**Perceptual-Motor Stage** Directionality Eye-hand coordination **Perceptual Stage** Form perception Constructive form Form reproduction	Mature stage
7 to 10 years	**Concrete Operations Phase** Additive composition, reversibility, associativity, identity, deductive reasoning Relationships Classification	**Perceptual Cognitive Stage**	**Specialized Movement Phase** Transition stage
11 years and over	**Formal Operations Phase** Intellectual maturity Symbolic operations Abstract thinking Propositional thinking	**Cognitive Perceptual Stage** **Cognitive Stage**	Application stage Life-long utilization stage

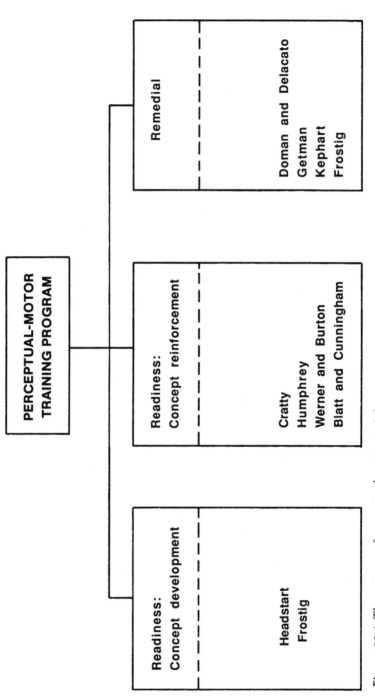

Figure 13.1 Three types of perceptual-motor training programs

experience and learning. When we speak of children being perceptually ready to learn, we are, in fact, referring to a point at which they have sufficiently developed their basic perceptual and conceptual learning tasks. Perceptual readiness for learning is a developmental process, and perceptual-motor activities play an important part in helping young children achieve a general stage of readiness. Specific perceptual readiness skills, such as visual perceptual readiness for reading, "may" be affected by the quality and quantity of the perceptual-motor experiences engaged in by children, but this has not been conclusively demonstrated in controlled research studies.

The reading process (as well as other important tasks) involves a number of abilities, an important one of which is visual perceptual ability. The reading process may be considered in terms of three basic areas: language, skill, and perception. Considerable research has been conducted in the first two areas, but the third has only begun to be explored. The perceptual phase of reading involves the identification and recognition of words on a printed page. Form and shape perception may be enhanced through movement as may be directional awareness of up, down, left, and right. All are important factors associated with word identification and recognition.

The period of the greatest amount of perceptual-motor development is between ages 3 and 7. These are the crucial years preceding and during the time that children begin to learn to read. They are perceptually ready to read when they have developed a sufficient backlog of information that enables them to encode and decode sensory impressions at a given point in time with the benefit of previous learning experiences of high quality and high quantity. A sufficient enough number of children enter the first grade lagging in perceptual abilities to warrant offering programs in readiness training that utilize perceptual-motor development activities as one of many avenues for intervention.

PERCEPTUAL-MOTOR RESEARCH FINDINGS

Research efforts are continually being made in an attempt to document the virtues of perceptual-motor training programs on readiness and remedial aspects of perceptual and cognitive development. Each new research effort stimulates new questions and problems. The available results are inconclusive, but there is ample evidence to suggest that perceptual-motor training programs are making a limited but positive contribution to the motor and perceptual development of children (Kavale and Mattson, 1983). In reviewing the literature, one may discover several generalizations that lend support to and seem to have specific implications for the educator and parent concerned with the prevention and remediation of perceptual-motor learning disabilities. However, the meta-analysis study of Kavale and Mattson (1983) clearly demonstrated that perceptual-motor training programs are ineffective in remediating learning difficulties of any nature. Field practitioners often disagree with this conclusion and are quick to assert that they have seen, with their own eyes, children make dramatic improvements in their schoolwork. In recognition of this dichotomy between "statistical causality" and "practical causality," some tentative conclusions that may be drawn are:

1. Not all learning difficulties are perceptual-motor in nature. Some may be due to problems in perceptual functioning. Others may be due to problems in concept formulation.

2. Perceptual-motor deficits may or may not lead to learning disabilities in a given child. Despite this fact, diagnosis and remediation of problems is worthwhile if only for the expanded competencies, both physical and emotional (self-concept), that result from such remediation.

3. Diagnostic tools for assessment are, at this time, in a rather primitive state. Distinct elements in the perceptual-motor spectrum have yet to be identified. Diagnostic tests cannot yet validly isolate separate factors.

4. Low-level functional deficits (perceptual-motor tasks) seem to be associated with high-level functional deficits (perceptual-cognitive tasks). This is to say that children who perform poorly on tasks of high complexity (reading and arithmetic) also tend to perform poorly on low complexity tasks (laterality, directionality, midline). This link, however, has not been proven to be causal, and must therefore be assumed to be casual.

5. Intramodal abilities develop before intermodal abilities. This means that children learn to use each of the senses separately before they interrelate them and use more than one mode at a time.

6. The most efficient learning mode seems to be vision, although learning is enhanced when information is presented to or processed by two or more modes at the same time. That is, the child is likely to learn more if presented information visually and auditorily at the same time than if presented information through only one mode at a time.

7. Not all children are at the same perceptual level on entering the first grade. Perceptual development is a process of both maturation and experience, and children therefore develop at their own rates.

8. Adequate perception (auditory, visual, tactile, kinesthetic) is prerequisite to success in school. Inaccurate perceptions lead to

difficulties in academic concept formation. Perceptual readiness is an important aspect of total readiness for learning.

9. Perceptual abilities can be improved through specialized training programs

10. A program of perceptual-motor assessment can be useful at the preschool or kindergarten level to identify potential readiness lags in children and to adjust the curriculum to their strengths and weaknesses.

11. Deprivation of perceptual-motor experiences at an early age may hinder the development of the child's perceptual abilities.

12. Perceptual-motor training programs enhance the development of auditory, visual, and tactile-kinesthetic perceptual abilities in children.

13. Perceptual-motor activities should be included as part of readiness training programs.

14. Developmental physical education programs provide many of the movement experiences that contribute to the development of the child's perceptual-motor abilities.

In conclusion, when we say that a child is "ready" to learn, we are, in fact, referring to a point at which the child, through maturation and learning, has sufficiently developed the perceptual and motor abilities to be able to benefit measurably from higher-order perceptual and cognitive tasks. Movement experiences serve as a vehicle by which these capabilities are developed and refined. Myers and Hammill (1982, p. 416), in their recommendations for needed perceptual-motor research, insist that three basic questions be addressed:

1. Identifying the characteristics of children for whom training has been demonstrated to be beneficial.
2. Determining the optimal amount and type of training necessary to produce real perceptual and/or motor growth.
3. Demonstrating that perceptual-motor processes can actually be improved as a result of training.

Children learn by doing. The physical educator plays an important role in the development of the young child's perceptual-motor abilities through a varied program of movement experiences that values the worth of each child as an individual.

ASSESSING PERCEPTUAL-MOTOR DEVELOPMENT

During the past several years, numerous measures of perceptual-motor development have been constructed. Generally, these tests were developed as measures for children who had been classified as "slow learners," "brain-damaged," or "neurologically impaired." They have been used with varying degrees of success. A list of selected tests of perceptual-motor functioning may be found at the conclusion of this chapter. The classroom teacher and physical education teacher are the first to pick up subjective cues of possible perceptual-motor difficulties in preschool and primary grade children. The validity of these subjective observations must not be discounted or minimized. On the contrary, the careful daily observation of children's behavior can be very valuable and reliable in detecting potential lags in development. It is suggested that the teacher refer those students suspected of a developmental lag to the school psychologist for testing and specific delineation of the problem. The results of the testing should be shared with both parents and teachers with whom the child comes in contact. In this way they can form an effective team to eliminate or diminish the difficulty. The checklist of cues that follow may aid the teacher in more accurate, informal assessment of children with a potential perceptual-motor problem.

Checklist of Possible Perceptual-Motor Dysfunctions

The checklist in Table 13.3 is designed to serve only as a subjective indicator of possible perceptual-motor difficulties. There is very little interrelationship among these variables and there is no predictable pattern for determining difficulties. Failure in several of these items may lead the teacher to seek further information through more objective evaluative procedures.

SUMMARY

Perceptual-motor training programs possess many of the same elements as any quality physical education program. Many of the movement skills taught in the perceptual-motor curriculum, whether it be a readiness or a remedial program, parallel those taught in regular preschool and elementary school physical education classes. The goals of each program are obviously different. Whereas a primary goal of the physical education program is to develop movement control through practice and instruction in a variety of movement activities, the goal of the perceptual-motor program is to enhance perceptual-motor abilities through practice and instruction in a variety of movement activities.

Perceptual-motor training programs that purport to enhance academic achievement or to promote specific readiness for schoolwork do so amid considerable controversy and lack of research support. Public testimony and opinion have served for years as the basis of support for perceptual-motor training programs. This is inadequate in today's world of accountability. But the value of perceptual-motor experiences to a

Table 13.3 Checklist of Possible Perceptual-Motor Dysfunctions

1. Has trouble holding or maintaining balance._____
2. Appears clumsy._____
3. Cannot carry body well in motion._____
4. Appears to be generally awkward in activities requiring coordination._____
5. Does not readily distinguish left from right._____
6. In locomotor skills, performs movements with more efficiency on one side than the other._____
7. Reverses letters and numbers with regularity._____
8. Is unable to hop or skip properly._____
9. Has difficulty making changes in movement._____
10. Has difficulty performing combinations of simple movements._____
11. Has difficulty in gauging space with respect to the body, and collides with objects and other children._____
12. Tends to be accident-prone._____
13. Has poor hand-eye coordination._____
14. Has difficulty handling the simple tools of physical education (beanbags, balls, and other objects that involve a visual-motor relationship)._____
15. Has persistent poor general appearance._____
    (a) Shirt tail always out._____
    (b) Shoes constantly untied._____
    (c) Fly constantly unzipped._____
    (d) Socks bagged around ankles._____
    (e) Hair uncombed._____
16. Is inattentive._____
17. Does not follow directions; is able to follow verbal but not written directions, or vice versa._____
18. Has speech difficulties._____
    (a) Talks too loudly._____
    (b) Talks too softly._____
    (c) Slurs words._____
19. Poor body posture._____
20. Has hearing difficulties._____
    (a) Frequently turns head to one side._____
    (b) Holds or prefers one ear over the other._____
21. Has difficulty negotiating stairs._____
22. Daydreams excessively._____
23. Is excessively messy in work._____
    (a) Goes out of the lines._____
    (b) Inconsistency of letter size, etc._____
    (c) General sloppiness._____
24. Is unable to copy objects (words, numbers, letters, etc.)_____

general state of readiness should not be dismissed. Enhancement of body, spatial, directional, and temporal awareness as a means of guiding the child toward improved movement control and efficiency in fundamental movement is worthwhile. Practice in perceptual-motor activities will enhance perceptual-motor abilities. Whether these abilities have a direct effect on academic performance is questionable. One can be assured, however, that they do play an important role in developing and refining the child's movement abilities.

A comparison of the Phases of Motor Development with Kephart's developmental sequence and Piaget's cognitive phases of development was presented in Table 13.2. Careful review of these models reveals the interrelated nature of the perceptual, motor, and cognitive processes. The magnitude of this relationship and the conditions necessary for improved functioning in each area await further well-controlled scientific research.

CHAPTER CONCEPTS

13.1 Development of perceptual abilities depends, in part, on movement.

13.2 All voluntary movement involves an element of perception.

13.3 Perceptual and motor abilities do not necessarily develop at the same time and at the same rate.

13.4 Vision is the primary perceptual modality. The auditory, olfactory, and gustatory modalities are important but have not been studied as closely as visual perception.

13.5 Visual, tactile, and kinesthetic perception are of particular importance to the movement behavior of the child.

13.6 The extent of the role of movement in visual perceptual development is unknown. Movement has been shown as a sufficient condition for developing selected visual perceptual abilities, but it has not been proved necessary.

13.7 The child restricted or behind in perceptual development often encounters problems developing perceptual-motor abilities.

13.8 Practice in perceptual-motor activities will enhance perceptual-motor abilities.

13.9 There is insufficient evidence to support the claim that practice in perceptual-motor activities will enhance academic achievement.

13.10 Bodily, spatial, directional, and temporal awareness are four perceptual-motor components that may be enhanced through quality developmental physical education programs.

13.11 Perceptual-motor programs may be thought of as readiness and remedial in nature. Ample testimony is available to support both, but research evidence is lacking.

13.12 Both formal and informal assessment instruments have been devised to assess perceptual-motor abilities. These subjective instruments must be thought of only in terms of providing clues to possible developmental difficulties and not as a means of labeling children.

TERMS TO REMEMBER

Visual-Motor Adjustment
Perception
Visual Perception
Static Visual Acuity
Dynamic Visual Acuity
Figure-Ground Perception
Depth Perception
Monocular Depth Cues
Binocular Depth Cues
Retinal Disparity
Visual-Motor Coordination
Visual Tracking
Object Interception
Coincidence-Anticipation
Perceptual-Motor
Sensory Input
Sensory Integration
Motor Interpretation

Movement Activation
Feedback
Temporal World
Spatial World
Body Awareness
Spatial Awareness
Egocentric Localization
Objective Localization
Directional Awareness
Laterality
Directionality
Temporal Awareness
Rhythm
Perceptual-Motor Training
Readiness Development Programs
Concept Development Programs
Concept Reinforcement Programs
Remedial Training Programs

CRITICAL READINGS

Bower, T. G. R. (1977). *The Perceptual World of the Child.* Cambridge, MA: Harvard University Press.
Sage, G. H. (1984). *Motor Learning and Control: A Neuropsychological Approach.* Dubuque, IA: Wm. C. Brown, (Chapter 9).
Williams, H. G. (1983). *Perceptual and Motor Development.* Englewood Cliffs, NJ: Prentice-Hall, (Chapter 4).

14

Childhood Self-Concept Development

CHAPTER COMPETENCIES

Upon Completion of This Chapter You Should Be Able To:

* List and describe sociocultural correlates that may affect motor development.

• Distinguish similarities, differences, and relationships among various terms used in the study of self concept.

• Describe the developmental aspects of self-concept.

• Demonstrate how movement competence is related to self-esteem.

• Analyze similarities and differences of movement competence on social status in males and females.

• List the consequences of a negative self-concept.

• Propose means of enhancing self-esteem through movement.

• Describe problems associated with assessing self-concept.

Do you remember when you were a child with nothing to do but play for hours and hours each day? Do you remember the excitement of that first climb to the top of the monkey bars, your first successful two-wheeler ride, or your first swim all the way across the pool? We all can remember how good it felt as children to succeed and can probably remember a time or two when we did not. Those childhood successes and failures may seem remote and meaningless to us now, but they once were important events in our lives that had an influence on what and who we are today. Many of these events centered around our early play experiences, because how children feel about themselves is greatly determined by their play experiences, both successful and unsuccessful.

Children are active, energetic, emerging beings. Much of their life is spent in play and in active exploration of their ever-expanding world. The so-called play world of children occupies a large portion of their day and is of central importance to them. It is an important avenue by which children come to learn more about themselves, their bodies, and their potential for movement. The development of many basic affective concepts have their roots in the carefree, exhilarating world of play.

Self-concept is an important aspect of children's affective behavior that is influenced through the world of games, play, and vigorous movement. Because the establishment of a stable, positive self-concept is so crucial to effective functioning in our lives, its development is too crucial to be left to chance. The important contribution that movement and vigorous physical activity can make to forming a positive self-concept should not be overlooked; we should be genuinely interested in the development of a good self-concept in our children. In the past, the important link between physical activity and self-concept has often been given only lip service. In this chapter we will examine self-concept development and the potential for movement to enhance self-concept.

WHAT IS SELF-CONCEPT?

The topic of "self" has been a central focus of the psycho-social literature for almost one hundred years. The now classic work of William James (1890/1963) represents the underpinnings upon which much, if not most, study of the developing self is based. In self study, a variety of terms have been used with "self" as a hyphenated prefix (Figure 14.1). As a result, there has been considerable confusion over meanings, similarities, and differences. For our purposes we will attempt to clarify these often subtle differences prior to viewing the role of movement in the establishment of a positive view of self. It should be noted that there is a considerable overlap and cross-use among these terms as they are commonly used in the literature today.

Self-concept, as used here, is the umbrella term under which several other variations of self are categorized. Self-concept is generally viewed as one's awareness of personal characteristics, attributes, and limitations, and the way in which these qualities are both like and unlike others. Self-concept is one's value-free view of self. On the other hand, *self-esteem* is the value one attaches to his or her unique characteristics, attributes, and limitations. Weiss (1987, p. 88) indicated that "self-esteem represents the evaluation and effective component of one's self-concept: that is, it refers to the qualitative judgements and feelings attached to the descrip-

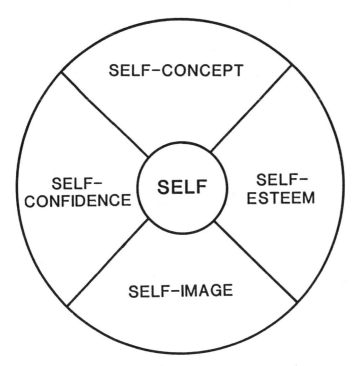

Figure 14.1 Terms commonly used to describe one's perception of self

tions one assigns to self." Whereas self-concept is merely one's perception of self, self-esteem is the value one places on those perceptions.

James was the first to attempt to decipher the elusive meaning of self-esteem. His now famous formula concluded that one's feelings of self-worth (self-esteem) are equal to the ratio of one's accomplishments to one's potential for achievement (i.e., self-esteem = $\frac{success}{potential}$). Therefore, the closer the success-to-potential ratio is to 1.0, the nearer one is to his or her ideal self. Perhaps Coopersmith (1967, p. 5) defined self-esteem best when he stated that "self-esteem is a personal judgement of worthiness that is expressed in the attitudes the individual holds toward himself." Although linked, self-esteem is not the same as self-confidence.

Self-confidence is a term used to denote one's belief in his or her ability to carry out some form of mental, physical, or emotional task. It is one's anticipated ability to master particular challenges and to overcome obstacles or difficulties. Self-confident persons are ones who believe they can cause things to happen in accordance with their desires. Self-confidence as used here means the same as Bandura's (1982, p. 39) term "self-efficacy." Namely, "the conviction that one can successfully execute the behavior required to produce the [desired] outcome."

It is important to note that self-confidence may be unrelated to self-esteem in some situations. For example, one may not have a sufficient level of self-confidence to attempt a difficult or potentially dangerous gymnastics trick but may possess a high level of self-esteem. In support of this notion Dickstein (1977, p. 13) stated that "self-confidence involves carrying off a particular task or fostering a role. Level of self-confidence at any one moment may be unrelated to an overall level of self-esteem." One must conclude, however, that the perceived importance of the activity or task by the individual or by significant others (peers, parents, teachers, coaches, etc.) may actually forge a link between self-confidence and self-esteem (Dickstein, 1977). If the task is viewed as important to self and to others, then competence in executing the task will have an impact on self-esteem. Therefore, the term "competence" becomes an important construct in the development of self-esteem.

The notion of *competence* as related to self-concept was first introduced by White (1959) and later expanded upon by Coopersmith (1977), and Harter (1978). Competence may be viewed as one's actual ability to meet particular achievement demands. Competence refers to one's level of mastery which may range from incompetent to varying degrees of competent. Competence, then, is an important factor in the development of one's self-concept. More specifically, the perception of one's competence (*perceived competence*) in a given situation and its perceived importance may have a significant impact on one's actual competence, self-confidence, self-esteem, and self-concept (Figure 14.2).

SELF-CONCEPT: GENERAL OR SPECIFIC?

A question that has intrigued theorists and researchers for decades is the general nature or specificity of one's self-concept. That is, is self-concept a global trait, or can it be differentiated into various components? A strong case can be made for both views, and research can be cited to support both positions. Therefore, it seems entirely possible that one possesses both a differentiated concept of self and a global self-concept. In support of this Rosenberg (1979, p. 20), in insisting that the two are not identical, stated that: "Both exist within the individual's phenomenal field as separate and distinguishable entities and each can and should be studied in its own right." Rosenberg (1982, p. 536), in a later paper, makes the telling point that: "Although widely overlooked in self-esteem studies, it is fairly obvious that a persons' global self-esteem is not based solely on his assessment of his constituent qualities. His self-esteem is based on his self-assessments of qualities that count." In other words, global self-concept is the product of one's perception of his or her

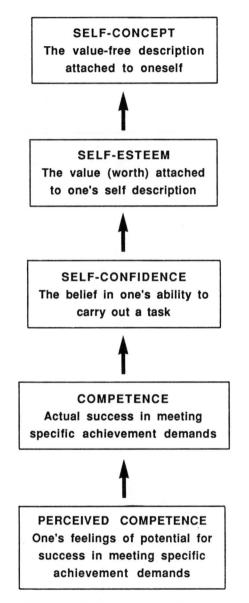

**A HIERARCHIAL VIEW
OF SELF-CONCEPT DEVELOPMENT**

SELF-CONCEPT
The value-free description
attached to oneself

SELF-ESTEEM
The value (worth) attached
to one's self description

SELF-CONFIDENCE
The belief in one's ability to
carry out a task

COMPETENCE
Actual success in meeting
specific achievement demands

PERCEIVED COMPETENCE
One's feelings of potential for
success in meeting specific
achievement demands

Figure 14.2 A hierarchial view of self-concept development

competence in areas that have personal meaning. It is unaffected by one's self-assessment of competence in areas that have little or no personal meaning. It follows, therefore, that if being good at games, play activities, and sports is important to children, then success in these areas will have an impact on their global self-concept. If, however, these attributes are not perceived as being personally meaningful, then they will have little impact.

Today, in North American society, being good in games, play activities, and sports is of high positive value to both boys and girls. Competence in these areas is important in terms of social acceptance and status within the peer group (Anastasiow, 1965; Greendorfer and Lewko, 1978). Moreover, adults frequently give children the impression that their competence in physical endeavors is closely linked to their acceptance and value within the family (Snyder and Spreitzer, 1973) or team (Greendorfer and Lewko, 1978; Snyder and Spreitzer, 1979) unit. It is reasonable to conclude that, in a society which places high positive value on success in games and sport, one of the important component parts of global self-concept is *movement competence* and that movement competence plays a crucial role in positive self-esteem development. Harter (1978, 1981) and Harter and Connell (1984), in studying the developmental aspects of self-concept, attempted to isolate three self-evaluative dimensions of competence. The Perceived Competence Scale for Children (Harter, 1982; Harter and Pike, 1984) subdivides perceived competence into cognitive and physical (movement) domains, along with a measure of social acceptance and general self-worth. Using this scale, Harter (1982) found that children in grades 3 through 9 made clear distinctions among categories. Harter and Pike (1984) did not find the same to be true with younger children (ages 4 to 7). These children tended to lump cognitive and physical competence together into a category of "general competence" and to view social acceptance (by the peer group and mother) as important. Also, they did not possess a concept of general self-worth. It appears, therefore, that the notion of movement competence has significant implications for children from about the third grade onward. Prior to that time, children tend to view themselves as either competent or incompetent with little distinction between the physical and cognitive domains.

What makes people different from each other and uniquely themselves is their self-concept and view of the world as they know it. The sum of their experiences and their feelings about these experiences contributes to this mental model. We find out about ourselves in many ways. By choosing, trying things out, experimenting, and exploring, we discover who we are, what we can do, and what we cannot do. Not only do we discover who we are, but, through our experiences, contribute to the making or formation of our unique identity. Each new choice adds something to our backlog of experience and hence to our world and to ourselves.

DEVELOPMENTAL ASPECTS OF SELF-CONCEPT

Self-concept is learned, and its development begins at least at birth. Some authorities argue that the emotional state of the expectant mother, ranging from a relaxed, happy pregnancy to one that is tension-filled and traumatic, may have a dramatic effect on the unborn child. Yamamoto (1972, pp. 181-182) stated that:

> Some studies have suggested that stress experiences by a pregnant mother can alter the movements of the fetus from normal to hyperactive—the mother should know that a physically healthy child has a greater chance for adequate psychological development, since the concept of a child's physical self plays an important part in the entirety of the self-concept.

The early months of life mark the first tangible beginnings of self-concept development. The tenderness, warmth, and love displayed between parent and child convey the first feelings of "I am loved" and "I am valued." The infant's sense of well-being is affected by the emotional state of the parent and attention to his or her physical needs. The fulfillment of psychological needs is just as important; the infant needs to establish a sense of trust, security, recognition, and love. Trust is a basic issue to be resolved in the early mother-infant relationship. Mothers and fathers create a sense of trust in their children by combining sensitive care of their baby's needs with a firm sense of personal trustworthiness. Erikson (1963, 1980) was among the first to recognize the importance of establishing a sense of trust during the early months of life. His stage of "trust versus mistrust" is rooted in the child's developing a sense of being loved and valued in a world that has constancy and permanence.

The toddler experiences the satisfaction of mastering the art of walking succssfully or solving a problem with a new toy. This development of a sense of autonomy is an important facilitator of a positive self-concept, influenced greatly by adults central in the life of the child. These individuals have a unique opportunity to selectively reinforce the child's learning about herself or himself. This is done through consistent acceptance, with respect, concern, and provision for freedom and independence within carefully defined limits. Much of what the young child learns is imitative, and this learning is not restricted to overt action. Feelings and attitudes can also be learned through imitation. As a result, the type of model that central adults project determines many of the attitudes and feelings that the child develops. It should be noted that published studies on self-concept development in young children are quite rare and that problems in theory and methodology make generalizations from those that do exist unwise (Wylie, 1979).

Gradually, the child develops a greater sense of independence. During the sixth or seventh year, the child begins to shift his or her frame of reference from the home and family to the school and teacher. The sphere of "significant others" that have an impact on the developing self expands. Teachers and the peer group begin to exert greater influence. The teacher becomes a primary model for the child, and there is a great desire to please. Martinek and Zaichkowsky (1977) found that the teacher's expectations of the child's performance level had a definite impact on self-concept from the second through the sixth grades. A study by Zaichkowsky et al. (1975) revealed that the teacher's level of expectancy for children in a physical activity was positively correlated with self-concept scores. Furthermore, Schempp et al (1983) found that an atmosphere which encouraged children's decision-making promoted positive self-concept and attitude development as well as creativity and motor skills. In other words, those expected to do well who were also involved in decision-making had higher self-concepts than those expected to do poorly who were not involved in decision-making. The implications of these findings are enormous when applied to the teacher/learner, or coach/athlete dyad.

Older children feel good about the accomplishment of new and difficult tasks and the newly-found sense of independence that accompanies performing meaningful work and earning money. The thoughtful parent recognizes the importance of the peer group at this level and the importance of assisting in the gradual establishment of a sense of mature independence. Self-concept can be enhanced continually throughout life through the pride of accomplishment and the sense of being needed, loved, and valued.

Our conviction of personal worth and effectiveness develops chiefly through successful experiences in coping, according to Maynard (1973). For one to have confidence he must be able to cope. One must be willing to accept himself along with others who are different. Children who cope are adaptable rather than rigid in their behavior. They are diligent, can concentrate on a task, and can work through difficulties. Confidence in oneself is developed both through the joy of finding what one does well and of doing anything really well. Movement skill fitness development are important avenues by which self-confidence may be enhanced. It is especially important for most children, because much of their daily life experiences are centered around the need for efficient and effective movement.

Movement plays an important role in enhancing or limiting self-concept development in children, because it is a central focus in their lives. High positive value is placed by both boys and girls on competence in physical activities, and this is an essential factor in global self-esteem (Harter, 1982; Weiss, 1987).

SOCIAL STATUS AND MOVEMENT COMPETENCE

The relationship between children's social status and their movement competence has been a subject of interest to researchers for many years. Numerous studies point out that there is a link between high positive peer group acceptance and ability in games and sports, especially in boys. Tuddenham (1951) pointed out that central in the boys' constellation of values is athletic skill, predicated upon motor coordination, strength, size, and physical maturity.

Skill level is often controlled by factors that are outside the child's influence. Such things as physical stature, health-related conditions, and lack of experience and quality instruction make it impossible for many children to meet the values of their peer group. As a result, they often suffer feelings of inferiority, rejection, and poor self-image. Tuddenham (1951) stated that personal insecurity and social maladjustment often have their roots in this area.

When considering the effect of skill level on the social status of young girls, the available literature presents a somewhat different picture. The results of Tuddenham's (1951) classic study indicated that girls are less dependent than boys on the possession of specific physical skills. Cratty (1967) indicated, however, that it seems important for girls to be moderately skillful in motor performance between the approximate ages of 5 and 14 years, but after that superior motor performance in other than a few "acceptable" sports (golf, tennis, horseback riding, etc.) can detract from a girl's popularity. The tremendous changes in the role of women in our society and the recent surge of interest in all forms of competitive athletics for girls and women may soon prove Tuddenham's and Cratty's researches to be generally outdated. The upsurge of interest in participation in traditionally male activities, along with increased interscholastic competition for girls, has cleared the way for change in the social status of the physically active female. The majority of literature has shown little in the way of gender differences between boys and girls in terms of self-concept. (Felker, 1974; Erhartic, 1977; Martinek and Zaichowsky, 1977; Piers, 1969). But Harter, (1982) using the Perceived Competence Scale for Children, found that boys' perceptions of their competence in sports and outdoor games was greater than girls'.

The playground, gymnasium, and play environment of children provide an excellent medium for positive self-concept development. A child's perceived competence as well as actual competence in the physical, cognitive, and affective domains has been theorized to be an important facilitator of positive self-concept development (Harter, 1978). With regard to the physical domain, Roberts et al. (1981) tested fourth and fifth graders and Harter (1982) tested sixth graders that were either nonparticipants or participants in organized youth sport programs. The results of their independent investigations indicate that participants perceive themselves as more competent in games and sports than nonparticipants. Ulrich (1987), however, found somewhat different results in her study of younger children (grades K-4). She compared children's perceptions of physical competence, their actual motor competence, and their participation in youth sport programs. Her results revealed that the perceived physical competence of young children was not significantly related to their participation in organized sport. Their actual motor competence, however, was significantly related to sport participation. It seems, therefore, that, whereas older children are clearly influenced by their perception of physical competence and participation, younger children are not. Reasons for this difference are yet unexplained.

CONSEQUENCES OF A POOR SELF-CONCEPT

A poor self-concept is reflected in the feelings of "I can't," "I'm always wrong," or "I'm no good." Children who feel bad about themselves and the world they know are not likely to feel better about the part of the world they do not know. As a result, they often reflect the attitude of caring little to explore that world. This is simply because it does not look inviting and appears hostile and full of possibilities for humiliation and defeat. Holt (1970) makes the point that this hostile and threatening new world becomes one that does not lure the child out but thrusts in on him or her, invading those few fairly safe places where even a small sense of who and where he is are threatened. Children with a negative self-concept come to view the world they do not know as even worse than the world they are familiar with.

Children who feel themselves to be of little worth due to repeated failure often fall back on the protective strategy of deliberate failure. Deliberate failure serving as a self-protective device can be explained by the principle that you cannot fall out of bed when you are sleeping on the floor. In other words, children who view themselves as complete failures will not even be tempted to try. They avoid the "agony of defeat" because they feel that the "thrill of victory" is a hopeless cause.

Children with poor self-concepts are also negatively affected by what they think others think of them (Yawkey, 1980). Children, as well as adults, tend to live up to the expectations of others, or at least to what these expectations are perceived to be. Teachers are of tremendous importance in shaping children's basic attitudes toward themselves in relation to school. Durng the elementary years a significant correlation exists between a child's perception of his teachers' feelings toward him and his own self-image. Teachers who place a great deal of emphasis and value on self-concept tend to be associated with students who hold a positive view of themselves. The use of such terms as "stupid," "dumb," "always wrong," "bad boy/girl," "trouble-maker," and "lousy" all have tremendous impact on children. These spoken words, as well as our unspoken indications of disapproval, disgust, anger, and surprise, have an effect on what children think others think of them. Given enough negative information, the child soon learns the role that he or she feels expected to play. Children with a negative self-image tend to live up to their perceived negative role. As a result, a cycle of failure and perceived expectations of failure is established.

Children with a poor self-image often are very little cheered when now and then they do succeed. Their perception of themselves as nonachievers and the idea that others perceive them in the same manner is a difficult cycle to break when success is infrequent. This may be explained with the analogy of the person who is usually ill and suddenly starts to feel well. Unlike the usually healthy people who think they will soon be well, the sick person thinks that this good feeling surely cannot last. It is much the same with children. Even when the normal pattern of failure is broken occasionally with success, they still have the feeling that it cannot last and that things will certainly go wrong soon.

The influence of a poor self-concept on the learning process can be tremendous. Brookover et al. (1967) concluded from their extensive research on self-concept and achievement that the assumption that human ability is the most important factor in achievement is questionable and that the student's attitudes limit the level of achievement in school. Students' perceptions of themselves as "learners" or "nonlearners" often have a dramatic effect on high or low academic achievement. Lecky (1945) demonstrated that low achievement is often due to children's definitions of themselves as nonlearners because they resist learning when it is, in their view, inconsistent for them to learn. Children who feel they cannot achieve experience a situation in which their actual ability to achieve is reduced or negated. On the other hand, children with a success-oriented outlook find that they can plunge into a project or take on a new challenge with little past experience and more often than not be successful.

In summary, the consequences of a poor self-concept can be devastating. Children with low self-esteem often display little interest in their expanding world. They often fail deliberately and perform poorly as both a protective device and an attempt to live up to perceived expectations. Children with poor self-concepts are little cheered by occasional successes. They often view themselves as nonlearners and perform poorly academically while possessing average or above-average intelligence. The consequences of negative feelings toward oneself are tremendous. They are associated with high anxiety, underachievement, behavior problems, learning difficulties, and delinquency. The establishment of a stable, positive self-concept is too important to be left to change. The role of movement in self-concept development must not be minimized.

MOVEMENT AND SELF-CONCEPT ENHANCEMENT

Limited research has been conducted in the area of movement and self-concept. It has long been considered a "sloppy" area in which to do study, for a variety of reasons. First, it is difficult to isolate the possible variables that influence the self. Second, the criterion measures of self-concept that are used are often suspect in terms of validity. Third, the manner of construction of numerous tests has often been "weird," according to McCandless (1976). Research in the area of movement and self-concept is now beginning to reflect a concern for these difficulties and to deal effectively with them within the scope of the particular investigation. Several investigations into the effects of movement on the self-concept of children are just coming into view.

Martinek and Zaichkowsky (1977) found that children given a chance to share in the decision-making process concerning the conduct of a physical education class actually developed more positive self-concepts. Erhartic (1977) and Martinek and Zaichkowsky (1977) also found that there is little correlation between children's motor abilities and their self-concepts. Ulrich (1987) found similar results.

Wallace and Stuff (1973) administered a perceptual-motor training program conducted by classroom teachers over a one-year period for thirty minutes per day. The most frequently reported change by the teachers was in behavior areas. The data from the rating scales that were dispensed revealed a significant positive change in self-concept.

Exceptional children were studied by Johnson et al. (1968) in a clinical physical education program. A specially constructed self-concept scale was administered before and after the six-week, hour-per-day program. The results of the experiment revealed that the discrepancy between ideal self and actual self decreased in several areas. The children showed a great desire to work in groups and an increased willingness to be with certain family members.

Clifford and Clifford (1967) reviewed the effects of the Outward

Bound Program in Colorado. The stated purpose of the program was to build physical stamina and push each individual to his or her physical limit. Self-concept measures dealing with ideal self (what I would like to be) and actual self (what I am) were administered before and after the month-long program. At the conclusion of the program, the gap between ideal self scores and actual self scores was lessoned with a positive change occurring in the actual self-concept.

Collingswood and Willett (1971), working with obese teenage boys, found that a specially designed gymnasium and swimming program had positive effects on self-concept. Postsession scores of self-image were significantly increased, and the ideal self versus actual self discrepancy significantly decreased.

In a study to investigate the influence of competitive and noncompetitive programs of physical education on body image and self-concept, Read (1968) found significant differences in self-concept scores between those identified as "consistent winners" and "consistent losers." The consistent winners had significantly higher self-concept scores than did the consistent losers. The subjects who were neither consistent winners nor losers did not drastically change in body image or self-concept.

Although the above-cited research investigations pointed to a relationship between improved movement skills and an enhanced view of self, none demonstrated a causal relationship between skill improvement and self-concept enhancement. The question still remains: does increased competence lead to improved self-esteem? Or, does one's level of self-esteem influence achievement? Physical educators and coaches, for the most part, have adopted the behavioristic point of view that improved levels of movement competence lead to enhanced self-esteem.

MOVEMENT TECHNIQUES FOR ENHANCING SELF-ESTEEM

Children who have difficulty performing the many fundamental skills basic to proficient performance in games and sports encounter repeated failure in their everyday play experiences. As a result, they often encounter difficulties in establishing a stable view of themselves as worthy beings. Taylor (1980, p. 133) stated that "one of the best and easiest pathways to a strong self-concept is through play. Play offers opportunities to assist the child in all areas of development. Its importance can be found in how he [the child] perceives himself, his body, his abilities and his relationships with others." The question now becomes: (1) What can we do? and (2) How can we utilize the movement activities of children and aid them in the formation of a stable, positive self-concept?

During the past several years, this author has conducted a motor development program designed to make positive contributions to the self-concept of children from ages 4 to 12 years. The four-day-per-week "Challengers" program caters to children who are experiencing difficulty in their everyday play world. A large percentage of the children are referred to the program because of problems in school adjustment, peer relations, self-confidence, and emotional immaturity. The others do not possess any apparent difficulties in these areas. The results of the informal research show positive increases (as measured by the Piers-Harris Children's Self-Concept Scale [Piers, 1969]) in self-concept in a significant majority of the children taking part in the program. Throughout the operation of the "Challengers" program, a concentrated effort has been made to apply common-sense principles through movement to the enhancement of the developing self. The following paragraphs are a delineation of these principles.

Success

The most important thing we can do is help children develop a proper perspective on success and failure in their daily lives. Because of the egocentric nature of children, it is very difficult for them to accept both success *and* failure. Success is that feeling of "I can," "I did it," or "Look at me" that we love to see in children. It is the sense of accomplishment that accompanies mastering a new skill, executing a good move, or making a basket. Failure is that feeling of "I can't," "I don't know how," or "I am always wrong." It is the feeling of frustration and hopelessness that often follows failure to either master a skill or execute a move.

We need to help children develop a balance between success and failure. We need to bolster their sense of self-worth so that, when things go poorly and they fail to achieve something, they will not be completely defeated. This backlog of successful experiences will help develop that "I can" attitude. Success is very important, particularly at the initial stages of learning. We need only look at ourselves and our tendency to continue those activities we are successful in. This basic principle of learning theory is applicable to both children and adults. We need to take the importance of success into consideration when working with young children by using teaching methods that emphasize success.

The use of problem solving or guided discovery in the learning of new movement skills enables all children to experiment and explore their movement potentials. It enables the children to become involved in the "process" of learning instead of being solely concerned with the "product." In other words, it is a child-centered approach that allows a vareity of solutions or correct answers. Both teacher and children are more concerned about individual solutions to the problem than about finding the best way. The astute teacher of young children recognizes that there is no best way of performing at this level of development. The astute teacher is more interested in helping children gain greater knowledge of their bodies and how they move, and in fostering more mature patterns of movement. For example, the teacher may structure a movement problem or challenge such as, "How can you balance on three body parts?" or "Who can balance on three body parts?" The number of possible solutions is great and so is the range of difficulty. As a result, several solutions are possible and all children gain increased knowledge of how they can move and balance their bodies. The teacher, through questioning or movement challenges, also avoids imposing a predetermined model of what the performance should be and how it should look.

Individualizing instruction is another way of emphasizing success for each child. Individualized instruction takes into account the uniqueness of each learner and provides all with opportunities to achieve at their own particular level of ability. Although it is often difficult to put individualization into practice because of large classes, limited staff, time, and facilities, teachers should try whenever possible. The typical nursery school program does a tremendous job of individualizing instruction through incorporation of an open classroom approach with a variety of interest centers. Too often, however, on entering the first- or second-grade classroom, children are faced with the rigid structure of the traditional classroom and a gymnasium program that assumes all children to be at the same level in interests, abilities, and motivation for learning. The unquestionable fact is that all children are not "typical" first-graders. Within any given class, the children can be functioning at levels passing through both ends of the spectrum of that particular grade level in cognitive, affective, and motor abilities. Greater attention to recognizing individual needs and interests and abilities will do much to strengthen the success potential of each child.

Traditional methods of teaching movement are valuable, especially at higher skill levels, but the teacher often dominates and requires that all students perform at a certain level or emulate a particular model of performance (Schempp et al. 1983). Some children may have considerable difficulty accomplishing the desired level of performance. Teacher-dominated methods are often limited in providing success-oriented experiences for everyone. Although these methods should be a part of the movement activity program, they should not be stressed too early in the learning process. They should attempt to allow individual differences in readiness rates and abilities for learning new movement skills.

Movement programs that make use of problem-solving approaches and recognize the value of individualizing instruction whenever possible make positive contributions to self-concept development. But what actually is involved in using these success-oriented approaches?

Through the use of developmentally appropriate movement experiences that are challenging and properly sequenced, we can help children. We can also help in the formation of a good self-image by helping them establish reasonable expectations of their abilities and by communicating our expectations (Figure 14.3).

Developmentally Appropriate Activities

Children are not miniature adults ready to be programmed to the whims and wishes of adults. They are growing, developing beings with needs, interests, and capabilities that are quite different from those of adults. Too often, we fall into the trap of trying to develop miniature athletes out of 6- and 7-year-olds without first developing the children's fundamental movement abilities. Too often, we force children to specialize in the development of their movement abilities at an early age. They become involved in competitive athletics before they are ready to handle the physical and emotional demands that competition can bring. Competition is not an evil or something to be excluded from the lives of children, but it must be kept within the proper perspective. Coaches and parents need to be fully cognizant of the children they are dealing with and the

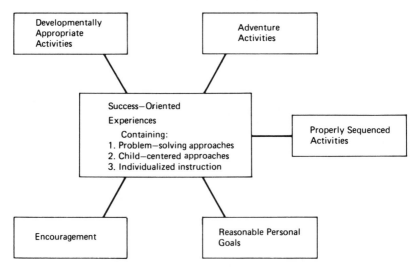

Figure 14.3 Five important factors to consider when utilizing success-oriented experiences to enhance self-concept development

fact that winning is not everything, as proponents of that often-quoted phrase "Winning isn't everything, it's the only thing" philosophy would have us believe. Parents and coaches must have as their objective the balanced, wholesome, and healthful development of children. The needs, interests, and capabilities of each child must be carefully considered. Developmentally appropriate activities must be sought as means of aiding children in establishing a realistic concept of their abilities.

Tasks need to be challenging, yet within the ability level of the child. This balance between difficulty and challenge was noted by Harter (1974), who coined the term *"optimal challenge."* An optimal challenge is one in which the task difficulty is carefully matched to one's developmental level. Weiss (1987, p. 97) indicated that: "Tasks that are too difficult result in frustration and anxiety, whereas those not challenging enough result in boredom and reduced motivation." Furthermore, the challenge has to be one that is valued or respected by the child, otherwise little sense of accomplishment will result, a fact which Coopersmith (1967, p. 242) noted when he stated that: "The degree of self-esteem an individual actually expressed would thus reflect the extent to which his success approached his aspirations in areas of performance that were personally valued."

Adventure Activities

We can have an impact on the self-concept of children in the area of adventure or pseudo-dangerous activities. Weissbourd (1987) noted that a positive sense of self is linked to the child being given opportunities to be adventurous in exploring his or her environment. Children need to experience the thrill offered by climbing, balancing, and crawling through objects. They need the feeling of mastery that comes from succeeding at activities that challenge their courage and imagination. They need to experience the adventure of hanging by their knees, balancing on a beam, climbing a ladder, or crawling through a tunnel. Adventure playgrounds and child-oriented play spaces play an important role in the child's search of self (Bruya, 1988; Moore et al., 1988).

The teacher, through voice inflection and the use of the young child's imagination, can also help create an atmosphere of challenge and adventure. Imaginary obstacles may be put in the path of successful completion of an activity. Such things as "sharks" beneath the balance beam, which has been transformed into a "narrow log" across a "shark-infested pond," or a story play depicting a bear hunt, or a trip to the circus stimulate children's imaginations. Through adventure activities, both real and imagined, children have an opportunity to learn more about their own bodies and have the thrill of successfully overcoming a challenge.

Sequencing of Tasks

A third factor involved in using a success-oriented approach to enhancing self-concept is the sequencing and difficulty of a movement task. The proper sequencing of movement activities is crucial in determining a child's sense of success or failure. For example, it seems perfectly logical to first learn a tripod or frog stand followed by a headstand, and then to learn a handstand, rather than proceeding in the reverse order. Yet we often do just that when, as adults, we try to make miniature athletes out of 6- and 7-year-old children. Too often, parents and teachers neglect the development of fundamental movement abilities before proceeding to higher-level skills. Instead of looking at the development of movement skills from the point of view of the child, we too often look at movement from our point of view, namely as athletes. We skip the basics and go directly to high-level skill development. It is much better to begin at a lower level where the chances for experiencing success are greater, and then to proceed to develop skill upon skill in a logical sequential progression. Success at the initial stages of learning will not only encourage continued performance, but will tend to generate success at later stages. Children who attempt a difficult task without the proper basic skills may not succeed and may give up entirely. It is important that we analyze the movement activities children engage in and determine logical sequences for accomplishing them.

Coakley (1987, p. 54) noted that when children are involved in physical activities they cite four facets of interest:

- action
- personal involvement in the action
- close scores and challenges matching their level of skill
- opportunities to reaffirm relationships with friends

Strikingly absent from this list is the winning or losing of the contest. Children are interested in the game for the sake of game, challenges and fun, not for who wins or loses. In fact, Coakely suggested that children will readily accept playing with "handicaps" in order to keep games close and interesting. Such modifications as playing left handed or counting to ten before rushing the passer serve to equate those of greater or lesser ability levels. Those with greater skill levels are challenged to do their best with an increased level of difficulty, while those who possess low levels of skill can compete on equal footing with their peers. It is important to keep this concept in mind when establishing developmentally appropriate activities, that the game be kept just that, a game.

Exactly scorable tasks such as archery or bowling may be difficult to deal with in the initial stages of learning unless modifications and provisions are made for success-oriented experiences. Cratty (1968, p. 30), stated that "tasks which have performance limits (e.g., a bullseye in archery) will be more likely to produce feelings of failure when projected goals are not achieved." It would be better, in archery for example, to eliminate the target during the initial stages of learning, or to enlarge it or move it closer in order to maximize the opportunities for success.

Caution should also be taken not to introduce competition too early in the learning process. Because competition necessitates winners and losers, it gives too accurate an indication of relative success or failure during the early phases of learning. It may be better to postpone competitive situations until the child can make a sound appraisal of his or her ability.

Reasonable Expectations

A fourth area in which we can have an influence on children's developing self is in helping them establish reasonable expectations of their abilities. This is especially true with young children because of their black and white world of good or bad and right or wrong that allows little room for anything but these two extremes. It is important that we help children develop an attitude about personal success that is based on the extent to which they feel they have reached some goal and not on the absolute scores obtained. Children need to learn how to set reasonable goals for themselves, and we can help them by providing goals not so high that attaining them is unrealistic, but high enough to ensure quality effort and a reasonable chance for success. For example, lowering the basket or reducing the size of the basketball will provide children with more opportunities for success than insisting on the use of a regulation ball and putting the standard at the regulation 10-foot height. It must be remembered, however, that once reasonable success through quality effort is ensured, new goals need to be established. This must be done in order to keep the activity challenging. Frost (1972, p. 21), reinforces this by stating that "when tasks are too easy and success too cheap, little development takes place. When tasks are too difficult and achievement impossible, frustration and reinforcement of a negative self-concept are likely to follow."

Encouragement

A fifth way to influence the developing self is by communicating our expectations to the child. We must communicate how we feel about the child's accomplishments. Bloom (1985), in a study that examined the environments of Olympic swimmers, found that the predominant feature in their future success was that when they were young, they were provided with a great deal of encouragement by their families and coaches. Self-concept development is based in part on what we think others think of us. For children, these significant others center around the home and school. It is important to use positive encouragement in order to communicate our feelings about their accomplishments, whether they be large or small. Positive encouragement must be used judiciously because children will soon read the meaninglessness of inappropriate praise. We can communicate our feelings to children by praising a job well done with a pat on the back or a smile. We need to communicate the feeling of "you are loved" and "you are worthwhile." One way to encourage these feelings is to recognize that it is often not so much what we say to children that influences their feelings about themselves as how we treat them. Children value themselves to the degree that they are valued. The way we feel about our children actually instills (or destroys) self-confidence and a sense of self-worth. Children build their pictures of themselves from the words, attitudes, body language, and judgments of those around them.

By providing children with a nurturing climate of acceptance and experiences of success, negative attitudes can be changed to high self-esteem. It is important that when we do make specific statements about things that disturb us or that we dislike about a child's behavior, we restrict our comments to the behavior instead of making generalized criticism of the child as a person. For example, it is much better to say "I am worried about your difficulties with sharing" rather than "nobody likes a stingy person." Similarly, it is dangerous to label children as "stupid," "bad," or "motor moron." They often believe the labels that are attached to them and inadvertently act out their expected role. We should not link a personal lack of worth with undesirable behavior. We should not make children feel they are personally worthless just because such things as their schoolwork and sports abilities do not meet our expectations.

There is no place for devastating remarks in teacher-child communication. The teacher's role is not to injure but to prevent injury and to heal. Positive encouragement on the playground, in the classroom, and at home plays an important role in helping children develop a stable, positive self-concept.

ASSESSING SELF-CONCEPT IN CHILDREN

Problems in accurately assessing self-concept have plagued psychologists for years. The validity of a vast majority of measures of self is questionable, and the reliability of the information is often subject to criticism (Wylie, 1979). In spite of these obvious limitations, a number of self-report measures have become available in recent years. The basic assumption underlying any self-report measure is that the respondent is the only individual qualified to reveal his or her feelings and that these responses provide an accurate and truthful indication of how that person feels.

The problems that surround self-concept assessment in children are many. Zaichowsky et al. (1980, p. 157) have indicated that "attitudes toward the self do not become generalized until about 8 years of age. Up until that time they are more a function of the immediate situation." This, coupled with the additional problems of reading level, comprehension, and the testing environment makes it questionable whether the assessment of self-concept prior to ages 8 or 9 can be of practical, let alone research, value. Nevertheless, a variety of self-concept measures suitable for use with children have been devised. A list of selected self-concept measures may be found at the end of this chapter. The Perceived Competence Scales for Children devised by Harter (1982) and Harter, and Pike (1984) hold particular promise.

SUMMARY

Self-concept is an important aspect of the affective development of children. The concept that children have of themselves is based on their feelings about themselves and what they think others think of them. Their self-concept is in the developmental stages and is profoundly influenced by all that happens to them in their daily life experiences. It is important that adults make an effort to ensure the development of a positive, stable self-concept in children, because once it is firmly established, it becomes increasingly difficult to make radical changes. Combs and Snygg (1959, p. 130) have alluded to the stability of self-concept beyond its developmental stages:

> Once established in a given personality, the perceived self has a high degree of stability. The phenomenal self with the self-concept as its core represents our fundamental frame of reference, our anchor to reality; and even an unsatisfactory self-organization is likely to prove highly stable and resistant to change. This stability has been repeatedly demonstrated in modern research.

Because of the importance of vigorous play in the lives of children and the high value placed on physical ability by children and adult, movement can serve as an important facilitator of a positive self-concept. We must be sure, however, to apply sound principles of growth and development to this important task. We need to provide children with success-oriented experiences that minimize the failure potential.

In order to do this, we must employ developmentally appropriate movement experiences that are within the ability level of the individual. We must be sure that the learning of new movement tasks is properly sequenced, based on sound progressions from the simple to the complex. We must also help children establish reasonable goals for their performance within the limits of their abilities. We also must provide encouragement and incorporate adventure activities into their lives.

Although movement is only one avenue by which a positive self-concept may be fostered, we must recognize that it is an important one for most children. The development of a positive self-concept is too important to be left to chance. We must do all that we can to assure its proper development.

CHAPTER CONCEPTS

14.1 The child's self-concept begins developing at birth. Movement plays an important role in its development.

14.2 Adult expectations have a significant impact on self-concept development in children.

14.3 A negative self-concept can have devastating effects on all aspects of the child's life.

14.4 Significant others play an important role in self-concept reinforcement.

14.5 Once formulated, a negative self-concept is difficult to alter without special effects by parents, teachers, and friends in a nonthreatening environment.

14.6 Self-concept has been shown to be enhanced in children participating in success-oriented physical education programs.

14.7 Children on athletic teams identified as consistent winners tend to have higher self-concepts than children on teams identified as consistent losers.

14.8 Success-oriented experiences play an important role in developing positive self-concepts in children.

14.9 Developmentally appropriate activities, adventure activities, properly sequenced experiences, and positive reinforcement are all important factors in self-concept development.

14.10 Self-concept is difficult to measure, especially in children.

14.11 Attitudes toward oneself do not become generalized until about 8 years of age.

TERMS TO REMEMBER

Self-Concept
Self-Esteem
Self-Confidence
Competence
Perceived Competence
Movement Competence
Movement Confidence

CRITICAL READINGS

Harter, S. (1983). "Developmental Perspectives on the Self System." In, Mussen, P. H. (Ed.) *Handbook of Child Psychology*. New York: Wiley, pages 274-385.

Weiss, M. R. (1987). "Self-Esteem and Achievement in Children's Sport and Physical Activity." In, Gould, D. and Weiss, M. R. (Eds.) *Advances in Pediatric Sport Science: Volume II, Behavior Issues*, Champaign, IL: Human Kinetics.

Wylie, R. (1979). *The Self-Concept*. Lincoln, NB.: University of Nebraska Press. (Chapter 2).

SELECTED MEASURES OF SELF-CONCEPT IN CHILDREN

Harter, S. (1982). "The Perceived Competence Scale For Children." *Child Development*, 53, 87-97.

Harter, S. and Pike, R. (1984). "The Pictoral Scale of Perceived Competence for Young Children." *Child Development*, 55, 1969-1982.

Martinek, T. and Zaichkowsky, L. D. (1977). *Manual for the Martinek-Zaichkowsky Self-Concept Scale for Children*. Psychologists and Educators, Jacksonville, IL.

Piers, E. V. (1969). *Manual for the Piers-Harris Children's Self-Concept Scale*. Counselor Recordings and Tests, Nashville, TN.

SECTION IV
ADOLESCENCE

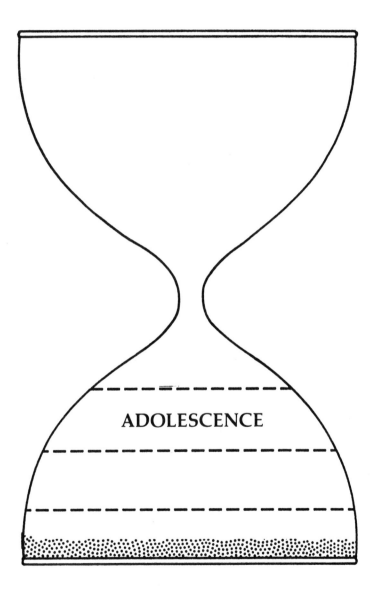

ADOLESCENCE

15

Adolescent Growth, Puberty, and Reproductive Maturity

CHAPTER COMPETENCIES

Upon Completion of This Chapter You Should Be Able To:

* Describe and interpret the normal curve and displacement and velocity graphs of human growth.

* Describe variations in biological maturity within and across genders.

* Discuss characteristics of the adolescent growth spurt.

• Analyze factors associated with the onset of puberty.

• Describe hormonal factors that impact on puberty.

• Chart the sequence of events leading to reproductive maturation.

• Discuss the concept of adolescent reproductive sterility.

• List and describe the stages of pubic hair growth and its use as a maturity assessment technique.

The period of time that makes up adolescence is affected by both biology and culture. It is affected by biology in that the end of childhood and the onset of adolescence is marked by the beginnings of sexual maturation. It is affected by culture in that the end of adolescence and the beginning of adulthood is marked by financial and emotional independence from one's family. As a result, there has been a constant reshuffling of the adolescent years over time. The net result is that in North American society today the period of adolescence is significantly longer than it was 100 or even 50 years ago. The earlier onset of *puberty* (the start of sexual maturation) coupled with a lengthening period of dependence on famiy has caused us to view adolescence in a much broader perspective.

Secular trends in biological maturation over the past 100 years have dramatically lowered the average age of puberty. Economic and sociocultural trends over that same period, however, have dramatically extended the average age of adolescence. The net result is that adolescence is no longer described solely by the teen years. It has been extended, in both directions, beyond that point. Whereas adolescence used to be considered roughly the period of time from 13 to 18 years of age, it is now considered to begin as early as age 11 and not to end until about age 20 or beyond.

During adolescence tremendous changes occur. The adolescent growth spurt, the onset of puberty, and sexual maturation are the primary biological markers of adolescence. Each of these will be discussed in the sections that follow.

ADOLESCENT GROWTH

The onset of adolescence is marked by a period of accelerated increases in both height and weight. The age of onset, duration, and intensity of this growth spurt is genetically based and will vary considerably from individual to individual. One's *genotype* (growth potential) establishes the boundaries for individual growth, but the individual's *phenotype* (environmental conditions) will have a marked influence on achievement of this potential.

In accounting for an adolescent's growth potential, his or her genotype will play the determining role in linear body measures, skeletal maturation, sexual maturation, and body type. One's final adult standing height, trunk, arm, and leg lengths are ultimately determined by genetic factors. Similarly, bone ossification, the onset of puberty, and the manner in which fat is distributed around the body are all products of one's genotype. Each of these may be modified to a certain extent, but one cannot go beyond his or her inherited potential. On the other hand, the environment working in concert with heredity will influence how close one comes to his or her genetic potential. Such things as body weight, skinfold thickness, and circumferences are all subject to significant modification.

Height

Because of the interacton of one's genotype with the environment there is considerable variability in the growth process during the adolescent period. There is, however, a definite period of accelerated growth at the end of childhood that is known by a variety of terms. To some it is the "adolescent growth spurt," to others it is the "period of preadolescent acceleration," and to still others it is known as the "circumpubertal period" (Krogman, 1980). This period of "growing like a weed" begins prior to sexual maturation. We will, therefore, refer to it as the "preadolescent growth spurt."

The *preadolescent growth spurt* is a time period that lasts about 4½ years (Thissen et al. 1976). Males, on the average, begin their growth spurt around age 11, reach their peak velocity by age 13, and taper off by age 15. Females are about two years advanced, beginning their spurt around age 9, peaking in velocity at age 11 and tapering off by age 13 (Tanner, 1978). It is not uncommon to show a one-year incremental gain in height of 6 to 8 inches or more during the period of peak velocity. Further growth continues at the end of the preadolescent growth spurt but at a much slower rate. Males reach their mature adult height around age 19. Females attain their maximum height around age 17 (Krogman, 1980).

It should be noted that the preadolescent growth spurt is highly variable from individual to individual (Table 15.1). Some will have completed the process before others have begun. The results are clearly evident in the typical youth sport setting where "midgets" and "giants" are frequently grouped together with little or no consideration given for biolog-

Table 15.1 Height in Inches of Youths Aged 12-17 Years by Gender and Age at Last Birthday[1]

Gender and Age	Mean	Percentile						
		5th	10th	25th	50th	75th	90th	95th
Males								
12 years	60.0	54.6	55.7	57.8	60.0	61.9	64.0	65.2
13 years	62.9	57.2	58.3	60.4	62.8	65.4	68.0	68.7
14 years	65.6	59.9	60.9	63.2	66.1	68.1	69.8	70.7
15 years	67.5	62.4	63.7	65.7	67.8	69.3	71.0	72.1
16 years	68.6	64.1	65.2	67.0	68.7	70.4	72.1	73.1
17 years	69.1	64.1	65.7	67.2	69.2	70.9	72.6	73.7
Females								
12 years	61.1	55.8	57.4	59.5	61.2	63.0	64.6	65.9
13 years	62.5	57.8	58.9	60.7	62.6	64.4	66.0	66.9
14 years	63.5	59.6	60.5	61.9	63.5	65.2	66.7	67.4
15 years	63.9	59.6	60.3	62.0	63.9	65.8	67.2	68.1
16 years	64.0	59.7	60.7	62.4	64.2	65.6	67.2	68.1
17 years	64.1	60.0	60.9	62.3	64.3	65.9	67.4	68.1

[1]Source: U.S. Public Health Service. Vital and Health Statistics, Series 11, No. 124, Height and Weight of Youths, 12-17. United States: January 1973.

ical maturation. Remember, development is age-influenced but it is not age-dependent. Overreliance on chronological age as a guide for youth sport team selection is unwise and inconsistent with what we know about motor development and quality education. We must, therefore, devise methods that use means other than chronological age for equating and grouping athletes for sports.

Figure 15.1 provides a longitudinal view of the growth patterns of two individuals (my children, David Lee and Jennifer). From childhood through adolescence, annual height, weight, and girth measurements have been taken. Although a longitudinal view of just two individuals does not provide a complete picture of the growth process, Figure 15.1 does provide us with a typical growth curve of two individuals. Note that, at age 9, Jennifer, an average maturer, was actually taller than her brother at that age, but that, by age 10, David Lee was 4 inches taller than his sister at that age. Notice also that between ages 9 and 11, David Lee (an early maturer) grew 12 inches in height, whereas his sister grew only about 3 inches during the same period. Jennifer's preadolescent growth spurt was at its greatest velocity between 11 and 12 years of age where she grew 3 inches before slowing down at menarche and plateauing by age 16. Similarly, David Lee's velocity curve slowed down although he continued to make small annual incremental height gains to age 19.

Events within the preadolescent growth spurt are interdependent. For males, the period of most rapid growth coincides with the appearance of secondary sex characteristics such as the emergence of axillary and pubic hair (Tanner, 1962). For females, the peak velocity in growth tends to occur prior to menarche. Females with an early growth spurt tend to reach menarche earlier than those with a later growth spurt (Tanner, 1970).

The attainment of maximal adult height is of interest to most adolescents. Males are frequently concerned about being too short, females about being too tall. A number of prediction formulas are available, and mature adult height is correlated with height prior to the preadolescent growth spurt. Therefore, if a child was in the fiftieth percentile prior to puberty, he or she is likely to remain at the same percentile after puberty. Krogman (1980) recommends the following formula for predicting approximate adult height:

Males: 2 × height at age 2 = adult height

Females: 2 × height at 1½ years = adult height

It should be remembered that attainment of adult height is dominated by one's genotype and under normal circumstances only minimally

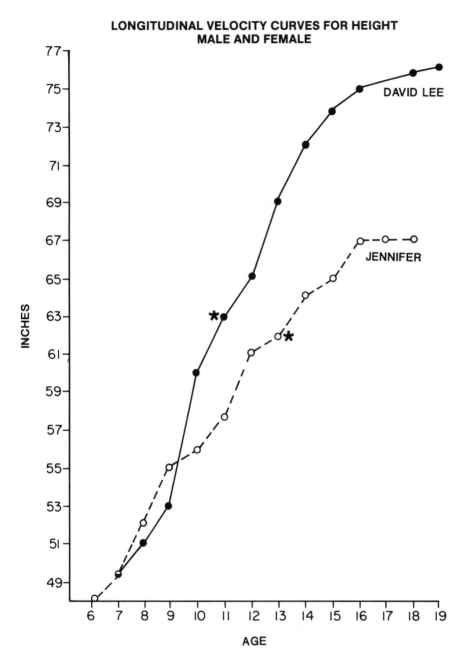

Figure 15.1 Longitudinal velocity curves for height for a single male and a single female from childhood through adolescence (*=date of menarche for Jennifer, onset of axillary hair development for David Lee)

influenced by the environment. On the other hand, one's attained adult weight is strongly influenced by environmental factors. Krogman (1980) indicated that early maturers tend to be shorter as adults than predicted from their stature as a child and late maturers tend to be taller. Table 15.1 provides a percentile equivalent chart for height in inches for males and females 12 to 17 years of age. This chart may be used to predict adult height and to determine an individual's percentile equivalent in comparison with other youth from the United States. For example, a male at the twenty-fifth percentile at age 12 (57.8") will probably remain within that percentile and can expect to attain a height of about 67" by age 17. This would make him about 2 inches shorter than the average 17-year-old American male (69.1") and about 3 inches taller than the average American female (64.1"). Conger and Peterson (1984, p. 94) indicated that once an early maturer and his or her late-maturing age-mate has passed the period of accelerated preadolescent growth, "their comparative standings in height are most likely to return to those of preadolescence." The genetic influence on stature is strong and, unless significant long-term changes are made in diet and lifestyle during the growing years, there will be little variability from the predicted growth channel.

A new and frightening potential for both growth retardation and enhancement has surfaced in the last few years. Steroid use by adolescents during the growing years has been found to have permanent effects on stature (Taylor, 1987). Steroid use by prepubertal children may cause the epiphyses of the long bones to prematurely fuse (American College of Sports Medicine Position Statement on the Use and Abuse of Anabolic-Androgenic Steroids in Sports, 1977). On the other hand, certain steroid products have been safely prescribed by physicians for years to stimulate growth in males with uncomplicated short stature. Taylor (1987) reported that:

> Clear evidence that heavy steroid use can reduce the ultimate height of adolescents is lacking. It is safe to say only that self-prescribed use of supratherapeutic doses of steroids by adolescents can have powerful effects on maturation processes and that these effects may lead to either increased or decreased adult stature (p. 147).

Further research is necessary to determine the long-term effects of steroid use on adolescent stature. The dosage, duration, and types of steroids used must be investigated before conclusions can be drawn.

Weight

Weight changes during adolescence are great. For both males and females, increases in weight tend to follow the same general curve followed by height increases. Skeletal maturation, increases in both muscle and fat tissue, and organ growth all contribute to the weight gains of adolescence. Over-reliance on adolescent weight curves is unwise because weight reflects a combination of developmental events and as a result is limited in its information value. For example, failure to gain weight or to actually lose it may be a reflection of an adolescent's increased attention to diet and exercise and not a cause for alarm. Failure, however, to make incremental gains in height would be a cause for concern. Weight gain throughout the period of adolescence will be affected by diet, exercise, gastric motility, and general lifestyle factors as well as by hereditary factors. We know that American youth have a greater percent of body fat than their counterparts of 20 years ago (NCYFS, 1985;

Table 15.2 Heights and Weights of American Children

Age	Males Height (in.) M	S.D.	Weight (lbs.) M	S.D.	Females Height (in.) M	S.D.	Weight (lbs.) M	S.D.
Birth	20.0	1.0	7.6	1.3	19.7	1.0	7.5	1.1
3 mos.	23.5	1.0	13.0	1.8	23.05	1.0	12.0	1.4
6 mos.	26.3	1.0	17.4	2.05	25.05	1.0	16.3	1.85
9 mos.	28.15	1.1	20.55	2.35	27.5	1.0	19.0	2.15
1 yr.	19.7	1.1	23.0	3.0	29.3	1.0	21.6	3.0
2 yrs.	34.5	1.2	28.0	3.0	34.1	1.2	27.0	3.0
3 yrs.	37.8	1.3	32.0	3.0	37.5	1.4	31.0	4.0
4 yrs.	40.8	1.9	37.0	1.3	40.6	1.6	36.0	5.0
5 yrs.	43.7	2.0	42.0	5.0	43.8	1.7	41.0	5.0
6 yrs.	46.1	2.1	47.0	6.0	45.7	1.9	45.0	5.0
7 yrs.	48.2	2.2	54.0	7.0	47.9	2.0	50.0	7.0
8 yrs.	50.4	2.3	60.0	8.0	50.3	2.2	58.0	11.0
9 yrs.	52.8	2.4	66.0	8.0	52.1	2.3	64.0	11.0
10 yrs.	54.5	2.5	73.0	10.0	54.6	2.5	72.0	14.0
11 yrs.	56.8	2.6	82.0	11.0	57.1	2.6	82.0	18.0
12 yrs.	58.3	2.9	87.0	12.0	59.6	2.7	93.0	18.0
13 yrs.	60.7	3.2	99.0	13.0	61.4	2.6	102.0	18.0
14 yrs.	63.6	3.2	113.0	15.0	62.8	2.5	112.0	19.0
15 yrs.	66.3	3.1	128.0	16.0	63.4	2.4	117.0	20.0
16 yrs.	67.7	2.8	137.0	16.0	63.9	2.2	120.0	21.1
17 yrs.	68.3	2.6	143.0	19.0	64.1	2.2	122.0	19.0
18 yrs.	68.5	2.6	149.0	20.0	64.1	2.3	123.0	17.0
19 yrs.	68.6	2.6	153.0	21.0	64.1	2.3	124.0	17.0
22 yrs.	68.7	2.6	158.0	23.0	64.0	2.4	125.0	19.0

Source: Krogman W. M. (1980) *Child Growth*. Ann Arbor: The University of Michigan Press, p. 34

1987). This increase in percent body fat can be attributed to the sedentary lifestyle and permissive eating patterns of a significant proportion of our society.

By age 10, males have attained approximately 55 percent of their final adult weight, and females have attained 59 percent (Heald and Hung, 1970). Prior to age 10 the average weights of both males and females are almost identical, with males being only slightly heavier. During the preadolescent growth spurt, however, females are frequently heavier than their male age-mates. Females tend to weigh more than males until about age 14 whereupon they begin to level off in weight gain. Males continue to make significant gains in weight until about age 22 (Krogman, 1980). Figure 15.2a&b depicts growth in weight from childhood through adolescence. Table 15.2 provides a table of average weights and heights for both males and females from birth to age 22. Note the small standard deviations (S.D.) for height and the increasingly large S.D. with age for weight. Both are a clear indication of the relative influence of both genotype and phenotype on height and weight, respectively.

The reader is cautioned to disregard height-weight tables published prior to 1960. Secular trends in both height and weight have been repeatedly documented and reported in the literature (Krogman, 1980; Gortmaker et al., 1987; Ross et al., 1987).

The reasons for this are many and include changes in the health and nutritional status of youth, socio-economic factors, genetic factors, and changes in activity patterns. Whatever the case, weight is a factor of considerable importance to the adolescent. Constant media bombardment and our obsession with the "perfect body" has raised the weight consciousness of the typical adolescent to the point of obsession. Care must be taken to help the adolescent understand the changing nature of his or her body and not to overstep the fine line between a healthy regard for one's weight and an obsessive preoccupation with weight gain. The problems of anorexia nervosa, and bulimia are as much a sign of the times as they are emotional disorders of individuals overly concerned with weight.

Heart and Lungs

Dramatic changes in height and weight are easily observable during the period of adolescence, but what about other less apparent but equally important changes? Growth of the heart and lungs is dramatic and is a primary factor in the increased functional capacity of the adolescent.

The heart increases in size by about one-half and almost doubles in weight during adolescence (Maresh, 1948). Females have slightly smaller hearts than males during childhood, begin accelerated growth of the heart earlier, and attain a significantly smaller total growth by the end of

CROSS-SECTIONAL VELOCITY CURVES FOR HEIGHT CHILDHOOD-ADOLESCENCE

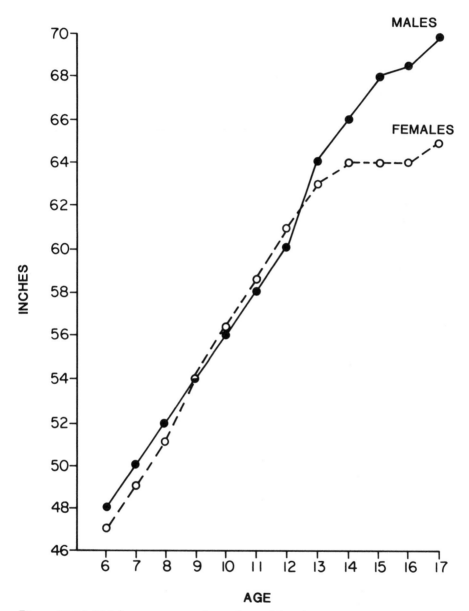

Figure 15.2A Height mean scores for males and females 6-17

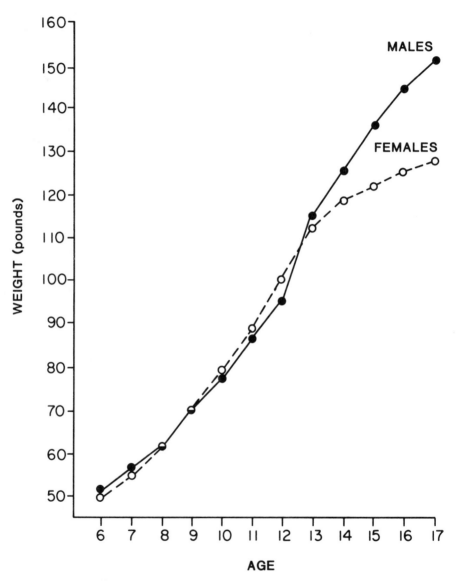

Figure 15.2B Weight mean scores for males and females 6-17 (Data for both courtesy of: Chrysler—AAU Physical Fitness Program [1987] Indiana University, Bloomington, IN)

adolescence. Although heart rate is related to overall body size, we tend to see a gradual lowering of heart rate throughout the entire growth process. By age 17 male heart rates are, on the average, about 5 beats-per-minute slower than females heart rates (Eichorn, 1970). On the other hand, systolic blood pressure rises at a steady rate throughout childhood and accelerates rapidly during puberty before settling down to adult values by the later period of adolescence (Katchadourian, 1977).

Growth of the lungs parallels heart growth during adolescence. Both the size of the lungs and their respiratory capacity increases rapidly during puberty after a period of slow steady growth during childhood. Respiration rates decrease throughout childhood and puberty for both males and females. However, *vital capacity* (the amount of air that can be taken in with a single breath) increases much more rapidly in boys from about age 12 onward even though males and females are almost identical in this measure prior to puberty (Katchadourian, 1977). Dramatic gender differences may be attributed to the larger heart size of males and traditionally more aerobically-active lifestyles.

Physical differences between males and females are just that, differences and nothing more. Ascribing superiority or inferiority to one gender over the other on the basis of biological differences is absurd. On the other hand, those who deny the relevance of any basic physical gender differences apart from reproductive functions are naive. There are fundamental genetic differences between males and females irrevocably established at conception. These differences are heightened during the adolescent period and assert themselves in significant differences in height, weight, body proportions, and functional capacity of the heart and lungs. Such differences can only be expressed in terms of population averages and there is considerable overlap between the sexes. The only way in which males and females are truly unique is in reproductive functions. To understand this uniqueness we must understand the process of puberty and sexual maturation.

PUBERTY

The onset of puberty is generally termed *pubescence*. Pubescence is the earliest period of adolescence, generally about 2 years in advance of sexual maturity. During pubescence, secondary sex characteristics begin to appear, sex organs mature, changes in the endocrine system begin to occur, and the preadolescent growth spurt begins.

The highlight of puberty in females is marked by a clearly distinguishable event, menarche. *Menarche*, or the first menstrual flow, generally occurs between the ages of 12½ and 13½ in the average North American female (Wieczorek, and Natapoff, 1981). The development of mature ova follows menarche by as much as two years, so female puberty is not actually complete until sexual maturity has been attained.

The highlight of puberty in males is less distinct. In a clinical sense, it is marked by the first *ejaculation*, (the sudden discharge of semen) but, as with menarche, this milestone does not truly mark reproductive maturity. Only when live sperm are produced is reproductive maturity attained. This usually begins to occur between 13 and 16 years of age (Wieczorek, and Natapoff, 1981).

Onset of Puberty

During the period of infancy and childhood, both boys and girls develop at highly similar rates. There is little difference in height, weight, heart and lung size, or body composition. By age 10 children have attained about 80 percent of their adult height and a little over half of their adult weight. But as the second decade of life begins, there are dramatic changes not only in measures of growth but in sexual maturation as well. The onset of puberty marks the transition from childhood to sexual adulthood. Exactly when this process begins and what starts the process is not clearly understood. We do know that the timing of the process is highly variable and may begin as early as age 8 in females and age 9 in males, or as late as age 13 and 15 for girls and boys, respectively (Katchadourian, 1977). Clearly, the general sequence of events that mark puberty are much more predictable than specific dates on which they will occur.

Sequentially, for males the preadolescent growth spurt coincides with enlargement of the penis and is preceded by testicular growth. This is generally followed by the first apperance of pubic hair. *Axillary hair* (hair under the arms) formation soon follows, along with a deepening of the voice. Mature sperm formation and sexual maturation occur shortly after, followed by acne, facial hair, and increased body hair.

The sequence of puberty for females in also predictable. There is a close correlation between the female growth spurt and breast development (Katchadourian, 1977). Budding of the nipples occurs prior to budding of the breasts. Breast bud development coincides with the beginning of pubic hair formation. This is followed by growth of the genitalia. Axillary hair formation and menarche soon occur followed by mature ova and the capacity for becoming pregnant. A tendency toward acne and slight deepening of the voice are the final events of female sexual maturation. Table 15.3 provides a visual representation of the sequence of events marking puberty and an approximate timetable of appearance. It should be noted that many events of puberty overlap and may not occur in self-specific time frames.

Table 15.3 Sequence of Events Marking Puberty

Males	Females	Approximate Age of Onset
First Testicular Growth	Beginning of Growth Spurt	9-10
	Budding of Nipples	10-11
Beginning of Growth Spurt	Budding of Breasts	11-12
Start of Pubic Hair Growth	Start of Pubic Hair Growth	
	Growth of Genitalia	
	Peak of Growth Spurt	12-13
	Axillary Hair Formation	
	Menarche	
Penile and Testicular		13-14
Peak of Growth Spurt		
Axillary Hair Formation	Mature Ova Production	14-15
Deepened Voice	(End of Puberty)	
Mature Sperm Production	Acne	15-16
(End of Puberty)	Deeper Voice	
	Mature Pubic Hair & Breast Development	
Acne, Facial Hair	Cessation of Skeletal Growth	16-17
Body Hair		
Mature Pubic Hair Development		
Cessation of Skeletal Growth		18-19

Hormonal Influences

The onset of puberty may be influenced by a variety of factors, but genetics play the dominant role. For example, Chinese females achieve menarche earlier than females of European origin (Conger and Peterson, 1984), and the events of puberty are much more closely related between identical twins than between nonidentical twins, and in nonrelated agemates (Tanner, 1978). Environmental factors may also have a dramatic impact on puberty. Although incompletely understood, stress, nutritional status, general health, and metabolism all appear to affect the onset of puberty and duration in some yet-unexplained manner.

The endocrine system plays a critical role in the growth and maturation process. Malina (1986, p. 24) reports that: "Endocrine secretions are themselves strongly influenced by genetic mechanisms." He further states that: "The nervous system, in turn, is intimately involved in regulating endocrine secretions" (Malina, 1986, p. 24). Therefore, there appears to be a complex interaction among the endocrine system, the nervous system, and the gonads leading to puberty. The hormones from the endocrine system are responsible for "translating the instructions of the genes into the reality of the adult form" (Tanner, 1978, p. 112).

The pituitary gland, located below the brain, appears to be of critical importance. When the *hypothalamus* (a central regulating nerve center in the brain) matures, hormones are secreted by the hypothalamus which, in turn, stimulates the anterior pituitary gland to begin releasing *gonadotropic (GnRH) hormones*. The hormones released by the anterior pituitary gland have a stimulating effect on other endocrine glands, resulting in the release of other growth and sex hormones. The release of sex-related hormones initiates maturation of the gonads. *Androgens* (female hormones) account for initiation of the events of female puberty. Malina (1986) quotes Wierman and Crowley (1986) as stating that:

> At this time, however, no definite statement can be made as to the precise trigger (or triggers) of sexual maturation. Although the final common pathway of this effects is clearly mediated by modulation of hypothalamic secretion of GnRH, little else is clear (p. 235).

REPRODUCTIVE MATURATION

The onset of the preadolescent growth spurt and puberty marks the transition from childhood to reproductive maturity. The bodily changes and appearance of secondary sex characteristics are frequently a cause for heightened interest in one's body and a dramatically increased level of self-consciousness. If young adolescents appear preoccupied with matters of sex it is because a whole host of dramatic and rapid changes are occurring right before their eyes. The young adolescent frequently feels like a spectator in his or her own growth process. Each day seems to bring about changes that are whispered about, giggled over, and closely scrutinized. The wise adult will be sensitive to these physical changes and the impact they have on the social and emotional development of the individual. The journey from childhood to reproductive maturity follows a predictable pattern for both males and females. The student of motor development will want to be knowledgeable about these events and will learn to recognize physical changes that offer cues to physical maturity. Many of these have been discussed in the previous sections on growth and puberty. This section will, therefore, focus on a brief overview of sexual maturation in females and males, and a reliable technique for maturational assessment.

Females

Breast growth marks the first visible step of the female journey to sexual maturity. *Breast development* begins around age 11 and is completed around age 15, although it may begin as early as age 8 and not end until age 18 (Katchadourian, 1977). Breast development has been described by Tanner (1962) and is depicted in Figure 15.3. These stages can be useful as reliable developmental landmarks of maturity.

Pubic hair is usually the second sign of progress toward sexual maturity. On the average, hair growth begins between 11 and 12 years of age and the triangular adult pattern of growth is established by age 14 (Katchadourian, 1977). Tanner's (1962) stages of pubic hair development provide useful indices of development (Figure 15.4).

Changes in the *female genitalia* are usually the third step toward reproductive maturity. The external sex organs (i.e., the vulva, mons, labia, and clitoris) all increase in size and become sensitive to stimulation. Because of the female's anatomy, changes in her exterior genitalia are not as useful as indices of pubic hair growth, and breast development for clinically assessing maturity.

The internal sex organs of the female also undergo considerable change. The uterus and ovaries increase in weight—the uterus dramatically. According to Katchadourian (1977, p. 59), "the uterus develops an intricate and powerful musculature." The vagina increases in size, and the ovaries, although structurally complete at birth, continue to moderately gain weight throughout adolescence.

The average age of menarche for North American females is about 12½ (Conger and Peterson, 1984). It may range from as early as 9 years of age to as late as 18 (Katchadourian, 1977). Menarche is often mistakenly considered the marker of the onset of puberty. It is, in fact, one of the later events that characterizes puberty and the period of adolescence. Menarche occurs after the peak of the growth spurt and about two years after the start of breast development. Menarche does not mark the beginning of reproductive maturity. Generally, up to 1½ years may pass from the first menstrual cycle until the young female is physiologically capable of conception (Conger and Peterson, 1984). This lag is known as the period of *relative sterility of puberty*. It is, however, unwise to assume that this is a period safe from conception. Individual differences are great between menarche and reproductive maturity, and no safe period should be assumed.

Males

Puberty begins in males with growth of the *testes*. Increased testicular growth begins around 11½ years of age and may range from ages 10 to 14 (Tanner, 1962). Growth continues until somewhere between ages 14 and 18 (Katchadourian, 1977). As the male reproductive gland, the testes produce *sperm* and male sex hormones. The ability of the male to ejaculate seminal fluid is largely a function of the prostate gland which becomes

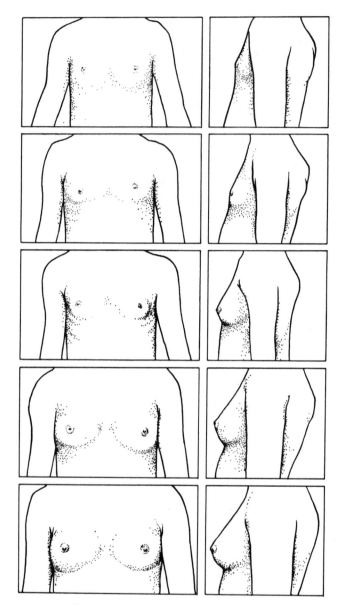

Figure 15.3 Tanner stages of breast development: (1) prepubertal flat appearance like that of a child; (2) small, raised breast bud; (3) general enlargement and raising of breast and areola; (4) areola and papilla (nipple) form contour separate from that of breast; (5) adult breast—areola is in same contour as breast. [Redrawn from J. M. Tanner, *Growth at Adolescence*, 2d ed., Oxford: Blackwell, 1962]

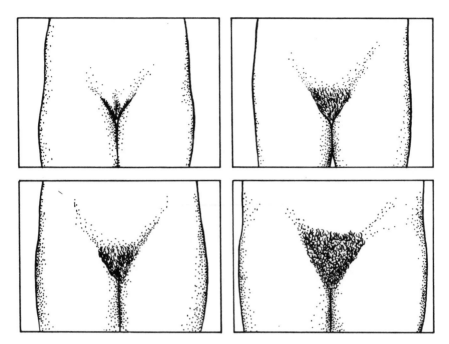

Figure 15.4 Tanner stages of female pubic hair development: (1) prepubertal (not shown) in which there is no true pubic hair; (2) sparse growth of downy hair mainly at sides of labia; (3) pigmentation, coarsening, and curling with an increase in the amount of hair; (4) adult hair, but limited in area; (5) adult hair with horizontal upper border. [Redrawn from J. M. Tanner, *Growth at Adolescence*, 2d ed., Oxford: Blackwell, 1962]

much larger during puberty. Ejaculation is a psychological as well as a physiological event and occurs most frequently in the young male through both nocturnal seminal emissions and masturbation beginning anywhere from age 11 to age 16 (Conger and Peterson, 1984). Mature sperm are not contained in the ejaculate until approximately ages 15 to 17.

Pubic hair growth begins early in adolescence. It may begin as early as age 10 or as late as age 15. As with female pubic hair growth, Tanner (1962) developed a five-stage pubic hair scale for males (Figure 15.5). Mature (stage 5) pubic hair distribution continues until the mid-twenties in males, and the area is less clearly defined than in females.

The external *male genitalia*, the penis and scrotum, change little in appearance throughout childhood. Penis growth begins about a year after the first onset of testicular and pubic-hair growth. The scrotum first becomes larger followed by lengthening and then thickening of the penis

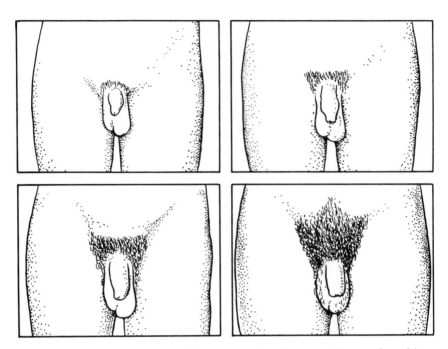

Figure 15.5 Tanner stages of male pubic hair development: (1) prepubertal (not shown) in which there is no true pubic hair; (2) sparse growth of downy hair mainly at base of penis; (3) pigmentation, coarsening, and curling with an increase in amount of hair; (4) adult hair, but limited in area; (5) adult hair with horizontal upper border and spread to thighs. [Redrawn from J. M. Tanner, *Growth at Adolescence*, 2d ed., Oxford: Blackwell, 1962]

(Tanner, 1962). See Figure 15.6 for the Tanner Stages of male genital development. Masters and Johnson (1970) note that the size and shape of a male's penis is unrelated to physique, race, and virility.

Secondary sex characteristics such as axillary hair, facial hair, and deepening of the voice are all associated with progress toward reproductive maturity. Axillary and facial hair usually begin to appear about two years after the growth of pubic hair. Facial hair, an important badge of manhood, first begins to appear on the upper lip. It then starts to grow on the upper cheek in an area parallel with the lower ear and under the lower lip. In the final stage of facial hair growth, it spreads to the lower face and chin creating a full beard (Katchadourian, 1977). Axillary hair appears in concert with facial hair, and body hair continues to spread until well after puberty.

Maturity Assessment

A *maturity assessment* is a means of assessing how far one has progressed toward physical maturation. A variety of techniques are available

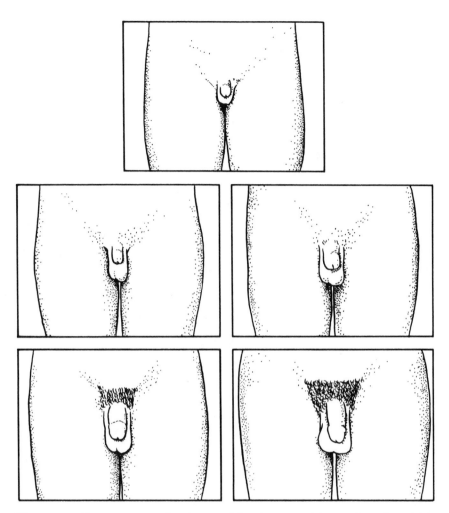

Figure 15.6 Tanner stages of male genital development: (1) prepubertal in which the size of the testes and penis is similar to that in early childhood; (2) testes become larger and scrotal skin reddens and coarsens; (3) continuation of stage 2, with lengthening of penis; (4) penis enlarges in general size, and scrotal skin becomes pigmented; (5) adult genitalia [Redrawn from J. M. Tanner, *Growth at Adolescence*, 2d ed., Oxford: Blackwell, 1962]

including circumpubertal, skeletal, and dental assessments that measure the progress of a particular body part or system toward maturity. Unfortunately, these maturity assessments are seldom used as a routine aspect of the preparticipation physical examination of the young athlete. Such a situation is unfortunate because young athletes could be more equitably equated for competition. Instead, chronological age is used as the most frequent measure of maturity. Throughout our discussion of growth we have continually referred to the individuality and extreme variability of the process, particularly during later childhood and early adolescence. Such a situation is, however, understandable. Most maturity assessments are expensive, time consuming, and inconvenient. Nevertheless, some means of equating youth for participation and competition needs to be devised in order to reduce the incidence of athletic injuries.

Caine and Broekhoff (1987) present a convincing argument for including standardized maturity assessment as part of the preparticipation physical examination that every youth should have prior to sports participation. They argue that maturity assessments can be used to match adolescents for contact sports and to determine when youth are experiencing their growth spurt (and are, therefore, more susceptible to injury). Caine and Broekhoff (1987) argue that use of the *Tanner stages* of circumpubertal maturation can be easily and effectively used. They cite that sociocultural mores and embarrassment are obstacles that can be overcome. Asking parents to assess the circumpubertal maturity of their children, or asking the young athlete to rank his or her maturity with reference to the Tanner scales can yield useful information. Duke et al. (1980) and Kreipe and Geivanter (1983) both reported moderate to high correlations between self assessed Tanner stages and physician assessed Tanner stages. Yet, according to Caine and Broekhoff (1987), to date, only one state, New York, includes a maturity assessment as part of the preparticipation health examination.

The benefits of maturity assessment are obvious. First, it can aid in injury reduction serving as a basis for matching athletes for contact sports. Second, it can serve as a means of limiting or disqualifying individuals for participation in contact sports. Third, it can be used to identify rapid growth periods, and used as a basis for reducing training regimens in long-term high intensity sports such as cross country, swimming, gymnastics, and ballet (Caine and Broekhoff, 1987).

SUMMARY

Due to biological and cultural factors adolescence has gradually expanded to roughly encompass the second decade of life. Dramatic growth increments, the onset of puberty, and reproductive maturation are highlights of the adolescent period.

Adolescent growth in height and weight follows a predictable pattern although there is considerable variability in the onset and duration of the preadolescent growth spurt. Wide variations in stature are typical among preadolescents and have many ramifications for athletic participation and social acceptance.

The onset of puberty is generally considered to coincide with the start of the growth spurt. It is influenced by a variety of genetic factors operating in concert with environmental factors such as nutrition, illness, climate, and emotional stress.

Puberty and reproductive maturity are not the same thing. Reproductive maturity occurs somewhat after the onset of puberty. Furthermore, menarche in females and the ability to ejaculate in males does not mark reproductive maturity. The production of ova and sperm that are capable of conception is the hallmark of reproductive maturity.

Maturity assessments can be used as an effective aid for equating young athletes for competition and reducing the risk of injury. Circumpubertal assessment measures offer an easy, reliable, and valid means of maturity assessment.

CHAPTER CONCEPTS

15.1 The period of adolescence has lengthened due to the combined effects of biology and culture.

15.2 Secular trends in biological maturation have lowered the average age of puberty.

15.3 The beginning of the growth spurt marks the first observable indicator of the onset of puberty.

15.4 The age of onset, duration, and intensity of the growth spurt is controlled by one's genotype.

15.5 The phenotype influences achievement of one's growth potential.

15.6 The preadolescent growth spurt lasts for about 4½ years.

15.7 Females begin their growth spurt about 2 years prior to males.

15.8 It is possible to predict adult height with reasonable accuracy.

15.9 Steroid use can affect the growth potential of the preadolescent and adolescent in yet-unexplained ways.

15.10 Changes in weight roughly approximate the curve for height, but weight is much more influenced by environmental factors.

15.11 Excessive weight is of great concern to many, but today's youth are more fat than their age-mates of 20 years ago.

15.12 Pubescence marks the beginning of reproductive maturity.

15.13 Menarche is the primary event of female puberty but it does not mark reproductive maturity.

15.14 Female reproductive maturity occurs up to 2 years after menarche.

15.15 The ability to ejaculate seminal fluid is a highlight of male puberty.

15.16 Male reproductive maturity requires mature sperm production.

15.17 The onset of puberty is regulated by heredity and may be influenced by nutrition, illness, climate, and emotional stress.

15.18 Secondary sex characteristics appear in a predictable sequence although there is considerable variability in the rate.

15.19 Hormonal influences are the unexplained trigger for the onset of puberty.

15.20 The journey to reproductive maturity is marked by many primary and secondary sex changes.

15.21 Maturity assessment based on the Tanner scales offers a reliable, valid, and easy device for equating athletes, limiting training, and reducing injuries.

TERMS TO REMEMBER

Puberty

Genotype

Phenotype

Preadolescent Growth Spurt

Vital Capacity

Pubescence

Menarche

Ejaculation

Axillary Hair

Hypothalamus

Gonadotropin (GnRH)

Androgens

Breast Development

Pubic Hair

Female Genitalia

Relative Sterility of Puberty

Testes

Sperm

Male Genitalia

Secondary Sex Characteristics

Maturity Assessment

Tanner Stages

CRITICAL READINGS

Conger, J. J. and Petersen, A. C. (1984). *Adolescence and Youth*. New York: Harper and Row, (Chapter 8).

Katchadourian, H. (1977). *The Biology of Adolescence*. San Francisco: W. H. Freeman.

Krogman, W. M. (1980). *Child Growth*. Ann Arbor: The University of Michigan Press.

Malina, R. M. (1986). "Physical Growth and Maturation." In Seefeldt, V. (ed.) *Physical Activity and Well-Being*. Reston, VA: AAHPERD.

Malina, R. M. (1988). "Competitive Youth Sports and Biological Maturation." In *Competitive Sports for Children and Youth*, Brown, E. W. and Branta C. F. (Eds). Champaign, IL: Human Kinetics.

Wells, C. L. and Plowman, S. A. (1988). "Relationship Between Training, Menarche, and Amenorrhea." In *Competitive Sports for Children and Youth*, Brown, E. W. and Branta, C. F. (Eds). Champaign IL: Human Kinetics.

16

Specialized Movement Abilities

Specialized movement skills are merely mature fundamental movement patterns that have been further refined and combined with one another to form sport and other specific and complex movement skills. Specialized movement skills are task-specific; fundamental movements are not.

Most children have the potential to perform at the mature stage in most fundamental movement patterns by age 6 and to begin the transition to the specialized movement phase. That is, they are developmentally mature enough in terms of their neurological makeup, anatomical and physiological development, and visual perceptual abilities to have the necessary equipment for functioning at the mature stage in most fundamental movement skills. There are a few obvious exceptions to this generalization: making contact with a moving object (as in striking), and volleying. These tasks require sophisticated visual tracking abilities. Many lag behind, however, in their movement capabilities because of poor or absent instruction, little or no encouragement, and a general lack of opportunity for regular practice. We are all familiar with teens and adults who throw a ball at the elementary stage or jump for distance using the pattern of movement characteristic of the 2- or 3-year-old child. We can logically expect the young child to perform at less than the mature level. It is not logical, however, for the older child, the adolescent, or the adult to perform fundamental movements at less than the mature level. Failure to develop mature forms of fundamental movement will have direct consequences on the individual's ability to perform task-specific skills at the specialized movement phase. Progress through the transition, application, and lifelong utilization skill stages in a particular movement task is dependent on mature levels of performance at the fundamental movement pattern phase (Figure 16.1). For example, one whose fundamental striking, throwing, catching, or running abilities are not at the mature level cannot expect to succeed in the game of softball. There is a definite *proficiency barrier* (Seefeldt, 1980) between the fundamental movement pattern phase and the specialized movement phase of development. The transition from one phase to another depends on mature patterns of movement being applied to a wide variety of movement skills. If the patterns are less than mature, ability will, by necessity, be adversely affected.

This chapter focuses on the specialized movement skill phase of development. Two important points should be kept in mind. First, even though one may be cognitively and affectively ready to advance to this phase, advancement depends on successful completion of specific aspects of the previous phase. Second, progress from one phase to another is not an all-or-none proposition. One is not required to be at the mature stage in all fundamental movements prior to advancing to subsequent stages. The 12-year-old, for example, who specialized early in gymnastics may be performing at a highly sophisticated level in several locomotor and stability movements and at the same time be unable to throw, catch, or kick a ball with the proficiency expected for his or her age and developmental level.

DEVELOPMENTAL SEQUENCE OF SPECIALIZED MOVEMENTS

After the child has achieved the mature stage in a particular fundamental movement pattern, little change occurs in the form of that

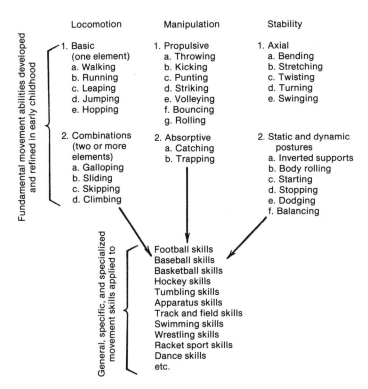

Locomotion	Manipulation	Stability

Fundamental movement abilities developed and refined in early childhood

1. Basic
   (one element)
   a. Walking
   b. Running
   c. Leaping
   d. Jumping
   e. Hopping

1. Propulsive
   a. Throwing
   b. Kicking
   c. Punting
   d. Striking
   e. Volleying
   f. Bouncing
   g. Rolling

1. Axial
   a. Bending
   b. Stretching
   c. Twisting
   d. Turning
   e. Swinging

2. Combinations
   (two or more elements)
   a. Galloping
   b. Sliding
   c. Skipping
   d. Climbing

2. Absorptive
   a. Catching
   b. Trapping

2. Static and dynamic postures
   a. Inverted supports
   b. Body rolling
   c. Starting
   d. Stopping
   e. Dodging
   f. Balancing

General, specific, and specialized movement skills applied to

Football skills
Baseball skills
Basketball skills
Hockey skills
Tumbling skills
Apparatus skills
Track and field skills
Swimming skills
Wrestling skills
Racket sport skills
Dance skills
etc.

Figure 16.1 Mature fundamental movement abilities must be developed prior to the introduction of sport skills

movement ability during the specialized movement phase. Refinement of the pattern and stylistic variations in form occur as greater skill (precision, accuracy, and control) is achieved, but the basic pattern remains unchanged (Wickstrom, 1983). Dramatic changes in the performance level, however, based primarily on increased physical abilities, may be seen from year to year. As the adolescent improves in strength, endurance, reaction time, speed of movement, coordination, and so forth, we can expect to see improved performance scores. Chapters 12 and 17 provide detailed discussions and comparisons of the physical abilities and the performance scores of children and adolescents, respectively.

Within the specialized phase, there are three separate but often overlapping stages. The onset of stages during this phase of development depends on cognitive and affective factors within the individual as well as on neuromuscular factors. Factors within the individual and conditions within the environment stimulate movement from one stage to another.

One's fundamental movement patterns are little changed after reaching the mature stage, and physical abilities influence only the extent to which one's sport-skill abilities are acted out in recreational or competitive situations. Therefore, *sport skills* are mature fundamental movements that have been adapted to the specific requirements of a sport, game, or dance activity. The extent to which these abilities are developed depends on a combination of factors. The three stages within the specialized movement phase are outlined here.

Transition Stage. This stage is characterized by the individual's first attempts to refine and combine mature movement patterns. There is heightened interest in sport, in pitting one's developing abilities against others', and in standards of performance and the skills of others. The child is interested in all sports and does not feel limited by physiological, anatomical, or environmental factors. Stress begins to be placed on accuracy and skill in the performance of games, lead-up activities, and a wide variety of sport-related movements. During this stage the individual works at getting the idea of how to perform the sport skill. Skill and proficiency are limited.

Application Stage. During this stage the individual becomes aware of physical assets and limitations and begins to narrow his or her focus from all sports to certain types of sports. Stress is now placed on developing higher levels of proficiency. During this stage practice is the key to developing higher degrees of skill. The movement patterns characteristic of the beginner during the previous stage become smoother. More complex skills are refined and begin to be utilized in official sports for recreation and competition.

Lifelong Utilization Stage. This stage is characterized by the individual's further limiting the scope of participation to a few activities that are engaged in frequently over a period of years. Further specialization and skill refinement occur here. Lifetime activities are chosen on the basis of abilities, ambitions, availability, and past experiences. Activity limitation is brought about by increased responsibilities and time demands. This is a fine-tuning stage. During this period the individual's performance is highly refined. Performance is highly reliable, appearing automatic and approaching the limits of the individual's capabilities.

It should be recognized that many individuals do not go through the development and refinement of specialized movement skills in the sequence presented above. Children are often encouraged to refine their skills in a particular sport at an early age. Early participation in sports is not detrimental, but too often this quest for specialization replaces quality physical education programs at the expense of the development of mature fundamental movement patterns and sport skills.

YOUTH SPORT

Under ideal conditions, the transitional movement skill stage begins at age 7 or 8. The child's growing interest in his or her performance capabilities and sport, coupled with increasing cognitive sophistication and improved group interaction, tends to cause a surge of interest in being involved in organized competition. The growth in youth sport participation over the past fifteen years has been phenomenal. A 1975 survey estimated the number of participants in nonschool-sponsored youth sports at 20 million (Athletic Institute, 1975). A Michigan study revealed that every community in the sample group provided some form of competitive activity for youth (Seefeldt and Gould, 1980). In fact, it would be difficult to find a sizable community in North America that does not provide competitive sport experiences for its youth through some form of nonschool-sponsored program. Youth sport is big, popular, and here to stay.

Youth sport can have detrimental as well as beneficial effects, all of which have been fully discussed over the years. See *The Handbook for Youth Sport Coaches*, (Vern Seefeldt, Ed., AAHPERD, 1987) for up-to-date, practical information. Youth sport provides an avenue by which those at the transition and application stages can further develop their abilities, get plenty of vigorous physical activity, and test developing skills against others in competitive situations. Competitive sport, however, should not be thought of as the only skill outlet for children. Participation in noncompetitive forms of cooperative recreation and dance and activities such as hiking, canoeing, fishing, and jogging also provide activity avenues for the individual.

Tables 16.1 through 16.9 provide an overview of several sport skills and the various fundamental locomotor, manipulative, and stability movements that are involved in the performance of these skills.

Changing a Well-Trained Technique

Oftentimes you will have an athlete that comes to you with a well-learned but improper technique of performing a skill. The athlete may be experiencing success with the technique, but you know that proper execution of the skill is more efficient and will result in more success. You are faced with the dilemma of determining whether to attempt to change the habit or peculiarity of your athlete's performance or to leave it alone and to permit its continuation. A well-learned technique is difficult and time-consuming to change because any new learning requires taking an unconscious advanced skill and returning it to the conscious level (beginning and intermediate stages). Under stress and in conditions where rapid decisions are required of the athlete, he or she is likely to revert to

Table 16.1 Basketball Skills

Fundamental Movements	*Specialized Movement Skills*	
Manipulation		
Passing	Chest pass	Shovel pass
	Overhead pass	Push pass
	Baseball pass	
Shooting	Lay-up shot	Jump shot
	Two-hand set shot	
Bouncing	Stationary dribbling	Bounce pass
	Moving dribbling	
Catching	Pass above the waist	Rebounding
	Pass below the waist	Pass to the side
		Jump ball reception
Volleying	Tipping	
	Center jump	
Locomotion		
Running	In different directions while dribbling	
	In different directions without ball	
Sliding	Guarding while dribbling	
Leaping	Lay-up shot	
	Pass interception	
Jumping	Center jump	Rebounding
	Tip-in	Catching a high ball
Stability		
Axial movements	Pivoting	
	Bending	
Dynamic balance	Compensation for rapid changes in direction, speed, and level of movement	
Dodging	Feinting with the ball	

the first or incorrect response. It is only after considerable practice that the incorrect response will be replaced by the correct action at the advanced fine tuning stage. In order to decide whether to make a change in the athletes technique the teacher/coach needs to:

1. Determine if there is sufficient time to make the change (in terms of weeks and months, not hours and days).
2. Determine if the athlete really wants to make the change.
3. Be certain that the athlete understands why the change is being made.

Table 16.2 Contemporary Dance Skills

Fundamental Movements	Specialized Movement Skills
Locomotion	
Walking	[1]"Contemporary dance is a form which utilizes
Running	a movement vocabulary specific to the par-
Leaping	ticular creative effort being expressed. The
Jumping	choreographer utilizes movement as a
Hopping	vehicle of expression. Therefore, fundamen-
Galloping	tal locomotor and stability movements serve
Sliding	as the means for conveying concepts and
Skipping	ideas."
Stability	
Axial movements	Bending, stretching, twisting, turning, reaching, lifting, falling, curling, pushing, pulling
Static and dynamic balance	Numerous balance skills requiring synchronizing rhythm and proper sequencing of movement

[1]Personal communication from Fran Snygg, Professor of Dance, Indiana University, 1988.

Table 16.3 Football Skills

Fundamental Movements	Specialized Movement Skills	
Manipulation		
Throwing	Forward pass	Lateral
	Centering	
Kicking	Place kick	Field-goal kicking
	Punting	
Catching	Pass above the waist	Over the shoulder
	Pass below the waist	Across the midline
	Pass at waist level	Hand-off
Carrying	Fullback carry	
	One-arm carry	
Locomotion		
Running	Ball carrying	
	Pursuit of ball carrier	
Sliding	Tackling	Blocking
Leaping and jumping	Pass defense	Pass reception
Stability		
Axial movements	Blocking	
	Tackling	
Static and dynamic balance	Blocking	Rolling
	Stances	Pushing
	Dodging a tackle	

Table 16.4 Softball/Baseball Skills

Fundamental Movements	Specialized Movement Skills	
Manipulation		
Throwing	Overhand throw for accuracy	
	Overhand throw for distance	
	Underhand toss	
	Overhand pitch	
	Underhand pitch	
Catching	Above-waist ball	Grounder
	Below-waist ball	Across midline
	Fly ball	Line drive
Striking	Batting	
	Bunting	
Locomotion		
Running	Base running	
	Fielding	
Sliding	Fielding	
	Base sliding	
Leaping	Base running	Fielding
Jumping	Fielding	
Stability		
Axial movements	Batting	
	Fielding	
	Pitching	
Dynamic balance	Compensation for rapid changes in direction, speed, and level of movement	

4. Be certain that the athlete realizes that performance will regress prior to improvement.
5. Provide a supportive, encouraging environment.
6. Structure practice sessions that will gradually bring the athlete from the initial to the intermediate and finally back to the fine tuning stage.

Knowing the Athlete

It is vitally important as the coach to know your athletes and to recognize that each comes to you with a varying set of physical, mental, emotional, and social capabilities. An awesome number of individual differences confront the coach and must be taken into consideration when

Table 16.5 Soccer Skills

Fundamental Movements	Specialized Movement Skills	
Manipulation		
Kicking	Instep kick	Inside of foot kick
	Toe kick	Outside of foot kick
	Heel kick	Dribbling
	Corner kick	Passing
	Goal kick	Goalie punt
Striking	Heading	
	Juggling	
Catching	Goalie skills	
Throwing	Throw-in	
	Goalie throw	
Trapping	Sole trap	
	Double-knee trap	
	Stomach trap	
	Single-knee trap	
	Chest trap	
Locomotion		
Running	With ball	
	Without ball	
Jumping and leaping	Heading	
Sliding	Marking	
Stability		
Axial movements	Goalie skills	
	Field play skills	
Dynamic balance	Tackling	
	Dodging opponent	
	Feinting with ball	

planning practice sessions. Some of these individual differences are easy to detect, others are not and may remain hidden. However, it is to your advantage to be aware of as many factors as possible in order that you may take them into consideration when planning training sessions and dealing with athletes as individuals. Some important points to remember are:

1. Athletes learn at differing rates.
2. Each athlete's potential for performance excellence varies.
3. Requisite fundamental movement abilities must be mastered prior to developing the sport skill.
4. Response to instructional approaches vary among athletes.
5. The responses to winning and losing vary among athletes.

Table 16.6 Track and Field Skills

Fundamental Movements	Specialized Movement Skills	
Manipulation		
Throwing	Shotput	Hammer
	Discus	
	Javelin	
Locomotion		
Running	Dashes	Pole-vault approach
	Middle distances	High-jump approach
	Long distances	Long-jump approach
Leaping takeoff	Low hurdles	Running long-jump
	High hurdles	Pole-vault takeoff
Jumping	High jump	
	Long jump	
Vertical jump	High jump	
Stability		
Axial movements	Pivoting and twisting (shotput, discus, javelin, and hammer)	
Dynamic Balance	Compensation for rapid changes in speed, direction, and level of movement	

Table 16.7 Racket Sport Skills

Fundamental Movements	Specialized Movement Skills	
Manipulation		
Striking	Forehand shot	Lob shot
	Backhand shot	Smash
	Overhead shot	Corner shot
	Sweep	Drop shot
Locomotion		
Running	Net rush	
	Ball retrieval	
Sliding	Lateral movement to ball	
Stability		
Axial movements	An aspect of all strokes (twisting, stretching, pivoting)	
Dynamic balance	Compensation for rapid changes in direction, level, and speed of movement	

Table 16.8 Volleyball Skills

Fundamental Movements	Specialized Movement Skills	
Manipulation		
Striking	Overhand serve	Spike
	Underhand serve	Dink
Volleying	Set-up	
	Dig	
Locomotion		
Sliding	Lateral movement	
Running	Forward	
	Backward	
Vertical jump	Diagonal	
	Spike	
Stability		
Axial movements	Found in general play (stretching, twisting, turning, falling, reaching)	
Dynamic balance	Rapid changes in speed, level, and direction of movement	

6. The responses to praise and criticism, reward and punishment vary among athletes.
7. The background of related sport experiences varies from athlete to athlete.
8. Differences in home life experiences influence athletes differently.
9. Deficiencies in certain areas can often be compensated for in other areas of performance.
10. The attention span and ability to concentrate vary among athletes.
11. The developmental level of athletes varies, resulting in dissimilar potential for learning and performance.
12. The physical abilities of athletes vary (particularly during the preteen and early teenage years).
13. Athletes will display greater or lesser degress of gross and fine motor skills depending on their background of experiences and inherited factors.
14. The ability to analyze, conceptualize, and problem-solve varies among athletes.

Table 16.9 Gymnastic Skills

Fundamental Movements	Specialized Movement Skills	
Locomotion		
Running	Approach	
Vertical jumping	Back flip	
	Front flip	
Skipping	Skip step	
Leaping	Various stunts	
Stability		
Axial movements	One or more found in numerous stunts and apparatus skills (bending, stretching, twisting, turning, falling, reaching, pivoting)	
Static balance	Integral part of all stationary tricks and landing on dismounts	
Inverted supports		Tip-up headstand
		Tripod handstand
Body rolling	Forward roll	Back walkover
	Backward roll	Front walkover
Dynamic balance	Compesation for changes in direction, level, and speed of movement	

TYPES OF SPORT SKILLS

Sport skills may be classified in a variety of ways. One classification scheme uses the terms "externally paced" and internally paced" as describing the nature and intent of the activity itself.

Externally Paced Skills

Externally paced skills involve making responses to changes in environmental cues. These environmental changes are generally rapid and unpredictable as with trap and skeet shooting. As a result, rapidity and flexibility in decision making are required of the athlete. Sports such as tennis, basketball, and football are examples of other externally paced activities. The coach needs to provide for practice sessions that promote rapid decision making and adaptive behaviors in a variety of game-like situations.

Internally Paced Skills

Internally paced skills, on the other hand, are those that require a fixed performance to a given set of conditions. The athlete is permitted the luxury of moving at his or her own pace through the activity and has time to recognize and respond to the conditions of the environment. Internally paced activities generally place a great deal of emphasis on accuracy, consistency, and repetition of performance. Target shooting, as well as bowling, golf, and archery are generally considered to be internally paced activities. The coach in these sports needs to provide ample opportunities for repetition of the activity under environmental conditions that duplicate, as nearly as possible, the actual competitive environment.

In both internally paced and externally paced sport skills the teacher/coach needs to:

1. Identify the type of activity (i.e. externally or internally paced).
2. Establish a practice environment that is consistent with the externally or internally paced nature of the activity.
3. Introduce externally paced activities under internally paced conditions first (i.e. control the environment and conditions of skill practice first).
4. Introduce situations that require responses to sudden and unpredictable cues in externally paced activities as skill develops.
5. Strive for greater consistency, duplication, and reduction of environmental cues for internally paced activities as skill develops.
6. Encourage the athlete to "think through" the activity in the early stages of learning.
7. Encourage the athlete to screen out unnecessary cues as skill develops.

STAGES IN SPORT SKILL LEARNING

All sport skill learning, whether internally paced or externally paced, involves a hierarchial sequence of learning. The sequential progression in the development and refinement of sport skills may be classified into three general stages. Each of these stages represents a period during which both the learner and the coach have specific identifiable tasks and responsibilities (Sage, 1984; Lawther, 1977; Gentile, 1972; Fitts and Posner, 1967; and Fitts, 1962).

Beginning Stage

The *beginning stage,* or "getting the idea" stage as it is sometimes called, is the first stage in sport skill learning. During this stage the movements of the athlete are generally uncoordinated and jerky. Conscious attention is paid to every detail of the activity. It is during this stage that the learner begins to construct a mental plan of the activity and is actively trying to understand the skill. Because of the conscious attention that is consistently given to the task itself, performance is poor. The movements of the athletes are generally slow, awkward, and take considerable conscious effort. The early onset of fatigue, due more so to the mental requirements of the task than the task itself, is often apparent. During this stage the learner tends to pay attention to all the information that is available and is unable to "screen" out the relevant from the irrelevant. Therefore, the athlete is often attracted by what is not important as much as by what is important.

The teacher/coach at the early stage of learning needs to be aware of the conscious cognitive requirements of this stage and understand that the intent, at this level, is only to provide the learner with the gross general framework idea of the skill activity. In order to do this the coach needs to:

1. Introduce the major aspects of the skill only (be brief).
2. Provide for visual demonstrations of the skill.
3. Permit the learner to try out the skill.
4. Provide plenty of opportunity for exploration of the skill itself and self-discovery of general principles of the skill.
5. Recognize that this is primarily a cognitive stage and that the learner needs only to get the general idea at this stage.
6. Compare the new skill, when possible, to a similar skill that the athlete may be familiar with.
7. Provide immediate, precise, and positive feedback concerning the skill.
8. Avoid situations that place emphasis on the product of one's performance at this stage. Focus, however, on the process.

Intermediate Stage

The *intermediate stage*, or "practice stage" as it is often called, begins after the athlete has obtained the general idea of the skill and is able to perform it in a manner roughly approximating the final skill. The learner at this stage has a better understanding of the skill. The mental plan of the skill becomes more fully developed. Conscious attention to the skill diminishes. More attention is devoted to the goal or product of the skill than to the process itself. The poorly coordinated, jerky movements so evident in the preceding stage gradually disappear. The athlete begins to gain a "feel" for the skill as kinesthetic sensitivity becomes more highly attuned. As a result, there is less reliance on verbal and visual cues and greater reliance on muscle sense.

The teacher/coach during the practice stage recognizes that the general idea is there and instead focuses on greater skill development. Practice conditions are devised that promote skill refinement and maximize feedback. In order to do this the teacher/coach needs to:

1. Provide numerous opportunities for practice.
2. Provide opportunities for skill refinement in a supportive, non-threatening environment.
3. Devise practice situations that progressively focus on greater and greater skill refinement.
4. Provide short, fast paced practice sessions with frequent breaks prior to longer sessions with few breaks.
5. Be able to analyze skill and to provide constructive criticism.
6. Structure quality practice sessions that focus on quality performance (i.e. "perfect practice makes perfect").
7. Provide frequent, precise, immediate, and positive feedback.
8. Allow for individual differences in the rate of skill development.
9. Focus attention on the whole skill whenever possible.
10. Practice at the rate and in the manner that the skill will be used during competitive performance of the activity.

Advanced Stage

The *advanced stage*, or "fine tuning" stage, as it is sometimes called, is the third and final stage of movement skill learning. The athlete who is at this stage has a complete understanding of the skill. The mental plan for the skill is highly developed and very little attention is paid to the cognitive aspects of the task. In fact, athletes at this level often have difficulty describing how they perform the activity. They often resort to a "let me show you," or a "do it like this" statement followed by actual performance of the skill. The athlete at this stage is refining and fine tuning the skill. In sports where movement is the key element, it is smooth, fluid, and highly coordinated. In sports such as archery where the absence of movement is most highly valued, there is a general appearance of ease, mastery, and total control. The athlete is able to scan out irrelevant information and is not bothered by distractions. There is excellent timing and anticipation of movements and the action appears automatic, although in reality it is a finely tuned skill requiring only a minimum of conscious cortical control.

Coaches of athletes at the advanced stage of movement skill learning have the responsibility to focus on further refinement, maintenance of the skill, and providing selected feedback. In order to do this the teacher/coach needs to:

1. Structure practice opportunities that promote intensity and enthusiasm.
2. Be available to provide encouragement, motivation, and positive support.
3. Offer suggestions and tips on strategy.
4. Structure practices that duplicate game-like situations.
5. Help the athlete anticipate his or her actions in game-like situations.
6. Know the athlete as an individual and be able to adjust methods to meet individual needs.
7. Provide feedback that focuses on specific aspects of the skill.
8. Avoid requiring the athlete to think about execution of the skill, which might result in "analysis paralysis."

Each of the stages in the movement skill learning process requires concerned, knowledgeable, and sensitive teaching. It is imperative that the teacher/coach understands the characteristics of the learner at each stage and is able to structure practice sessions that are most effective for maximizing performance. The acquisition of skill is a process that takes time. The teacher/coach is in a position to guide and direct the athlete in a manner that makes maximum effective use of the time available. Organized, quality practice sessions geared to the skill level of the learner are crucial to realizing the athlete's potential.

FOSTERING IMPROVEMENT*

By the third grade most children are at the transitional and application skill stages. The emphasis on skill improvement at this time results from the increase in the child's performance level potential. Both child and teacher become more concerned with the form, accuracy, and degree of skill used in performing a movement. Student needs are the general concepts upon which teachers formulate their teaching purposes. Probably the foremost concept is that the teacher's purpose is to help individuals improve. If teachers are concerned with improvement, they are aware of one's developmental needs and developmental potential. By condensing the factual knowledge of developmental needs and potential into the operational goal of improvement, teachers are not bogged down with where one should be theoretically. The danger in such concern with theoretics is that teachers will teach theoretical students rather than real students. The operational goal of improvement helps teachers see children realistically at whatever level they are performing. The teacher's

* A special thank you is extended to George Luedke, Southern Illinois University, Edwardsville, for his insightful contributions to this section.

function then becomes one of evaluating and directing the learning experiences in order to bring about new successes for students.

The operational goal of improvement encompasses three other concepts that guide teachers in reaching this goal. The first of these concepts is *movement control*. Here teachers are cognizant of the three categories of movement (stability, locomotion, and manipulation) and the Phases of Motor Development. Teachers are also aware of the need for variation and that learning moves from the general to the specific. By condensing this information into the concept of movement control, teachers again have a basis for analyzing their teaching effectiveness in this area of the child's growth and improvement.

The second concept under the goal of improvement is *emotional control*. Here teachers are concerned with students' understanding of themselves and others. Teachers rely heavily on their abilities to both communicate with students and teach them communication skills. These communication skills include self-discipline as well as experiences through which children can develop responsibility and self-control. The concept of emotional control gives teachers a guide for evaluating past experiences and designing new experiences.

The third and final concept is *learning enjoyment*. This concept also gives teachers a guide for evaluating and implementing their programs with student improvement in mind. The objective here is for teachers to develop within each child an eagerness to learn. Success-oriented experiences and opportunities to receive praise and recognition reinforce the child's view of learning. By making the development of learning skills enjoyable, teachers can foster intrinsic motivation within the student.

The overall goal of improvement, with its three emphases of (1) movement control, (2) emotional control, and (3) learning enjoyment, gives teachers a compact philosophical construct that can serve as an operational guide to teaching action.

This construct can and should be modified by the teachers. Its purpose is not to limit teachers, but to provide operational guidelines to assure that their teaching is meaningful. Every teacher must rely on some sort of philosophical construct in the teaching situation. A teacher, for example, who has taught a number of years in one school system has no doubt designed a program to meet his students' needs. Because he understands his student's needs and potentialities, he has certain performance expectations for them. If this teacher were to take a position in another school, he might temporarily lose his perspective of what to expect from new students. By not relying on a philosophical construct, he could impose performance expectations on new students based on knowledge of former students. The purpose of the suggested philosophical construct is to give teachers a basis for keeping their teaching realistic, practical, and meaningful.

SUMMARY

The refinement of specialized movement abilities may be viewed as a three-stage occurrence. In the transitional stage, it is crucial that a smooth shift be made from the mature fundamental movement pattern to corresponding sport skills. This transition will be hampered if the individual has not developed the mature pattern of movement necessary for performance of the sport skill. The teacher/coach must be alert to the proficiency with which the individual executes a sport skill and not give in to the temptation of ignoring incorrect form as long as the outcome is satisfactory. Too often the teacher/coach focuses on the product rather than on the process by placing more importance on the ball getting through the hoop, the batter reaching base, or the correct shooting or batting patterns being used. There is no reason not to use the mature, mechanically-correct pattern in the performance of a sport skill. Such use will, in the long run, enhance movement performance. But once the mature level has been achieved—once it has become relatively automatic through repeated application to numerous sport situations it is entirely appropriate to encourage unique individual variations in execution of the skill.

At the application stage attention is focused on greater degrees of precision, accuracy, and control. Performance scores generally improve at a rapid rate, and the individual is cognitively more completely aware of the specific advantages and limitations of his or her body. The individual at this level is also influenced by a variety of social, cultural, and psychological factors in the selection and continued involvement in specific sport, dance, and recreational activities. The lifelong utilization stage is a continuation and further refinement of the previous stage. It is the pinnacle of the phases and stages of motor development. This stage is closely aligned to the lifetime sport and recreational activities in which we all choose to actively take part. Failure to develop and refine the fundamental and specialized skill abilities of the previous stages will have a negative effect on one's reaching this stage.

The goal of the leader concerned with the motor development of children and youth is to foster improvement in such a way that there is an orderly and developmentally sound progression through the fundamental and specialized skill phases of development. Improvement in movement control, emotional control, and learning enjoyment serves as a practical philosophical construct around which to plan and implement meaningful experiences.

CHAPTER CONCEPTS

16.1 One's performance level potential increases during later childhood and the preadolescent period and results in greater emphasis on specialized movement skill development.

16.2 Specialized skill development in a specific sport often occurs prior to developing a sound base of fundamental movement abilities.

16.3 A sound base of fundamental movement abilities is essential to balanced motor development at higher skill levels.

16.4 The individual's developmental potential in the transition and application stages is based on the foundation of movement patterns previously established.

16.5 Both structured and unstructured movement experiences are necessary in developing specialized movement skills.

16.6 As performance comes closer to the expected performance model, more specific tasks and information become important. Selection of the best ways to perform a skill becomes imperative.

16.7 Emphasis on mature fundamental movement pattern acquisition is essential prior to learning specialized skills.

16.8 Activity selection and modification should be based on the teacher's knowledge of student capabilities and developmental needs.

16.9 Competition may be used to motivate children to put forth greater effort and concentration in practicing correct or best ways to execute skills.

16.10 Youth sport competition is an important element in the lives of millions of children requiring competent leadership and developmentally appropriate experiences.

16.11 Basketball, football, soccer, softball, volleyball, dance, and other sport-related activities all require the use of movement skills that are based on the three categories of movement (stability, locomotion, and manipulation).

TERMS TO REMEMBER

Specialized Movement Skill
Proficiency Barrier
Sport Skill
Transition Stage
Application Stage
Lifelong Utilization Stage
Internally Paced Skill

Externally Paced Skill
Beginning Skill Level
Intermediate Skill Level
Advanced Skill Level
Movement Control
Emotional Control
Learning Enjoyment

CRITICAL READINGS

Brown, E. W., and Branta, C. F. (1988). *Competitive Sports for Children and Youth: An Overview of Research and Issues*. Champaign, IL: Human Kinetics.

Eckert, H. M. (1987). *Motor Development*. Indianapolis, IN: Benchmark Press, (Chapter 10).

Haubenstricker, J. L. and Seefeldt, V. D. (1986). "Acquisition of Motor Skills During Childhood." In Seefeldt, V. (ed.) *Physical Activity and Well-being*. Reston, VA: American Alliance for Health, Physical Education, Recreation and Dance.

Keogh, J. and Sugden, D. (1985). *Movement Skill Development*. New York: Macmilliam, (Chapter 5).

Seefeldt, V. (ed.), (1987). *Handbook for Youth Sport Coaches*. Reston, VA: AAHPERD.

17

Physical Abilities of Adolescents

CHAPTER COMPETENCIES

Upon Completion of This Chapter You Should Be Able To:

* *Demonstrate knowledge of data available for performance scores and motor pattern changes over time.*

* *Describe gender differences and similarities in motor development.*

* *Discuss changes in movement dimension such as balance, timing, or force production/control.*

* *Demonstrate knowledge of major changes in body composition and physiological functioning in males and females.*

• *List and describe development aspects of health-related fitness during adolescence.*

• *List and describe developmental aspects of performance-related fitness during adolescence.*

Health-related and performance-related fitness changes rapidly during the period of adolescence. Both males and females are capable of making significant increments in all measures of fitness. This chapter will examine these changes. The first section is devoted to the components of health-related fitness. Results of the 1985 National Children and Youth Fitness Study (NCYFS) are the primary source of data because of the validity of the sample and the reliability of the data (Ross and Gilbert, 1985). It should be noted that all the figures discussed in this section are based on the mean sample scores for each health-related fitness item tested. There is considerable variability in performance scores on all items at all age levels.

The information presented in the discussion and figures on performance-related fitness are based on a synthesis of post-1960 studies reported by Haubenstricker and Seefeldt (1986). These data were selected because they represent the best representative sampling available of changes in motor skill performance over age.

The reader is encouraged to study carefully the figures and tables throughout this chapter. It will be of far more value to gain a conceptual grasp of the meaning implied in the slopes of the curves than to memorize specific data points.

HEALTH-RELATED FITNESS

The health-related fitness of youth has been a topic of considerable interest in recent years. It has been suggested that today's North American youth are unfit in comparison to both their age-mates of years ago and their peers from other nations (See Chapter 12). Such may be the case. Presently, however, no reliable data exist that permits us to make accurate comparisons across either generations or cultures. The problem exists primarily in sampling and data collection techniques. Prior to publication of the National Children & Youth Fitness Study (1985, 1987) large-scale, population-based field studies were based on *convenience samples*. That is, although thousands of children and youth were tested on a variety of fitness items, little attention was given to sampling procedures. As a result, the validity of the data obtained is questionable when generalizations are made across ages and across the population as a whole. For example, even when using large numbers, it is altogether possible that participants in some locations were more highly motivated by the testing than others. As a result, performance scores should tend to be biased in favor of more highly motivated participants. Furthermore, in convenience samples, little attention is given to geographical representation, rural versus urban settings, and private versus public school populations, all of which may have dramatic effects.

Another difficulty with nationally-normed fitness tests published prior to the NCYFS is inherent in the test administration itself. In other studies, data were collected by different examiners at each site—usually by a trained physical education professional. It is difficult, if not impossible, to assure consistency among testers. Therefore, *interrater reliability* (objectivity) and *intrarater reliability* (consistency) tends to be poor.

A third problem in comparing generational scores lies in the test items themselves. Comparison can only be made among items that are performed and administered in exactly the same manner. Changing the protocol even slightly for an assessment item may result in drastically inflated or deflated scores.

It is with these concerns in mind that I have chosen to use the NCYFS (1985) data as a basis for our discussion about the health-related fitness of adolescents. The NCYFS is based on a *stratified random sample* of 5,140 males and 5,135 females from 25 randomly selected counties in the United States. Over 88 percent (4,539) of the randomly selected males completed the test battery, and exactly 83 percent (4,261) females completed the testing (Errecart et al. 1985). The high participation rate and the definitive manner in which the sample was obtained contributed greatly to the validity and the ability to generalize from the results. Reliability of the NCYFS was insured by utilizing a highly-trained field staff of ten individuals who directly supervised administration of all the assessment measures given by trained teachers (Ross et al. 1985). The NCYFS represents the best field data available in terms of validity of the sample and reliability of the data. Each of the sections that follow discusses the various health-related components of fitness in respect to these data. Comparisons, where possible, are made with the 1980 AAHPERD Health-Related Physical Fitness Test (HRPFT). You will note that, in general, HRPFT scores are better than NCYFS scores. This may be due to sampling and test administration factors discussed earlier. When comparing the two tests (HRPFT and NCYFS), carefully observe the slope of the two curves. In most cases, the slopes are remarkably similar, thereby strengthening the validity of the data for both tests in terms of changes in performance over time. Care should be taken to note where age differences in the slopes of the two lines do exist. These differences may reflect differences in activity patterns between the two studies due to sociocultural shifts in activity levels over time (i.e., 1980-1985). Table 17.1 provides a synthesis of findings from the 1985 NCYFS.

Aerobic Endurance

Cardiovascular endurance (or aerobic endurance as it is frequently termed) is related to the functioning of the heart, lungs, and vascular system. One's aerobic capacity may be evaluated in the laboratory through a variety of stress tests that require the subject to exert an all-out effort in order to go into oxygen debt. These "max" tests, as they are called, are most generally performed on a treadmill or bicycle ergometer. The VO_2 max score is obtained as the result of exhaustive exercise. Although VO_2 max is the preferred method of determining aerobic capacity, population studies are non-existent using treadmill and ergometer tests. Instead, research has focused on *population samples* across age using field test estimates of aerobic endurance. As a result, the one-mile walk/run has emerged as the most popular field test item with adolescents.

Table 17.1 Common Measure of Health-Related Fitness and
A Synthesis of Findings

Health-Related Fitness Component	NCYFS (1985) Measures	Synthesis of Findings
Aerobic Endurance	1 Mile Walk/Run	Males and females both improve at a near parallel rate. Males are faster than females at all ages. Males continue to improve until late adolescence. Females regress and plateau from midadolescence onward. Males show rapid yearly increments until late adolescence.
Muscular Strength/ Endurance	Bent Knee Sit-Ups	Females improve at a less rapid rate than males. Females tend to plateau in performance during mid-adolescence. Males outperform females at all ages.
	Chin-Ups	Females average less than one chin-up throughout adolescence. Males demonstrate slow gains prior to puberty followed by rapid gains throughout adolescence. Males significantly outperform females at all ages.
Joint Flexibility	Sit-And-Reach	Females outperform males at all ages. Females make yearly incremental improvements until late adolescence. Males regress during early adolescence followed by rapid improvement.

Table 17.1 (continued)

Health-Related Fitness Component	NCYFS (1985) Measures	Synthesis of Findings
Body Composition	Skinfold Calipers	Females have a higher percent body fat than males at all ages.
		Female body fat percentages increase rapidly during early and mid-adolescence followed by a plateau in late adolescence.
		Males increase in percent body fat during late childhood and the pre-adolescent period.
		Males decrease in percent body fat during early adolescence and maintain low fat levels throughout adolescence.

Based on the 1985 National Children and Youth Fitness Study (NCYFS), and as depicted in Figure 17.1, males on the average continue to improve in their aerobic endurance until age 16, whereupon they regress slightly through age 18. These results are similar to mean-mile walk/run times on the 1980 AAHPERD Health Related Physical Fitness Test (HRPFT). The males tested in the HRPFT, however, regressed slightly between ages 10 and 11, followed by steady improvement through age 14. This in turn was followed by a general plateauing of scores through age 17. It is difficult to explain the discrepancy in the slope of the two curves (Figure 17.2) at age 11, but this may be a function of the sampling techniques employed. (The HRPFT used a convenience sampling technique, whereas the NCYFS utilized a stratified random sampling technique.) Nevertheless, the similar slope of the two curves demonstrates that males improve in their mile walk/run times with age. The fact that the boys in the NCYFS continued to improve until age 16 may reflect differences in aerobic activity patterns among boys between 1980 when the HRPFT norms were published and 1985 when the NCYFS was published. Note, however, that for both tests, males, with age, tend to plateau and even regress in their performance on the mile walk/run test. This should be viewed with concern in that it reflects a tendency toward

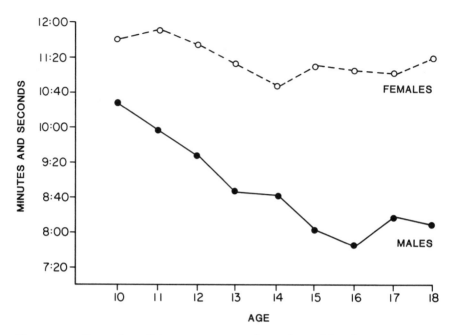

MILE WALK/RUN: MALES & FEMALES

Figure 17.1 One mile walk/run: mean scores for males and females 10-18 years, in minutes and seconds (*Source*: Ross, J. G., and Gilbert, G. G. [1985]. "The National Children and Youth Fitness Study: A Summary of Findings." *Journal of Physical Education, Recreation and Dance*, 56, 1, 46-50)

more sedentary activity patterns in the older adolescent. It is interesting to note that the drop in scores coincides with the age at which most males are eligible for their driver's license and gainful employment.

With regard to the performance of females on the mile walk/run test of aerobic endurance, the results are of similar concern. Although we might expect the male to outperform his female counterpart due to a variety of anatomical and physiological variables, we hope to see a descending slope (i.e., lower times) over a longer period of time. Based on the results of the NCYFS, the female is closest to her male counterpart on the mile walk/run at age 10, and the gap between males and females remains roughly parallel until age 14. It widens, however, at a dramatic rate from then on (Figure 17.1). Although females performing on both the NCYFS and the HRPFT tended to improve until around 13 or 14 years of age, it should be noted that there was a decided tendency to regress and plateau in performance—so much so that the 18-year-old female is at almost the same level as her 12-year-old counterpart.

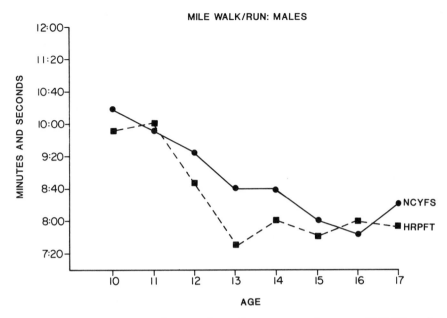

Figure 17.2 Comparison of one mile walk/run scores between NCYFS and HRPFT: mean scores for males 10-17 years, in minutes and seconds

Data from the HRPFT tend to support the data published in the NCYFS. Females in the HRPFT, however, peaked at an earlier age and regressed at a more rapid rate than those tested in the NCYFS (Figure 17.3). Perhaps there is room for cautious optimism in that comparison of the two slopes may indicate a tendency for females later in the 1980s to be more active aerobically than their peers of the early 1980s. The rapid rise of aerobic dance and other rhythmic exercise classes and their sustained popularity with females may be at least partially responsible for the less severe rate of regression.

Strength And Endurance

Bent-knee sit-ups and chin-ups are frequently used as field measures of abdominal *isotonic strength endurance*. They are isotonic in that the muscles go through a full range of motion while in a contracted state. They are related to the strength because a significant force is overcome, and they are related to endurance because a maximum number of repetitions is recorded. From 6 to 9 years of age, both boys and girls are similar in their performance scores on the bent-knee sit-up test. From age 10 onward, however, males improve at a much more rapid rate than their female counterparts (NCYFS, 1985). Figure 17.4 depicts males improving at a near linear rate from ages 11 to 16 with a tendency to level off and regress

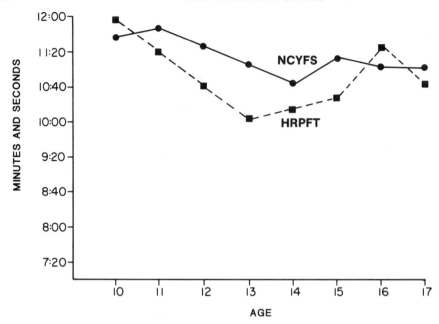

MILE WALK/RUN: FEMALES

Figure 17.3 Comparison of one mile walk/run scores between NCYFS and HRPFT: mean scores for females 10-17 years, in minutes and seconds

slightly from ages 16 to 18. This is clearly in conflict with the general notion (i.e., unsupported by data) that males peak in terms of strength shortly after puberty.

Figure 17.5 depicts chin-ups, a measure of upper trunk strength and endurance, providing additional support for the contention that strength increases at a near linear rate for boys from about age 12 (the approximate age of onset of male puberty) through approximately age 18. Comparing mean scores from published norms on bent-knee sit-ups in the HRPFT reveals similar conclusions, although the boys tested on the HRPFT outperformed their age-mates on the NCYFS (Figure 17.6).

In terms of female *upper body strength/endurance*, the data are somewhat different. Females appear to be weak in this area throughout childhood and adolescence. There appears to be no peaking-plateau-decline sequence as previously thought. There is, rather, a consistently flat curve indicating low levels of upper body strength/endurance at all ages. Females, however, seem to fare better on measures of abdominal endurance as measured by the NCYFS. Mean score values for the bent-knee sit-up test improve slightly with age. In terms of abdominal strength/endurance, older adolescents tend to score slightly higher than their

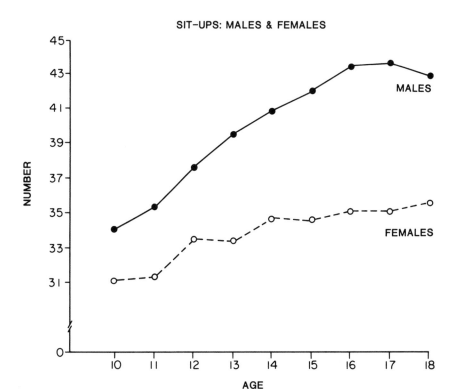

Figure 17.4 Bent-knee sit-ups: mean scores for males and females 10-18 years, number in 60 seconds (*Source*: Ross, J. G., and Gilbert, G. G. [1985]. "The National Children and Youth Fitness Study: A Summary of Findings." *Journal of Physical Education, Recreation and Dance*, 56, 1, 46-50)

younger counterparts. Mean score values for bent-knee sit-ups on the HRPFT revealed similar results, although females tended to perform at a higher level at all ages on the HRPFT (Figure 17.7).

In terms of strength and endurance, the sudden upsurge in performance by boys during adolescence may be explained by increased muscularity brought about by high levels of testosterone. Furthermore, the tendency for males at all ages to "go all out" on measures of fitness may account for the vast discrepancy between males and females. Perhaps because of greater amounts of fatty tissue in proportion to lean muscle mass females do not improve at such a rapid rate. The tendency for females to level off during midadolescence and later adolescence could also be a matter of motivation and lack of all-out test-taking cooperation instead of physiological factors. These are important points to consider. One must be careful not to imply that no matter how females try to improve their performance on measures of strength and endurance they

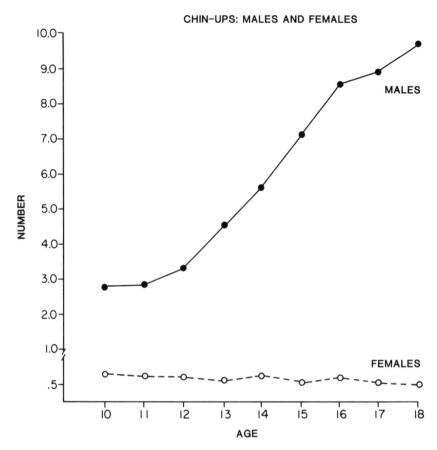

Figure 17.5 Chin-ups: mean scores for males and females 10-18 years, number completed (*Source*: Ross, J. G., and Gilbert, G. G. [1985]. "The National Children and Youth Fitness Study: A Summary of Findings." *Journal of Physical Education, Recreation and Dance*, 56, 1, 46-50)

will not be able to do so. In fact, the data using motivated females suggests the opposite.

The flexed arm hang, an *isometric strength endurance* measure, was administered to both males and females in the Manitoba Physical Fitness Performance Test (CAPHER, 1980). It, too, revealed developmental differences between the genders. Males tended to improve slightly from age 5 onward, with a preadolescent lull followed by rapid improvement through age 18. Females, on the other hand, improved somewhat until ages 11 or 12, whereupon they achieved a plateau until age 15 and showed a slight decline thereafter. Hunsicker and Reiff (1977) reported similar findings with American girls on the flexed arm hang. The per-

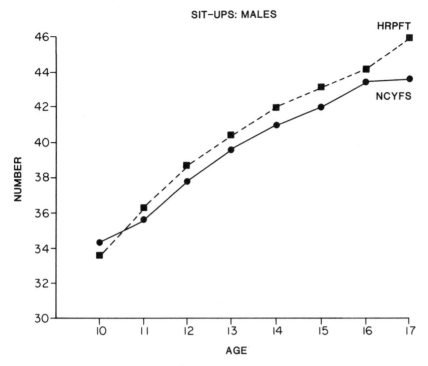

Figure 17.6 Comparison of bent-knee sit-up scores between NCYFS and HRPFT: mean scores for males 10-17 years, number in 60 seconds

formance of boys and girls was quite similar from ages 5 to 8 but began to diverge radically after that in favor of the boys.

The often dramatic differences exhibited between males and females and the span of years in which improved performances can be expected on measures of muscular strength and endurance should be examined carefully. Although males on the average can be expected to outperform females in measures of strength and endurance due to anatomical, physiological, and biomechanical advantages, there is not an adequate biological explanation of differences in the span of years over which relative improvement may be seen. A reasonable explanation may lie in social and cultural differences and child-rearing differences between males and females. Although our North American culture in recent years has radically changed its view of female involvement in vigorous physical activity, it is apparent that discrepancies in the opportunities, encouragement, and instruction remain.

Flexibility

The sit-and-reach test has become the standard field measurement

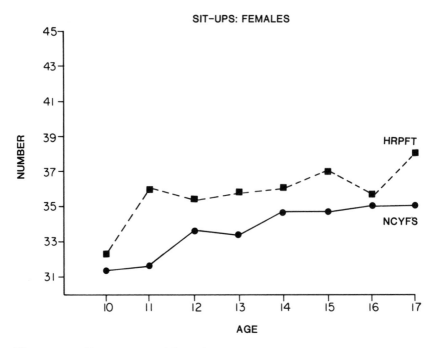

Figure 17.7 Comparison of bent-knee sit-up scores between NCYFS and HRPFT: mean scores for females 10-17 years, number in 60 seconds

of *joint flexibility*. Data from the NCYFS (1985) clearly indicate that, on the average, females make near linear improvements in sit-and-reach scores from ages 10 to 16, followed by a slight decline. Females at all ages outperform their male counterparts on this measure (Figure 17.8). Reasons for this discrepancy have not been adequately explained but may center around anatomical differences as well as sociocultural differences in activity patterns favoring joint flexibility in females.

It is interesting to note the slight drop in sit-and-reach scores for males around age 12. This may be associated with the prepubescent growth spurt during which time the long bones are growing at a faster rate than muscles and tendons. As a result, performance regresses until they catch up. Note also that males and females begin to plateau and regress slightly in their flexibility scores around age 17. Decreases in joint flexibility during this period are clearly associated with a general decrease in activity levels of the older adolescent, and not with aging. In fact, a high level of joint flexibility may be maintained well into adulthood and beyond if flexibility-promoting activities are maintained. In other words, "use it or lose it." Based on the NCYFS, loss of flexibility begins around age 17.

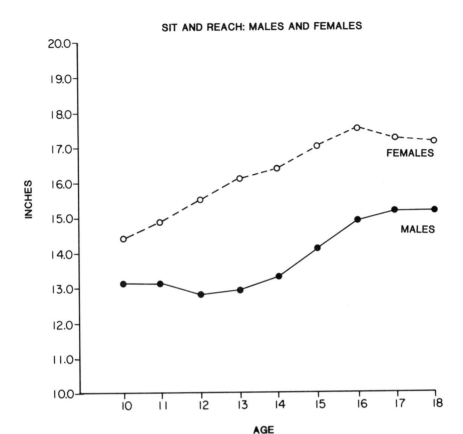

SIT AND REACH: MALES AND FEMALES

Figure 17.8 Sit-and-reach: mean scores for males and females 10-18 years, in inches (*Source*: Ross, J. G., and Gilbert, G. G. [1985]. "The National Children and Youth Fitness Study: A Summary of Findings." *Journal of Physical Education, Recreation and Dance*, 56, 1, 46-50)

Body Composition

Body composition (percent body fat) has only recently been considered a health-related aspect of fitness (AAHPERD, 1980). Previously, total body weight was used by insurance companies as an indicator of one's functional health. Total body weight is a poor predictor of body composition because it does not account for the distribution of one's body weight. Our total body weight is the sum of our muscle, skeletal, organ, and fat masses. Therefore, in order to accurately assess one's body composition, the percent of body fatness needs to be separated from the other components of one's total body weight.

Hydrostatic weighing is currently the most accurate method of determining percent body fat. It involves submerging the individual in water and calculating his or her underwater weight from which an accurate estimate of percent body fat can be calculated. Accurate hydrostatic weighing, however, is not a practical assessment measure for field-based assessments of body composition.

Bioelectrical impedance techniques hold great promise for the future (Katch, 1985). They are more convenient than hydrostatic weighing, but as of yet impedance techniques have not been perfected. Therefore, *skinfold calipers* have become the preferred method of estimating percent body fat. The reliability of the caliper technique has been frequently questioned (Bouchard, 1985), but when administered by trained personnel it may yield fairly accurate results. Body composition data from the NCYFS (1985) is based on the use of skinfold calipers.

Figure 17.9 illustrates tremendous developmental differences in body composition between males and females. Females show a sharp increase in body fatness from ages 10 to 11, followed by a less sharp but steady increase to age 15, which is in turn followed by a tapering off through age 18. The sharp rise between 10 and 11 years of age may be explained by the female prepubescent growth spurt which begins around this time. The steady increase until about age 15 is the result of the pubertal process of becoming a woman.

Males have a dramatically different pattern in terms of percent body fat during adolescence. The preadolescent shows a definite increase in body fatness from 10 to 12 years of age. The typically chunky sixth grader, upon entering his growth spurt, shows a dramatic decrease in adiposity and increase in muscle mass. Increases in male sex hormones account for this increase in muscularity and decrease in body fat. Males continue to display significantly lower levels of body fatness throughout the high school years.

It is interesting to note that, on the average, today's adolescents in terms of body fatness as measured by skinfold calipers are fatter than their counterparts of the 1960s. This suggests that there is indeed a *secular trend* (generational difference) toward increased fatness among different generations of American youth. Data published by the National Center for Health Statistics (NCHS) in the 1960s were the result of a national probability sample. When compared with the results of the NCYFS:

> It can be assured that the skinfold data from the NCYFS and NCHS projects are equally representative of the population of American youth, but at two different points in time. If we discount possible differences in measurement techniques, the differences in skinfold thickness may be explained by the passage of time: American children have become fatter since the 1960s. (Pate et al. 1985, p. 72)

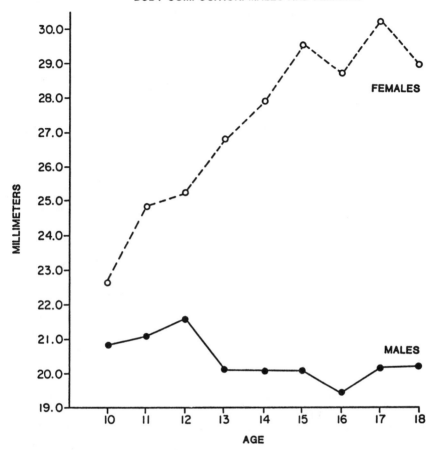

BODY COMPOSITION: MALES AND FEMALES

Figure 17.9 Sum of triceps and subscapular skinfolds: mean scores for males and females, in millimeters (*Source*: Ross, J. G., and Gilbert, G. G. [1985]. "The National Children and Youth Fitness Study: A Summary of Findings." *Journal of Physical Education, Recreation and Dance, 56,* 1, 46-50)

Although we may not be able to critically compare the previously discussed measures of health-related fitness generationally, we can make such a comparison in terms of percent body fat. The message is clear: "American children have become fatter since the 1960s." Regular vigorous physical activity can alter body composition. Exercise coupled with caloric regulation results in an increase in lean body mass and a decrease in percent body fat in children, adolescents, and adults. The extent to which body composition can be altered is dependent upon the degree and length of training. Alterations in body composition are not necessarily permanent. As activity levels decrease, body fat increases. Parizkova (1982) demonstrated that there is a significant relationship between one's level of physical activity and his or her percent of lean body mass. Also, Bar-Or (1983) noted that the intensity of activity is significantly lower in obese children. Clearly, increased levels of vigorous physical activity coupled with moderation in caloric intake are keys to reducing the trend toward increased fatness among our nation's youth.

MOTOR FITNESS

The *motor fitness* components of speed, power, agility, balance, and coordination are generally considered to be the performance-related components of fitness. These components differ considerably from the health-related components of fitness in that they are genetically dependent, resistant to major environment (experiential) modifications, and are relatively stable. Also, these abilities are closely related to skillful performance in a variety of sports.

Quantitative changes in a variety of gross motor skills has been studied by several investigators over the past several decades. As a result, we have a wealth of information on the performance abilities of males and females from childhood through adolescence. In fact, it is even possible to compare performance scores between generations and arrive at some tentative conclusions concerning secular trends in motor performance on selected skills. Haubenstricker and Seefeldt (1986) presented data summaries for four motor performance items that have been assessed by a variety of investigators prior to and since 1960. Three of these: running for speed, jumping for distance, and throwing for distance are summarized in the following sections and presented in Table 17.2

Running Speed

Running speed may be assessed across studies that use different distances by converting dash times (usually 30- to 60-yard-dashes) to units of yards covered per second. In order to further standarize measurements, Haubenstricker and Seefeldt (1986) reported that only those studies that utilized a stationary start were included. The results of these comparisons led them to conclude that:

> There is systematic improvement in the running speed of children during the middle and late childhood years. This improvement in running speed continues during the teenage years for males. The running speed of post-1960 females increases until age 15, after which time it appears to plateau. (p. 67-69).

Table 17.2 Common Measure of Motor Fitness and A Synthesis of Findings

Motor Fitness Component	Common Measures	Synthesis of Findings
Speed	30-60 Yard Dash	Boys & girls are similar throughout childhood. Boys outperform girls at all ages. Males make more rapid improvement after puberty than females. Males make significant annual gains throughout childhood & adolescence. Females tend to plateau in midadolescence.
Power Lower Trunk	Jump for Distance Jump for Height	Boys and girls are similar throughout childhood. Boys slightly outperform girls during childhood, but the gap widens significantly at male puberty.
Power Upper Trunk	Throw for Distance	Males make significant annual increments throughout adolescence. Females begin to plateau during early adolescence and regress by mid-adolescence.
Balance		Boys significantly outperform girls at all ages. Males make significant qualitative, as well as quantitative improvements with age; females don't. Males make rapid improvement at all ages but especially after puberty when they tend to plateau. Females and males improve with age throughout childhood & adolescence.

Table 17.2 (continued)

Motor Fitness Component	Common Measures	Synthesis of Findings
Static Balance	Stabilometer Stick Balance Foot Balance	Females tend to outperform males during childhood on both static & dynamic measures.
Dynamic Balance	Beam Walk	Males & females are similar on both static & dynamic measures throughout adolescence with no clear advantage for either.

Figure 17.10 graphically depicts changes in running speed from childhood through adolescence based on studies conducted after 1960. Running speed is similar in boys and girls—only slightly favoring the boys—throughout childhood. Beginning at about age 12, however, males begin to make more rapid improvements while their female age-mates begin to plateau in performance scores. Reasons for the early plateauing on the part of adolescent females may be explained, in part, in terms of early maturation and lower levels of personal motivation as compared to their late maturing and often more highly motivated male age-mates. Figure 17.11 illustrates comparable results in actual age changes in running the 100-yard-dash.

Jumping for Distance

Jumping for distance, a purported measure of muscular power (i.e., strength x speed), has been assessed in a large number of studies. Haubenstricker and Seefeldt (1986), in summarizing the post-1960 performance scores of children and adolescents 5 to 17 years of age (Figure 17.12), found that males only slightly outperform females and that there is steady improvement for both from ages 5 to 14. After that, females begin to level off in their performance and may even decline. Males, however, continue to improve at a linear rate to about age 17 (Figure 17.13). The discrepancy between males and females on the standing long jump begins to appear after age 12. The widening gap may be explained in a variety of ways. First, jumping for distance incorporates an element of strength. Males from puberty onward demonstrate dramatic strength gains whereas their female counterparts, because of low levels of circulating androgens, tend to level off in strength. Therefore, a widening of the gap at this time is to be expected. The tendency of females to regress in performance after age 14 may be explained by lack of motivation or an

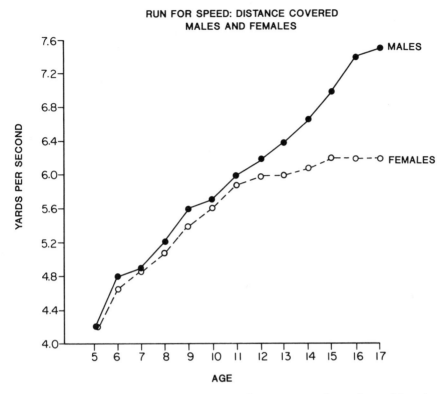

RUN FOR SPEED: DISTANCE COVERED
MALES AND FEMALES

Figure 17.10 Age changes in running speed: mean scores for males and females 5-17 years, from post-1960 studies (Adapted from: Haubenstricker, J., and Seefeldt, V. [1986] "Acquisition of Motor Skills During Childhood." In Seefeldt, V. [Ed.] *Physical Activity and Well-Being*. Reston, VA: AAHPERD)

increasingly sedentary lifestyle typical of later adolescence. Also, changes in body proportions and a lower center of gravity may help account for these changes.

Throwing for Distance

Throwing for distance is a frequently used measure of muscular power in the upper extremities. As in running for speed and jumping for distance, skill enters into the equation. In other words, those who perform the run, jump, or throw at the mature stage are likely to score better on performance measures that incorporate these skills. The contribution of a mature pattern is no more evident than in throwing for distance. Immature throwers are at a distinct disadvantage. Therefore, significantly lower mean performance scores for females throughout childhood and adolescence may be interpreted as just as much a factor of lower skill

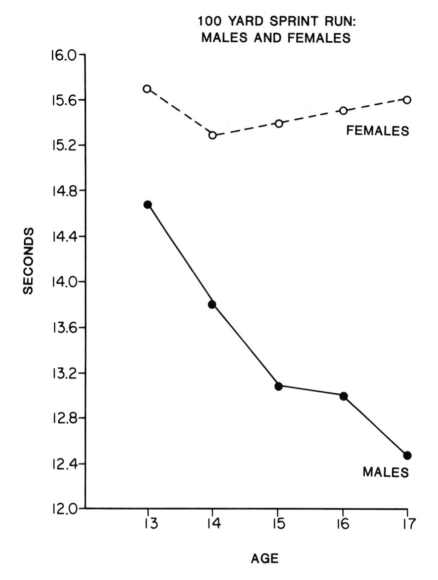

Figure 17.11 100 yd. sprint run mean scores for males and females 13-17 years, in seconds (*Source*: Ross, J. G., and Gilbert, G. G. [1985]. "The National Children and Youth Fitness Study: A Summary of Findings." *Journal of Physical Education, Recreation and Dance,* 56, 1, 46-50)

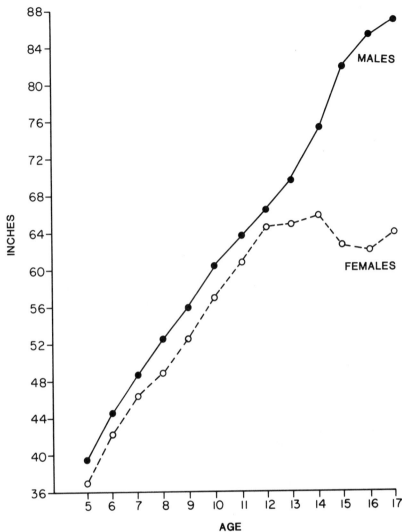

Figure 17.12 Age changes in standing long jump: mean scores for males and fe-
males 5-17 years, from post-1960 studies (Adapted from: Haubenstricker, J., and
Seefeldt, [1986] "Acquisition of Motor Skills During Childhood." In Seefeldt, V.
[Ed.] *Physical Activity and Well-Being*. Reston, VA: AAHPERD)

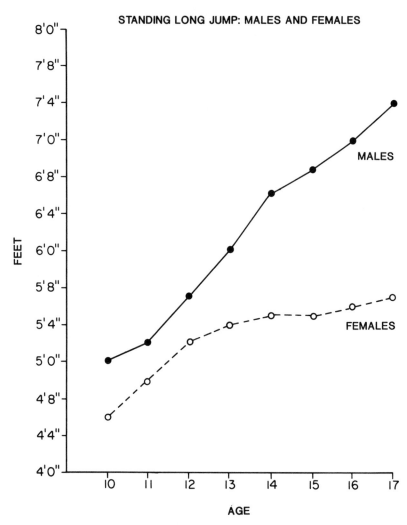

Figure 17.13 Standing long jump mean scores, for males and females 10-17 years, in feet (*Source*: Ross, J. G., and Gilbert, G. G. [1985]. "The National Children and Youth Fitness Study: A Summary of Findings." *Journal of Physical Education, Recreation and Dance*, 56, 1, 46-50)

levels as weakness in the upper arm and shoulder girdle area. Figure 17.12 clearly shows significant differences between males and females at all ages, and the gap only widens with age. Males experience a significant upsurge in performance scores around age 13, corresponding roughly with the onset of puberty. Females, however, demonstrate a much more gradual increase to age 15 followed by a tendency to regress slightly.

Reuschlein and Haubenstricker (1985) offer the best explanation for these dramatic differences between genders. In their study of the throwing patterns of fourth, seventh, and tenth graders, 51, 61, and 70 percent of the males, respectively, throw with "good form" at what may be considered the mature stage. But only 15, 19, and 23 percent of the females, respectively, threw at the mature stage.

Balance

Williams (1983), in her review of age and gender differences in bal-

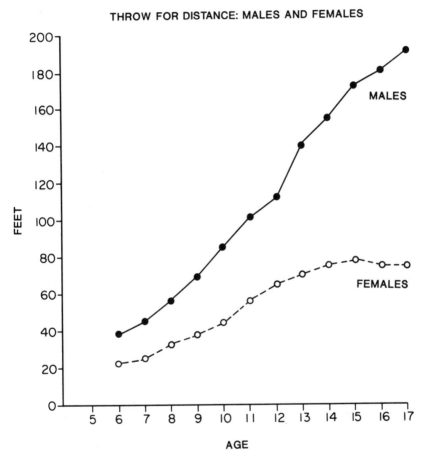

Figure 17.14 Age changes in throwing for distance: mean scores for males and females 6-17 years, from post-1960 studies (Adapted from: Haubenstricker, J., and Seefeldt, V. [1986] "Acquisition of Motor Skills During Childhood." In Seefeldt, V. [Ed.] *Physical Activity and Well-Being*. Reston, VA: AAHPERD)

ance performance, found that, in general, balance improves from age 3 to 18. Difficulty exists, however, in directly comparing the abundant information on balance that exists. A wide variety of measures have been used over the years to assess both static balance and dynamic balance and, as a result, comparisons between studies is not possible. It is possible, however, to conclude that balance tends to improve with age through childhood and adolescence. Furthermore, females tend to outperform males on measures of both static and dynamic balance during childhood, but appear to have no clear advantage during adolescence (Williams, 1983).

SUMMARY

The health-related and performance-related fitness of the adolescent undergoes dramatic changes from the beginning of the adolescent period to later adolescence. In general, boys and girls are similar throughout childhood on most measures of fitness. The onset of the preadolescent growth spurt marks the beginning of a rapid acceleration in fitness scores for males. This may be associated with a variety of physical as well as sociocultural factors. Females, on the other hand, do not display the same rapid improvement. There is a decided tendency for adolescent females to improve at a slower rate to about age 15 when they begin to plateau and sometimes regress in their performance.

Health-related fitness measures are susceptible to considerable improvement in both males and females. As activity patterns change (hopefully for the better) we can anticipate changes in the slope of the performance curves for both males and females. Highly motivated individuals are significantly better performers on all measures of fitness than they were indicated to be by the mean scores reported for population samples.

CHAPTER CONCEPTS

17.1 Adolescent males outperform their female counterparts on measures of aerobic conditioning at all ages.

17.2 Male and female differences in aerobic capacity remain roughly constant to age 14, at which time males continue to make rapid improvements while females plateau.

17.3 Convenience-based sampling techniques of aerobic endurance yield better scores across age for males and females than random samples of the population.

17.4 Field-based population studies of health-related fitness yield more valid and reliable data, thus giving a truer picture of the fitness of American youth.

17.5 The performance levels of boys and girls on measures of strength and endurance are similar during early and middle childhood.

17.6 Males tend to outperform females on most measures of muscular strength and endurance at all ages.

17.7 Males make rapid gains in muscular strength and endurance throughout adolescence.

17.8 Females tend to peak in their muscular strength and endurance at the onset of puberty with a tendency to plateau and regress slightly in later adolescence.

17.9 Females tend to be comparable to males in abdominal strength and endurance prior to puberty but males make significantly more rapid gains after that time.

17.10 Males significantly outperform females in measures of upper trunk strength and endurance at all ages, and the gap widens after puberty.

17.11 As a population, females are more flexible than males throughout the adolescent period as well as throughout childhood.

17.12 Males tend to regress in their flexibility during the prepubescent growth spurt.

17.13 Both males and females tend to plateau and regress in their flexibility during later adolescence. This phenomenon is associated with reduced activity levels rather than age.

17.14 Females steadily increase in percent body fat from the preadolescent period through adolescence.

17.15 Males increase in percent body fat during their preadolescent period followed by a sharp decline at puberty and a leveling off throughout adolescence.

17.16 American youth are more fat in the 1980s than their counterparts of the 1960s.

17.17 Boys and girls are similar in their performance abilities in running for speed and jumping for distance during childhood, with boys having only a slight advantage.

17.18 The gap between males and females widens considerably in favor of males from puberty onward in the run for speed and jump for distance.

17.19 Significant differences between males and females exist throughout childhood and adolescence in throwing for distance, and the gap widens with age.

17.20 The motor fitness abilities of children and adolescents are skill-related. Therefore, more skilled performers will perform better on the items measured and vice versa.

17.21 Developmental differences between males and females on measures of motor performance may be due to both physical and cultural differences between genders.

17.22 Adolescent males tend to exhibit near linear trends in performance measures that stress strength, speed, and skill.

17.23 Females tend to outperform males on measures of static and dynamic balance throughout childhood.

17.24 No clear pattern of male-female superiority appears to exist on measures of static and dynamic balance during adolescence.

17.25 Both dynamic and static balance appears to improve with age through adolescence.

17.26 Developmental differences between males and females on measures of health-related and performance-related fitness in no way imply superiority or inferiority of one gender over the other.

TERMS TO REMEMBER

Convenience Sample

Interrater Reliability

Intrarater Reliability

Stratified Random Sample

Aerobic Endurance

Population Sample

Isotonic Strength/Endurance

Upper Body Strength/Endurance

Joint Flexibility

Body Composition

Hydrostatic Weighing

Bioelectrical Impedance

Skinfold Calipers

Secular Trend

CRITICAL READINGS

Ross, J. G. and Gilbert, G. G. (1985). "The National Children and Youth Fitness Study." *Journal of Physical Education, Recreation, and Dance*, 56, 1, 43-90.

Haubenstricker, J. and Seefeldt, V. (1986). "Acquisition of Motor Skills During Childhood." In Seefeldt, V. (ed.) *Physical Activity & Well-Being*." Reston, VA: AAHPERD.

Williams, H. G. (1983). *Perceptual and Motor Development*. Englewood Cliffs, NJ: Prentice-Hall, (Chapter 9).

18

Adolescent Socialization

CHAPTER COMPETENCIES

Upon Completion of This Chapter You Should Be Able To:

* *List and describe sociocultural correlates which may affect motor development.*

* *Evaluate relationships between sociocultural correlates and motor development.*

● *Define the term "adolescence" in terms of biological and sociocultural factors.*

● *Demonstrate knowledge about the process of cultural socialization.*

● *Discuss the structure of socialization and its implication for the motor behavior of adolescents.*

● *List and describe the primary factors that influence cultural socialization.*

● *Discuss the role of sport and physical activity on cultural socialization.*

● *Describe the impact of physical activity and sport on affiliation, self-esteem, attitude formation and moral growth.*

The term *adolescence* is difficult to define. Not only is it a period of rapid physical change, but it is also a period of social and psychological transition from childhood to adulthood. Differential rates of social and psychological maturation are as clearly evident as the variability in physical maturation discussed in previous chapters.

The period of adolescence has lengthened in North America not only for biological reasons, but also because of fundamental societal changes. The introduction of compulsory education and the ever-extending length of time that individuals remain in school or college has increased the length of financial dependence for many. The shift from an agrarian to an industrialized, and now to a technological, society has also served to lengthen the period of adolescence. Adolescence is indeed a period of preparation for life, and as life has become more complex and complicated, the preparatory period has lengthened.

Adolescent behavior is essentially exploratory. This exploratory behavior should not be viewed as unimportant; it is this trait that helps youth adapt to the emerging reality of society and their place in it. It is inevitable that such a behavioral trait carries with it high risks. As a result, adolescence is often seen as a turbulent time full of heartaches and problems.

It is naive to assume that the period of adolescence will be as smooth and placid as childhood. Adolescents are not passive spectators to their growth process or to the world around them. This is a time of questioning, challenging, exploring, and critically examining the actions of both peers and adults. These traits are essential if the adolescent is to make a successful transition from childhood to adulthood. Adolescent development must not be stigmatized through demands for unquestioning obedience to authority. Wise adult leadership, positive role models, and nurturing guidance are essential to the healthy and productive psychosocial process of development.

To combat the rising and often life-threatening problems of adolescence, one must critically examine the causes prior to offering viable solutions. Teen alcohol and drug abuse, pregnancy, delinquency, and suicide are major problems among the teen culture of our society. The choices that are made in these areas as part of the exploratory process of adolescence have powerful implications and lifelong consequences. Problems in these areas frequently signals failure of the family, peers, school, and society at large to help adolescents make intelligent and responsible choices in their transition to adulthood.

In this chapter we will examine critical aspects in the process of adolescent socialization. Each of these areas may be influenced by the process of motor development.

THE STRUCTURE OF SOCIALIZATION

Cultural Socialization is a term that refers to the modification of one's behavior to conform to the expectations of the group. Sage (1986, p. 344) defines it as "the process by which persons learn the skills, attitudes, values, and behaviors that enable them to participate as members of the society in which they live." In other words, socialization is a lifelong process by which an infant becomes an adult in a cultural setting.

The structure of socialization is dependent upon three factors: status, roles, and norms. *Status* refers to one's position in society. Status is variable in that one may actually have several positions. Adolescents, for example, have different levels of status conferred upon them as sons or daughters, students, and athletes. They learn to play the role associated with the level of status that has been established. Therefore, a *role* is an individual behavior that one uses to carry out a status. It is the "job description" (status) interacting with the "interpretation of the job" (role). The manner in which one acts out his or her role as a son or daughter, student, or athlete is reflected by the status of that role and certain norms of behavior. *Norms* are standards of behavior expected of all members of a given society. Societal norms are the means by which cultural transmission occurs. Therefore, sons and daughters should "act" like sons and daughters, students should "act" like students, and athletes should "act" like athletes. These standards of behavior may change from society to society but remain relatively constant within a given society.

Socialization is an active process and should not be viewed as the mere internalization of status, roles, and norms. Although this is important, socialization is more than the passive stamping of society on the individual. We are dynamic, ever-developing beings and, as such, bring a wealth of individual differences to the process of socialization. Cultural socialization should be viewed as an interactive process between society and the individual with one intricately influencing the other.

INFLUENCING FACTORS

A variety of factors influence the process of socialization, including people, institutions, and activities. Each of these is briefly discussed in the following paragraphs.

People

Family members, the peer group, friends, and significant adults all play critical roles in the social development of the adolescent. The family structure has undergone dramatic changes in the last generation and is likely to continue to evolve in response to societal demands. Today, only about one family in four conforms to the traditional family stereotype of the two parent, one-marriage, multiple child family with mother as the primary caregiver and homemaker, and father as the sole wage earner (Conger and Peterson, 1984). Instead, a variety of family patterns may be found, including: two-income families, single-parent families, childless couples, blended families, and combined non-married households. As a result, the role of the "family" in social development has changed as the structure of the family has changed. Nevertheless, 98 percent of all children are still raised in "families" and 79 percent of these live with two parents (U.S. Department of Commerce Bureau of the Census, 1987).

The family remains the dominant agent of socialization throughout childhood and well into adolescence. It is responsible, among other things, for fostering a sense of autonomy, love, and trust in the adolescent. The family has a tremendous influence on socializing youth into physical activity and sport. The socioeconomic status of the family, for example, influences the activity choices of children and youth. Greenspan (1983) found that age-group swimmers, skiers, and gymnasts tended to come from upper-middle-class families but that young wrestlers, baseball players, and boxers tended to come from less economically privileged homes. Similarly, Greendorfer, (1977) and Greendorfer and Lewko, (1978) found that family members play a critical role in sport selection and involvement. Parental attitudes, encouragement, and personal participation were found to be important factors in activity selection.

As adolescence approaches and childhood wanes the influence of the family is frequently diminished by a rise in importance of the peer group. It must be remembered that increased importance of the peer group is a first giant step toward autonomy. The peer group serves as a buffer between the influences of the family and the influences of the "real" world. As a result, the peer group plays a powerful role in the life of the adolescent. With respect to socialization into physical activity and sport, the peer group is dominant during childhood, adolescence, and early adulthood (Greendorfer, 1977). Sport selection and participation is as much or more dependent on the need for group identity and affiliation than on the need for skill mastery and the opportunity to compete. The importance of the peer group during adolescence must not be minimized. Parents and coaches need to recognize that activity selection and participation is often less a matter of a desire to compete than it is a matter of wanting to fit in and belong.

Special friends and significant adults outside the family frequently play an important role in the process of adolescent socialization. At times these individuals may even overshadow the influence of the family and the peer group. The respected friend or the revered coach serve to influence the social development of the adolescent. Peer counseling and modeling behaviors of respected mentors offers promise as effective techniques for influencing behavioral changes in adolescents (Carnegie Report, 1987).

Institutions

Adolescents come into contact with a variety of societal institutions which all have impact on their socialization into the culture. The school is probably the primary institutional influencing agent if for no other reason than it occupies the greatest portion of the individual's day for the longest period of time. The school physical education program has the responsibility of developing fundamental and sport skills in the activities of the culture. It is charged with informing children about fitness and its importance and with helping them develop the skills necessary for maintaining a healthy, active way of life. The physical education program could be a significant socializing agent but is frequently misused and abused into having a reverse effect; Individuals are turned off to vigorous physical activity and skill development (Vogel, 1986; Seefeldt, 1987).

Youth organizations such as the YMCA, YWCA, Boys and Girls Clubs, and a host of youth sport leagues all play important roles in adolescent socialization. Youth sport programs are a significant cultural modifier in North American society today. It is estimated that more than 16 million children between 6 and 16 participate in more than 30 non-school sponsored sports programs (Martens, 1986).

Youth organizations such as the Boy Scouts and the Girl Scouts, along with the church, are also important institutions of socialization for many children and youth. These agencies serve to promote ethical and moral character. They help youngsters develop a set of values and a wholesome outlook on life and their responsibilities as citizens.

Activities

The activities engaged in by children and adolescents play an important role in cultural socialization. Children's play, games, and sports activities all play important roles in the socialization process. In fact, one of the often-stated objectives of physical education centers around the goal of social development through physical activities (Greendorfer, 1987). Although the research base for this claim is sparse, empirical evidence tends to support the notion that cultural attitudes and values can be transmitted (in some undefined and almost mystical way) through physical activity. The influence of physical activity on psychosocial development will be examined further in the section that follows.

PHYSICAL ACTIVITY AND SOCIALIZATION

The role of physical activity in the form of play, games, and sport cannot be denied. Growth and motor development does not take place in a vacuum but rather in a social setting that tremendously influences and is influenced by physical activity. The need for group affiliation and belonging is an often-cited reason for participation in peer play and sport (Greendorfer, 1987). So, too, is the enhancement of self-esteem through increased movement competence and confidence (Weiss, 1987). Physical activity as a socializing agent is also reported as a powerful influence on attitude formation (Sage, 1986) and moral development (Weiss and Bredemeier, 1986).

Affiliation

One of the most compelling forces of later childhood and adolescence is the need to belong. The need to be identified as part of a group, to have an identity as a member of the team or club, plays an important role in the adolescent's involvement in physical activity. The popularity of peer play and youth sport is in large part attributable to the need for affiliation. In fact, Coakley (1983, p. 438) reported that when asked why they are involved in peer play activity, adolescents frequently cited "reaffirmation of friendships." Oftentimes, winning is not the primary reason for engaging in peer play. When play is converted to organized sport, however, winning does become an overriding goal of activity involvement (Sage, 1986).

The need for affiliation, fun, and winning must be carefully considered in all sport programs. Certainly, athletes must have an opportunity to compete at the highest level of which they are capable, but fun and fellowship must not be omitted in the quest to be number one. Failure to stress fun and friendship has been associated as an important factor in the dramatic dropout rate in youth sport programs. It has been estimated that for all youth sports the annual dropout rate is about 35 percent (Gould, 1987). Overemphasis of competition is one of the most frequently-cited reasons for this high rate, along with burnout induced by overtraining and inadequate instruction.

Sport offers many potential benefits to its participants, but care must be taken to maintain a healthy balance between competition and cooperation. Recognition that the need for affiliation is one of the most influential factors for participation in play, games, and sport should alert teachers, coaches, and parents to its value as a socializing agent.

Self-Esteem

Self-esteem development begins at birth and is generally stabilized by the adolescent years (Wylie, 1979; Campbell, 1984). The nature of self-esteem development and the influences of physical activity on the developing self were discussed in Chapter 14 (Childhood and Self-Esteem). Historically, self-concept has been viewed as a global trait, but more recently it has been viewed as a trait that may be factored into several components representing the psychomotor, cognitive, and affective domains (Harter, 1982). Hence, the introduction of terms such as "movement competence," "movement confidence," and "perceived competence," all of which may foster the development of a positive self-concept.

Physical activity as part of the adolescent's total constellation of behavior provides one important avenue by which self-concept may be reinforced. Weiss (1986) cautions, however, that:

"A continuing controversy among educators pertains to the causal relationship between self-esteem and achievement. Specifically, does achievement or gains in competence lead to enhanced self-esteem, or does self-esteem influence achievement? That is, does a high level of self-esteem increase the likelihood for successful accomplishment?" (p. 103-104).

In terms of adolescent socialization, the question posed by Weiss, although interesting and in need of clarification, is moot. That is, regardless of whether self-esteem influences achievement, or achievement influences self-esteem, physical activity plays an important but largely undetermined role in the process of forming the stable, positive view of self so essential to the adolescent socialization process.

Attitude Formation

A major formation of socialization is the transference of the attitudes and values of one's culture. Basically, an *attitude* is a feeling of like or dislike about something. It is a learned behavior that has placed a value on something or someone. Kenyon (1968, p. 567) has defined an attitude as "a latent and nonobservable, complex but relatively stable behavioral disposition reflecting both direction and intensity of feeling toward a particular object, whether it be concrete or abstract." In other words, an attitude is an emotion, based on a knowledge or belief that results in either positive or negative behavior (Figure 18.1).

As learned behaviors, attitudes are acquired in a social context and, as such, may be taught, modified, shaped, and changed. Acquisition of an attitude involves three things: compliance, identification, and internalization (Kellman, 1958). *Compliance* is associated with doing something in the hope of getting a favorable response from someone else. Example: The young athlete, although not one to stretch out prior to a training run, does so because her coach is watching. *Identification* requires one to adopt the attitude or behavior of another. Example: The runner stretches out in preparation for her training run even in the coach's absence because she knows that is what the coach wants. *Internalization* deals with

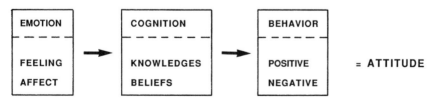

Figure 18.1 Components of an attitude

taking on a behavior as part of one's value system. Example: Our runner now stretches out prior to her training run because of her own desire to do so.

Physical activity in the form of peer play, games, and sport has the potential for shaping positive attitudes. Attitudes, when grouped together into the often-elusive constructs of character, sportsmanship, and fair play, contribute to the moral development and integrity of the individual.

Morality

Moral behavior within a sport context is called *sportsmanship*. It is commonly believed that participation in sport not only has the potential for developing character, but instills the moral ideals of the culture in the young athlete. Sport has great potential for developing moral behavior because of the variety of emotions engendered and the unpredictable situations that arise in practice and game situations. Sport provides an ideal setting in which to teach the qualities of honesty, loyalty, self-control and sportsmanship. Care should be taken to distinguish between the conventional aspect of sportsmanship and the moral aspect of sportsmanship. Weiss and Bredemeier (1986, p. 373) note that:

> Social-conventional behaviors are those which conform to prescribed social norms and are intended to maintain social organization.

Therefore, shaking hands and congratulating an opponent after a contest are not examples of moral behaviors but of accepted standards of conventional behavior. "Moral behaviors are those which are concerned with the physical or psychological welfare of others and the protection of rights and responsibilities" (Weiss and Bredemeier, 1986, p. 375). Refraining from lying, cheating, and intimidating opposing players are moral decisions governed by concern for the physical and psychological protection of the rights of others.

Moral development is the development of the conscience. Kohlberg (1981, 1984), a cognitive developmentalist building on the work of Piaget (1932), proposed a three-level hierarchical model of moral development that can be subdivided into six stages. The first level is known as *Preconventional Morality*. The Preconventional Level is characteristic of the preschool and primary grade child. The first stage within the Preconventional Level is the *punishment/obedience stage*. The child is egocentric, avoids punishment, and responds to power. Stage 2, or the *Naive Egotism Stage* is characterized by a "whatever feels good is okay" philosophy. The concept of "it is okay as long as you don't get caught" predominates at this level. At the *Conventional Morality Level* there is a real desire to win approval and to please others. It is frequently referred to as the *Good Boy/Nice Girl Stage.* Being liked and conforming to group norms are important individual goals at this stage. The next stage within the Conventional Level is the *Law and Order Stage* in which the individual recognizes that behavior is governed by the rules of society and that laws define what is right. Operation at the Conventional Level is typical of the childhood and adolescent period. In fact, it is suggested by some that most of us do not get beyond the fourth stage to the Postconventional Level. At the *Postconventional Morality Level* the individual is inner-directed rather than other-directed. The *Social Contract Stage* is a time when one recognizes that what is right is what is agreed on by the whole of society and that some laws are unjust and can be changed. Personal behavior at this level is not regulated by law but by a personal decision of what is right and wrong. The *Universal Ethical Principal* stage is the highest level of morality according to Kohlberg. At this stage right and wrong is determined by one's conscience within a logical, consistent and universal framework. The universal dignity and worth of all humankind is recognized (Figure 18.2).

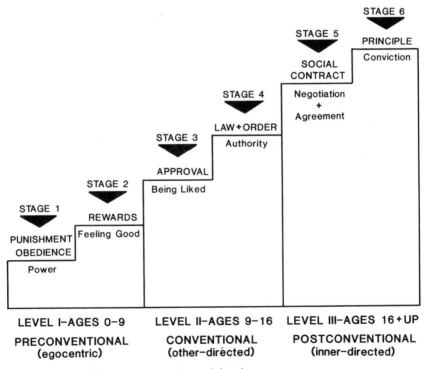

Figure 18.2 Kohlberg's stages of moral development

Moral development is not automatic but requires social settings where moral dilemmas can be provoked, worked out, and restructured based on one's own experiences. The environment of play, games, and sport offers an ideal social setting where all levels of moral behavior can be observed and developed and where real moral growth can occur. Unless the thought process is stimulated, dissonance will not occur. If dissonance does not occur, it is unlikely that moral growth will take place.

SUMMARY

Socialization is a lifelong process that is particularly important during the period of adolescence. Cultural socialization is influenced by status, roles, and societal norms of behavior. Adolescents are confronted with changing status and an increasing number of roles to play. They are shaped by society, and society is shaped by them.

A variety of societal factors shape the process of adolescent socialization. Other people, institutions, and activities serve as primary socializing agents. Physical activity is an important area of adolescent socialization. Participation in the games, play, and sport of one's culture provides a means for affiliation, self-esteem enhancement, attitude formation, and moral growth.

The process of development is continual and multi-faceted. As such, motor development influences and is influenced by the process of cultural socialization.

CHAPTER CONCEPTS

18.1 The period of adolescence has been extended at the upper end due to sociocultural factors.

18.2 Adolescence is a period of exploration and experimentation, both of which may have lifelong consequences.

18.3 To be socialized is to modify one's behavior to the expectations of the group.

18.4 Socialization is dependent on the interaction of status, roles, and norms.

18.5 A variety of factors influence the process of socialization. Among the most potent are the family, the peer group, and special friends.

18.6 Sport and physical activity has the potential for being a powerful socializing agent.

18.7 Games, play, and sport offer opportunities for affiliation and group identity formation.

18.8. Self-esteem and achievement are linked, but it is difficult to establish a causal relationship.

18.9 Attitude formation is a major function of socialization.

18.10 Formation of an attitude requires compliance, identification, and internalization.

18.11 Moral growth may be fostered through games, play, and sport.

18.12 Moral behavior in a sport setting is called "sportsmanship."

18.13 The conventional aspect of sportsmanship and the moral aspect of sportsmanship are not the same.

18.14 One's stage of moral development is age-related but not age-dependent.

TERMS TO REMEMBER

Adolescence

Cultural Socialization

Status

Roles

Norms

Attitude

Compliance

Identification

Internalization

Sportsmanship

Morality

Preconventional Morality

Conventional Morality

Postconventional Morality

CRITICAL READINGS

Bredemeier, B. J. and Shields, D. L. (1987). "Moral Growth Through Physical Activity: A Structural/Developmental Approach." In Gould, D., and Weiss, M. R. (eds.) *Advances in Pediatric Sport Sciences* (Volume 2: Behavioral Issues). Champaign, IL: Human Kinetics.

Coakley, J. J. (1987). "Children and the Sport Socialization Process." In Gould, D. and Weiss, M. R. (eds.) *Advances in Pediatric Sport Sciences*. (Volume 2: Behavioral Issues). Champaign, IL: Human Kinetics.

Gilbert, B. (May 16, 1988) "Competition." *Sports Illustrated*, 68, 20, 86-100.

Sage, G. H. (1986) "Social Development." In Seefeldt, V. (ed.) *Physical Activity and Well-Being*. Reston, Va: AAHPERD.

Weiss, M. R. and Bredemeier, B. J. (1986). "Moral Development." In Seefeldt, V. (ed.) *Physical Activity and Well-Being*. Reston, VA: AAHPERD.

SECTION V
PROGRAMMING

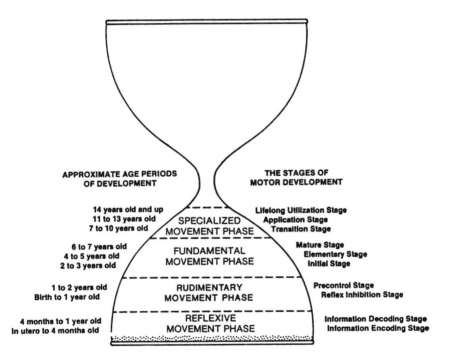

APPROXIMATE AGE PERIODS OF DEVELOPMENT		THE STAGES OF MOTOR DEVELOPMENT
14 years old and up	SPECIALIZED MOVEMENT PHASE	Lifelong Utilization Stage
11 to 13 years old		Application Stage
7 to 10 years old		Transition Stage
6 to 7 years old	FUNDAMENTAL MOVEMENT PHASE	Mature Stage
4 to 5 years old		Elementary Stage
2 to 3 years old		Initial Stage
1 to 2 years old	RUDIMENTARY MOVEMENT PHASE	Precontrol Stage
Birth to 1 year old		Reflex Inhibition Stage
4 months to 1 year old	REFLEXIVE MOVEMENT PHASE	Information Decoding Stage
In utero to 4 months old		Information Encoding Stage

19

Children's Play, Toys, and Play Spaces

CHAPTER COMPETENCIES

Upon Completion of This Chapter You Should Be Able To:

* *Apply motor development principles to equipment, play space, and living environments.*

* *Define the word "play" and discuss why people of all ages play.*

* *Chart the developmental aspects of play and show how they interact with the Phases of Motor Development.*

* *Discuss the role of toys in child development.*

* *Take a stand on the use of war toys in play.*

* *Demonstrate knowledge of toy safety and criteria for choosing toys.*

* *Be knowledgeable about the design developmentally appropriate indoor and outdoor play spaces.*

* *Provide a developmentally sound rationale for the design, inclusion and placement of play equipment in the indoor and outdoor play space.*

For children, play is essentially a learning medium, but for many it is often viewed as a frivolous pastime. It seems unnecessary among knowledgeable people to assert that play is valid as a learning medium as well as for its own inherent values, especially with the attention that the writings of Piaget (1957), Erikson (1963), and others have commanded in recent years and with the implications for developing cognitive and affective structures through play. More than 20 years ago Frank (1968, p. 433) noted that "within recent years there has been a strong movement to restrict the play of children, young and older, to adult-imposed patterns in order to promote formal learning, especially preparation for school." The situation has only been magnified since Frank's insightful statement. We must, therefore, continue to reassert the validity and the necessity for play in child development.

The greatest values of play in education are that it is interesting to children, holds their attention, arouses their enthusiasm, is fun, and contributes to the developing self. As a result, a primary distinction between the terms "work" and "play" is that play is engaged in simply for its own sake. Play does, however, through proper guidance, have numerous residual benefits that make it a desirable medium through which myriad psychomotor, cognitive, and affective competencies may be developed. Play is an effective learning medium because of the importance placed on it by children and its potential influence on all aspects of behavior. It is time that the validity of children's play be recognized for its own sake. To do this, we must pay more than lip service to its values. We must become sensitive to the play of children, and in doing so become familiar with the types of toys and play spaces that are conducive to children's optimal growth. This chapter will focus on three important aspects of children's lives: play, toys, and play spaces.

PLAY

The meaning of the word "*play*" is elusive and has various connotations to many people. Ellis (1973), in the excellent book *Why People Play*, explores in detail the questions on what play is and why people play. Play is usually considered pleasant and voluntary. With reference to children, the definition of play offered by Galambos (1970, p. 61), is perhaps the most appropriate for our discussion of motor development. Galambos considers play to be "direct, spontaneous activity by which children engage with people and things around them. It is imaginative, usually active; youngsters perform it with all their senses and use their hands or their whole bodies."

The following is a discussion of why children play and the developmental aspects of play. It should be read carefully to gain greater insight into the child's world of play.

Why Children Play

To children, play is serious business, and it is this seriousness of purpose that gives it its educational value. Play is the way in which children explore and experiment with the world around them as they build up relations with that world, with others, and with themselves. Children at play are discovering how to come to terms with their world, how to cope with the tasks of life, how to master new skills, and how to gain confidence in themselves as worthwhile individuals. Play provides a medium through which children can learn by trial and error. It provides a means through which they experience an endless number of real-life situations in miniature with a minimum of risks, penalties, and pain for mistakes. It is an excellent way in which to learn how to cope with the "real" world.

Play provides an avenue through which children gradually learn the difference between "mine" and "yours." It permits children to discover themselves before reaching out to others in their rapidly expanding world. Through play, children learn basic patterns of living. Their imagination and love for creative drama enable them to assume various roles, feelings, attitudes, and emotions.

Play is also necessary for the mental health of children. Children engage in play wholeheartedly, discarding all self-consciousness and restraint. They reveal their true nature through play and often provide the parent and teacher with subtle indicators of their emotional well-being. Immature children who have had limited play experiences often need to be taught how to play in a meaningful and constructive manner. These children exhibit their lack of ability to play through their wandering, constant boredom, and pleas that "there is nothing to do." Aggressive behavior is often exhibited through destructive play and is typified by children who always manage to break their toys or inevitably end up in a wrestling match with their peers. Children who are emotionally disturbed often prefer to play with things rather than interact with other children and are demanding of both adult attention and approval of their play. Well-adjusted children find it easy to slip in and out of various roles in dramatic play.

Play helps meets children's emotional needs to belong and to have status within a group and a feeling of personal worth. As a result, they generally play at things in which they do well (much the same as adults) and experience a reasonable degree of success.

Through active play children learn to move for movement's sake as well as for learning's sake. Directed play experiences can serve as an effective means by which they may develop and refine a variety of fundamental movement abilities. It also serves as a facilitator for enhancing physical fitness and motor abilities. The natural drive by most children to be active needs to be continually nurtured by both parents and teachers.

Developmental Aspects of Play

When viewing the play behavior of children, it is apparent that there is a predictable sequence of emergence of developmental aspects. The play of the infant and toddler is considerably different from that of the primary grade child. Increased complexity of the neuromuscular apparatus plus higher-order cognitive functioning and increased affective competencies make for characteristic forms of play at various ages. When observing play, however, one runs the risk of interpreting it within the context of one's own interests and understandings and failing to see it in its complete form. As a result, a narrow view of play is often developed. For example, an individual primarily interested in the motor development of children may view play from the perspective of gross motor activities, games, and sport. Individuals interested primarily in cognitive development often view play from the quiet activity aspect of problem solving and experimentation with new equipment, materials, and ideas. Persons primarily concerned with the affective domain often view play from the functions that it serves as a socializing agent, without regard to either its active or quiet forms. In actuality, play incorporates all aspects of development, whether motor, cognitive, or affective. We must, therefore, view play in light of its total contribution to the growth and development of children.

Play during the first year of life does not look much different from normal daily activity. The infant is constantly involved in using all of his or her senses and, when awake, appears to be in almost constant motion. The play of infants is centered around their own bodies, the bodies of others, and concrete objects. It involves the exploration and repetition of perceptual cues and is purposeful. Through play, the infant comes to grips with his or her world and develops a host of cognitive, affective, and psychomotor competencies. For example, the ever-popular game of "peekaboo" is enjoyed by all infants and may be viewed from a cognitive standpoint as a learning activity in which the child learns, through experience, the complex ideas of permanence, consistency, and reliability of objects, and that objects can reappear once they have disappeared. Peekaboo also has implications for affective development in that it provides a medium for the infant to learn to trust the world, to shape it, and to make things happen. From a psychomotor standpoint, it provides practice in controlling the musculature of the hands and proper sequencing of events in time.

The play of infants involves coming into contact with shapes, textures, colors, and sounds. A great deal of time is spent in looking, listening, grasping, sucking, teething, and exploring. In short, the play of infants is a sensorimotor experience that involves the broadening use of all of the senses in order to come to better know and to function better in the immediate world.

The toddler rapidly expands beyond the play of infancy. It is a time of reaching out into the world through ceaseless, joyful movement in an effort to order his or her world. The play of toddlers is primarily *egocentric*;

that is, it is confined to the individual and does not involve interaction in a constructive manner. Toddlers use their newly acquired mobility to explore space. They spend a great deal of time trying out their movement potentialities. They crawl, climb, scoot, walk, run, roll, and jump. They attempt to order their world by classifying objects and searching for patterns. They enjoy play with small manageable toys, lining them up, stacking them, and exploring them with their mouths. They play at classifying objects according to size, shape, color, and function. Toddlers also spend a great deal of time testing the limits of their world through imagination, imitation, and dramatic play. The *imitative play* world of toddlers enables them to make sense of experiences through dramatizing it in action. Toddlers enjoy loading and unloading objects of various sizes into containers. By doing so, they are developing concepts of volume and permanence. Stroking different-textured objects is a favorite quiet play activity of toddlers, and they often have a favorite cuddly toy or blanket. This may be viewed as an attempt by the child to find warmth and security at a time when many demands for more mature behavior are being made, such as with developing the self-help skills of feeding and toiletry.

The play of the preschooler is an elaboration of the earlier forms of play and also involves new aspects. Children at this age enjoy using and mastering a wide variety of materials. They thoroughly enjoy working with paints, sand, clay, water, and blocks. The use of these materials begins by being purely exploratory and then becomes more systematic, organized, and takes on concrete form. The imitative play of the toddlers gives way during these years to highly involved *sociodramatic play*, with a more mature grasp of what is real and what is fantasy. They enjoy acting out social situations, dressing as grown-ups, and travel play with cars, fire engines, and airplanes. Preschool children enjoy active play. They love to run and jump, throw and catch, and need little encouragement for active movement. They enjoy building things and progress from blocks to more advanced forms of construction.

Elementary grade children enjoy many of the same activities as preschoolers but exhibit increasing ability to work with others in small groups. Through *small group play* they are more interested in active games and table games with rules and regulations. They enjoy art and making designs in 2- and 3-dimensional form. Primary grade children enjoy drawing, painting, and molding as an expression of their creativity. Their imagination, however, is often less vivid than preschoolers, and care must be taken by adults to nurture it. Primary grade children enjoy discovery play, problem solving, and vigorous movement activities. Upper elementary grade children and beyond enjoy *large group play*. Team sport relays and activities that incorporate larger numbers are especially enjoyable.

There is considerable overlap between the play of toddlers, pre-schoolers, and elementary school children. Older children will often retreat to earlier forms of play in order to reestablish their security and self-confidence. Younger children likewise will often attempt the more sophisticated forms of play behavior of an older brother or sister, only to find that they do not possess the necessary gross or fine motor coordinations, nor the cognitive or affective capacity, for successfully engaging in that form of play. We return to the principle of readiness as the primary determinant of what, when, and how children play. We should view each child as an individual and structure play situations that are appropriate for that particular person.

Three hierarchical stages in the development of play behavior have been proposed by Reilly (1974), who views the development of play as having exploratory, competency, and achievement stages. *Exploratory play* roughly comprises the early childhood years. Every new thing the young child comes into contact with evokes curiosity, exploration, and play. *Competency play* is characteristic of the elementary school child. This represents a time for mastery over the environment. Practice, persistence, and the quest for mastery are characteristic of the competency stage. *Achievement play* places the individual within the competitive realm and achievement of the expectancies children and youth have for themselves as well as those others may hold for them.

Reilly's concept of the developmental aspects of play behavior is congruent with the Phases of Motor Development (Figure 19.1). The rudimentary movement phase corresponds nicely with exploratory play. Fundamental movement pattern development and refinement are congruent with mastery play, and the specialized movement phase parallels Reilly's achievement play.

TOYS

One of the most visible differences between today's modern schools and traditional classrooms is the number of objects made available for the purpose of helping children learn. Traditionally, schools have transmitted facts and concepts in an abstract way, by means of words, in an atmosphere removed from the everyday environment. In an effort to see that every child receives a socially useful and personally satisfying education, it has become apparent that this is not the only way for children to learn. For many it is not the best way, and for some, no way at all. Many children can learn better through activities that look suspiciously like play. Activities that involve toys, games, and manufactured and self-made puzzles; tools and materials; expressive media; models and replicas from the physical and social environment, concrete items that children

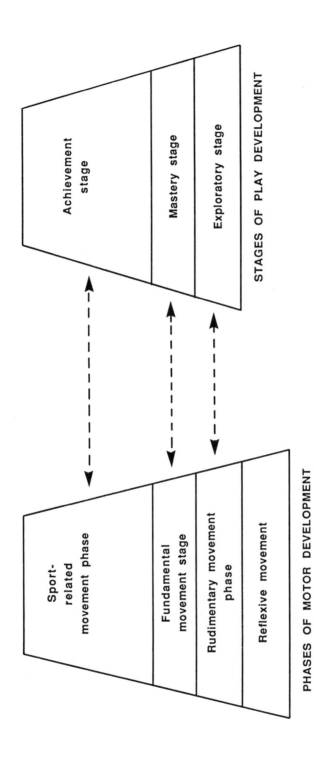

Figure 19.1 The relationship between the stages of play development and the Phases of Motor Development

can touch, handle, manipulate, and interact with are all being utilized with increasing frequency as an effective learning medium. In such ways they lay a solid foundation for abstract learning. This new emphasis is disturbing to many parents and some educators. "Why," they say, "the children are only playing. They can do that at home!" Such persons should be led to understand the many specific learning purposes for such "play" activities.

Toys and expressive media are often useful as tools for the various types of diagnosis that teachers make about the developmental stage, educational needs, and emotional health of their students. It is important, for example, for teachers to discover the maturational level of children entering the preschool or elementary grades. Observation of children's skills in using materials and their interaction with the materials and other children is revealing and valid to the knowledgeable observer. Toys such as building blocks are a good example. They give children power to construct and manipulate their world within their own frame of reference. Their building may be free in form and unstructured, or realistic and elaborated. In watching such activities, as well as in talking with children, the teacher receives clues to many of their perceptual, cognitive, and emotional needs.

The therapeutic value of letting children express themselves in activities like finger painting, clay modeling, pounding, playing with dolls and other people figures, and role playing with the help of costumes or puppets, has been commonly accepted. They are useful in determining whether the child's need to relieve anxieties and to express concerns is temporary or results from a more deep-seated problem involving motor or perceptual difficulties or the expression of hostilities, fears, or other symptoms of psychological and social maladjustment.

Another use of tangible objects in the educational process which teachers can apply with most children, is developmental. In determining whether a child's lack of readiness for academic work is due to age or to lack of stimuli in the home environment, object-oriented activities (toys) are a valuable aid. They encourage the desired learning in the cognitive, psychomotor, or affective area, or in a combination of these.

On the cognitive level, immature children must be encouraged to furnish their minds with the concrete experiences that are the necessary foundation for the increasing complexity and level of abstraction of their thoughts. Being deprived of these opportunities at home or at school may make it impossible for them to develop to their full potential for abstract thinking. Remediation by furnishing an environment rich in stimuli can do much to overcome the original deprivation. But the child's way of thinking may have been so affected that he or she will respond most easily to ideas demonstrated in a concrete way. An effective teaching strategy for such children is to give them solid, manipulable objects designed to demonstrate the desired concepts. Word games, cut-out letters, puzzles, and Cuisenaire rods are examples. Older children do better when ideas are presented with examples from their own experience. Such a presentation does not handicap the learning of children who are able to handle abstracts; it simply helps reinforce the concepts for them.

The development of movement abilities depends in large part on the availability of objects with which children may interact. They need things that can be folded, bent, nailed, glued, cut, sewed, stretched, bounced, poured, twisted, punched, tied, blown into, and crushed; surfaces that can be painted, carved, attached to, and washed; items to look at, listen to, sniff, taste, fondle, and stroke; and objects to climb, swing on, sit on, stamp on, jump over, and crawl through.

The ways that toys contribute to learning in the affective area are also many and varied. Games and toys help children learn to discriminate between and interrelate with their environment and with other people. The skills they develop as they interact give them a feeling of being able to cope and of being in control of themselves and their surroundings. Becoming familiar with objects from the outside world such as toy trucks, buildings, and household equipment, helps broaden their concepts in realistic terms. Trying out other roles through dolls, puppets, toys, or real objects similar to those adults use or wear also helps children explore and discover their own identity and provides a safe way to try out more mature or different real-life roles.

Toys are big business. According to Toy Manufacturers of America, there are approximately 150,000 different toys on the market, with about 5,000 new toys being introduced each year. Parents buy toys for a variety of reasons ranging from tradition to providing toys they never had. Some people buy toys and use them as bribes or rewards; hence toys are often used as a substitute for love and attention, to ease guilt, or to mold the child in the parents' image. For whatever purpose they are purchased, toys occupy many hours of the child's play and should be carefully selected.

Table 19.1 presents a list of appropriate types of gross and fine motor toys for children from infancy through the primary grades. It must be remembered that play materials must be safe, durable, and interesting to children.

War Toys

When reviewing Table 19.1 it should be noted that there are no *war toys* (guns, etc.) listed. It is my feeling that the use of toy guns is not a form of play to be encouraged by adults. The purchase of commercially manu-

Table 19.1 Appropriate Play Materials for Children

Infants (0-1 Year)

1. Teething ring	6. Mirror
2. Rattles	7. Shapes
3. Hedgehog	8. Crawligator
4. Textured ball	9. Crib mobile
5. Ball rattle	10. Buttons on a cord

Toddlers (1-2 Years)

1. First blocks	9. Washable doll
2. Nesting boxes	10. Bells and music box
3. Peg board	11. Squeaky toys
4. Stacking toys	12. Push and pull toys
5. Snap toys	13. Sand toys
6. Cuddly toys	14. Sturdy picture books
7. Stepstool	15. Simple inlay puzzles (3 to 6
8. Soft throwing toys	pieces)

Preschoolers (3-5 Years)

1. Picture books	13. Climbing equipment
2. Dress-up clothes	14. Balancing equipment
3. Shape, size, and texture toys	15. Striking toys
4. Miniature toys	16. Beanbags
5. Cardboard boxes	17. Woodworking equipment
6. Blocks	18. Wading pool
7. Dolls and puppets	19. Record player and records
8. Furniture	20. Musical instruments
9. Puzzles (8 to 20 pieces)	21. Blunt scissors, paste, and paper
10. Painting and coloring materials	22. Modeling clay
11. Pots and pans	23. Simple storybooks
12. Large balls	24. Floating bath toys

Elementary Grades (6-10 Years)

1. Large and small balls	11. Sports equipment
2. Climbing rope or ladder	12. Building toys
3. Climbing frame	13. Storybooks
4. Balance beam	14. Chalkboard
5. Tumbling mat	15. Science toys
6. Jump rope	16. Globe
7. Bicycle	17. Dolls and puppets
8. Tinker toys	18. Playhouse
9. Flash cards	19. Water toys
10. Playing cards	20. Workbench and tools

factured toy guns is discouraged because of their realism. One need only visit a local toy store to see guns that smoke, "bang," look like machine guns, shotguns, and even the M14 rifle used in Vietnam. The use of guns purchased from the toy store serves no useful purpose. Some may argue with this, claiming that toy guns provide children with an avenue by which to work out their aggressions and that they will outgrow their need for violent expression. It does seem ludicrous, however, that in a society which claims to abhor killing and violence, we go to such great lengths to ensure realism in the toy guns made for children. If children truly outgrow their need for violent expression, why are the television channels and movie theaters filled with realistic scenes of violence and killing?

Children have a right and need to express themselves through fantasy play. Such things as "cops and robbers," "war," and "cowboys and Indians" are forms of fantasy play engaged in by children for generations. Children have a right to work out their aggressions, and they should be permitted to do so, but in a manner that does not encourage or promote realism. Perhaps the use of a "fantasy gun" (such as a stick or the index finger) in this form of fantasy play would reduce the realism created by commercially purchased toy guns.

Guns themselves are not an evil. The problem is in the way we condone and use them in our society. Whether in real life or in play, shooting someone is not a form of behavior to be viewed as the norm for society, even though it takes place during war and is an aspect of law enforcement. The use of toy guns should be discouraged among children.

Toy Safety

The *Child Protection and Toy Safety Act* was passed by the U.S. Congress in 1969. This law prohibits the sale of toys that may prove harmful to children. Any toy that presents an electrical, thermal, or mechanical hazard, or that may endanger the safety of children through sharp or protruding edges, fragmentation, explosion, strangulation, asphyxiation, electrical shock, or fire is not to be sold. The *Bureau of Product Safety*, a division of the Food and Drug Administration, prevents such products from entering the market and is responsible for recalling unsafe toys from the market.

Toy manufacturers have the responsibility to design toys in such a way that the materials used and the methods of construction make the toy as childproof as possible. That is, the toy should require a minimum of education of the user to make it safe. Ideally, no imaginable use or abuse of the toy by a child should make it unsafe.

The following is a listing of examples of toys that have been deemed unsafe by the Food and Drug Administration:

1. Sharp or protruding objects.
   Dolls of pliable plastic. The doll can be bent into positions in several directions. By doing so, however, sharp wires, serving as

joints, protrude from the ends of the doll's hands and feet. This could puncture a child seriously.

Large Ring Darts. The darts are 1 foot long and weigh about a pound. The child could easily lose an eye or receive puncture wounds on the body.

2. Fragmentation.

Clackers. Not long ago "clackers" were introduced to the toy market. This created great fun for children of all ages. These are quite dangerous, however, because the clackers may chip or fragment when struck together. These flying pieces could cause serious eye injury.

3. Explosive toys.

Cap Guns. These are a potential cause of deafness to children. Noises reaching 130 decibels are safe. Indoors, at a distance of 2 feet, the noise produced could expose children and others to a continuous sound level roughly fifteen times louder than that considered safe for continuous sound.

4. Strangulation.

Crib Mobiles. Stuffed animal characters are often suspended from the side of the infant's crib and over the crib. When one of the figures is pulled, the plastic bracket that supports the mobile often breaks near its base, sending the entire assembly into the crib. The strings could cause strangulation, and the broken bars could cause serious injury.

5. Asphyxiation.

Fringed Balloon Squeakers. The balloon is blown up and let go. As the air escapes from the balloon, a metal noisemaker lodged in the mouthpiece of the balloon makes a loud noise. If the child does not take the balloon out of the mouth, air escapes into the mouth and the noisemaker, because of the air pressure, acts as a missile that could shoot down the child's mouth and become lodged in the throat, causing asphyxiation.

6. Burns caused by electrical toys.

Ovens. A toy stove was recently introduced on the market. The stove reached temperatures of 200°F on the sides of the oven. On top it reached 300°F, and the inside of the oven rose to an unbelievable 660°F. Most kitchen ranges rise to temperatures under 180°F on the noncooking surfaces. A child could easily receive serious burns from such a toy.

7. Toxicity.

Rhythm Band Set. One such set includes toy musical instruments, one of which is a pair of maracas. The maracas, which contain pellets of poisonous lead, may come apart. The chance of inhaling the tiny pellets into the lungs also makes them a serious hazard to children.

8. Flammability.

Foam Balls. A popular brand foam ball was tested against the flammability standard set by the 1969 Child Protection and Toy Safety Act. Under the specified conditions, the ball not only ignited within the time limits specified for contact with a candle flame, but smoked profusely while burning and shed drops of burning substances.

When a toy is determined to be unsafe for children's usage, it can be banned, according to the decision by the Division of Children's Hazards. When a toy is banned, it means that the item cannot be sold in interstate commerce. It is also considered illegal to sell banned items that are already on store shelves.

Choosing Toys

Even though the Food and Drug Administration attempts to prevent the sale and use of toys determined to be unsafe, much of the burden of protecting children from the dangers of toys still rests with parents and teachers. A good deal of caution needs to be exercised in the purchase of toys. The following are among the most important questions to ask yourself when buying a toy for a child.

1. Is it safe?
2. Is it appropriate to the developmental level of the child?
3. Is it durable?
4. Is it fun (for the child)?
5. Will it stimulate the child's imagination?

A good toy is one that does not do all of the playing or "have all the fun" for the child. Many top companies list on the box or package the approximate age range of interest in the toy and its potential benefits. This information should be read carefully but used only as a general guide for purchasing the right toy for the particular child. A great deal of money is spent on toys, and we should be careful to get the most for our money. All too often a youngster will open an expensive new toy and proceed to play with the box rather than the toy. If the toy does not stimulate the interest or imagination of the child, no amount of encouragement will get him or her to play with it. Answering the five questions outlined above will do much to ensure the purchase of toys that children play with, learn from, and enjoy.

The following is a partial list of safety recommendations to take into consideration when selecting toys for children.

1. Toys should fit the child's age and physical skill.
2. For children under 3 years of age, avoid toys with small or easily removable parts (loose nuts, bolts, removable eyes, projections, needles, nails, etc.).
3. Look for toys that do not shatter or break easily.
4. Wait until a child is at least 8 years old before giving him or her chemistry sets, bows and arrows, and sharp-edged toys that might come into contact with the hands, clothes, or other parts of the body causing bruises, cuts, punctures, or fractures.
5. Only electrical toys with the Underwriters Laboratory (U.L.) seal should be purchased. This seal means that the toy is required to have a safely device that prevents the child from putting his hands in the heated area when the toy is hot. Cooking, melting, and molding toys should be used by older children and only under adult supervision.
6. All toys should be sturdy and durable.
7. Look for areas where the fingers can become pinched in slots, holes, on the underside of the wheels, and in wind-up mechanisms.
8. Darts, archery sets, or spring-loaded guns with rubber suction cups that can be removed may cause punctures. Avoid such toys.
9. Avoid crib or playpen toys that are suspended on strings.
10. Avoid purchasing helmets or play eyeglasses that can shatter. These could result in serious head and eye injuries.

PLAY SPACES

The play environment provided for children should be conducive to all aspects of their development. It should be safe, attractive, and provide a wide variety of stimulating and interesting activities. All too often the indoor and outdoor play spaces, for a variety of reasons, limit or discourage gross motor activities. As a result, there has, over the past several years, been a tremendous emphasis on the cognitive and affective aspects of the toys, games, and play equipment found in the indoor and outdoor play space. If we subscribe to the notion that the balanced development of children in the motor as well as the cognitive and affective areas of behavior is important, we must see to it that children's play environments also stimulate gross motor activity. Children have a basic need to be active. Through the proper design of play environments, as well as through the use of appropriate methods of teacher interaction, this need for activity will be successfully channeled to promote children's learning to move and, hence, their learning through movement.

Indoor Play Spaces

Historically, the indoor play space found in most nursery schools has been one of children's "interest centers." The environment has been designed around a variety of areas that are geared to the children's needs, abilities, and interests. The following is a list of the various interest centers typically found in nursery schools. It should be noted that inclusion of any or all of these areas into the indoor play space depends primarily on budgetary considerations and the availability of space.

1. *Block Area*. The block area requires plenty of space and should be carpeted, if possible, to reduce the noise factor.
2. *Housekeeping Area*. This interest center should be equipped with a toy sink, stove, refrigerator, table, and chairs. Dolls, doll beds, and dress-up clothing are also found in this area. The housekeeping area makes possible considerable dramatization and role playing.
3. *Book Area*. To be effective, this should be in a quiet part of the room. Books may be kept on shelves and/or a table. If possible, the area should be carpeted so children may sit comfortably on the floor if they desire.
4. *Creativity Area*. Easels with paint and paper should be available for children who want to paint.
5. *Science Area*. Here, materials should be easily displayed and seen by the children. Room to spread out leaves, stones, shells, and other, "collector's" items should be provided in this area. Magnets, magnifying glasses, a terrarium, and an aquarium might also be added. Space should also be provided for pets brought into the room.
6. *Water and Sand Area*. Ideally, a table with built-in sections for sand and water is the best kind of equipment for this activity. Also included should be shovels, small buckets, things that float, things that sink, funnels, straws, and soap.
7. *Music Area*. The music area is a must in any program. A record player, records, cassette tape recorder, a variety of musical instruments, and a piano will make this an ideal area.
8. *Carpentry Area*. The carpentry area should include a workbench with an attached vise. An assortment of tools, nails, and wood should be available.
9. *Nesting Area*. In this area the children should have an opportunity to "escape" from the hustle-bustle of the classroom. Nesting cubes, an old refrigerator carton, or collapsible tunnel make ideal nesting areas.

10. *Movement Center.* A movement center is an essential part of the indoor play space for preschool children and is discussed in detail in the following section.

The Indoor Movement Center. Contrary to popular belief, an indoor movement center requires little space. The author has developed several movement centers in nursery schools in areas no larger than 8 by 10 feet. The key to success in developing an indoor movement center is to first establish the specific objectives that you want the children to achieve through participation in this activity area. Then, taking the space limitations and safety factors into consideration, carefully design and construct the movement center around the objectives. For example, you may have as one of your primary objectives "to provide the children with opportunities to enhance their movement abilities in a variety of fundamental stability, locomotor, and manipulative abilities." Therefore, the movement center should contain equipment that will encourage practice in a variety of stability, locomotor, and manipulative activities. The following is a partial list of equipment appropriate for use in an indoor movement center which may be purchased or made by hand.

1. Stability
   (a) Balance beam
   (b) Balance board
   (c) Bounding board
   (d) Newspaper mats
   (e) Coffee-can stilts
   (f) Ladder
   (g) Inner tubes
2. Locomotion
   (a) Collapsible tunnel
   (b) Carpet squares
   (c) Ankle jump
   (d) Cubes
   (e) Portable climbing equipment
   (f) Climbing rope
3. Manipulation
   (a) Beanbags
   (b) Hoops
   (c) Yarn balls
   (d) Automobile tires
   (e) Targets
   (f) Suspended balls

The indoor movement center should also include a variety of sensory stimuli. Play equipment consisting of various textures, colors, and geometric shapes is encouraged. The use of mirrors with which children may observe their movements and portable equipment that may be used both indoors and outdoors is also recommended.

Outdoor Play Spaces

The opportunity for active movement in the outdoor play space should go well beyond the traditional recess period characterized by mass confusion, boredom, and fighting. The outdoor play area should first of all be designed for children in such a way that it stimulates their interest, imagination, and large muscle development. As simple as this sounds, one need only note the majority of outdoor play spaces at the nursery school and elementary school levels to see that they are not designed for children. All too often the outdoor play space is constructed with its primary objectives being to amuse children and require minimum upkeep instead of to encourage children's motor development. As a result, a typical outdoor play space often unfortunately consists of acres of blacktop and galvanized swing sets, teeter-totters, and slides.

Creative expression and imaginative interpretation should be primary criteria for selection of outdoor play equipment. Outdoor equipment should be abstract or neutral in its sculptural form in order to stimulate the child's imagination. It should stimulate a variety of locomotor, manipulative, and stability activities. Although individualistic in nature, outdoor play materials and equipment should encourage social contact. They should also stimulate imagination and cognitive processes through media that invite physical exploration and enjoyment.

In planning an outdoor play space, the following questions must be answered.

1. Is it safe?
2. Is it of real interest to children?
3. Is it developmentally appropriate?
4. Is it practical?
5. Is it economically feasible?
6. Can it be easily supervised?
7. Can it be maintained with a minimum of maintenance?
8. Can it be made available to the general public?

The outdoor play area should provide children with a variety of large and small muscle activities. It should contain a wide selection of equipment that promotes its use in a manner that is creative, challenging, and developmentally appropriate. The outdoor area should provide:

1. Large muscle activities to enhance all areas of children's motor development
   (a) Locomotion
   (b) Manipulation
   (c) Stability
2. Experiences with various media
   (a) Art
   (b) Woodwork
   (c) Dirt
   (d) Sand
   (e) Water
3. Places for seclusion and quiet activities
   (a) Tunnels
   (b) Nesting cubes
4. Opportunities to observe nature
   (a) Animals
   (b) Gardens
   (c) Trees and shrubs
5. Opportunities to dramatize real-life experiences
   (a) Playhouse
   (b) Junk car
   (c) Boat

The Outdoor Movement Center. The outdoor movement center is easily incorporated into the total outdoor play space. There should be ample space for children to move freely. Ideally, there will be a large grassy area and hillside for running, jumping, sliding, rolling, and climbing. There will also be a hard surface area for riding wheel toys and for activities with balls. Trees should be an integral part of the movement center, not only to provide shade but to encourage climbing. A variety of equipment that encourages gross motor activities should also be located in the outdoor play space. This equipment may be used in addition to or in conjunction with the equipment found in the indoor movement center. Climbing, striking, and balancing equipment should be an integral part of the outdoor area. The following is a partial list of suggested types of equipment designed to encourage the development of these abilities (Figure 19.2).

1. Climbing equipment
   (a) Teepee tower
   (b) Cargo net climber
   (c) Climbing frames
   (d) Barrel pyramid
   (e) Climbing towers

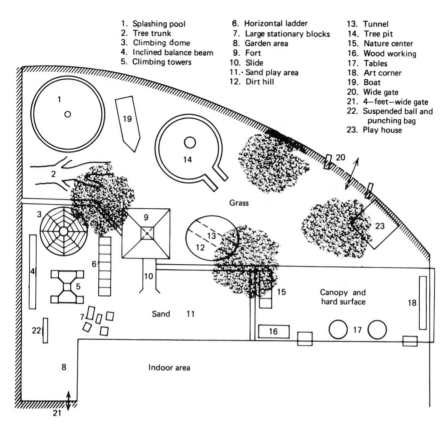

1. Splashing pool
2. Tree trunk
3. Climbing dome
4. Inclined balance beam
5. Climbing towers
6. Horizontal ladder
7. Large stationary blocks
8. Garden area
9. Fort
10. Slide
11. Sand play area
12. Dirt hill
13. Tunnel
14. Tree pit
15. Nature center
16. Wood working
17. Tables
18. Art corner
19. Boat
20. Wide gate
21. 4—feet—wide gate
22. Suspended ball and punching bag
23. Play house

Figure 19.2 Design for an outdoor play space

2. Striking equipment
   (a) Tetherball frames
   (b) Striking frames
   (c) Rebound nets
3. Balancing equipment
   (a) Inclined balance beams
   (b) Bouncing buddy
   (c) Telephone poles
   (d) Barrels
   (e) Spools

SUMMARY

The rapidly expanding world of children is one in which play, toys, and play spaces are in central focus for learning to move and learning through movement. As a result, it is important to have a clear understanding of what constitutes play, why children play, and the developmental aspects of play. The toys that we provide for children and their play environments are important to their total balanced development.

The selection of children's toys should be a matter for considerable thought and careful attention by parents and teacher. A variety of questions should be answered prior to the purchase of any toy, whether it be large or small, expensive or inexpensive, or for active or quiet play.

The indoor and outdoor play environment for children should be carefully designed. It should be conducive to gross motor development as well as to social interaction and cognitive growth.

Play, toys, and play spaces are important to children. This fact alone should be reason to see that the learning experiences within children's environments respond to their interests, needs, and developmental capabilities.

CHAPTER CONCEPTS

19.1 The evolution of play behavior follows a developmental sequence.

19.2 Play is the work of children. It is a primary means by which children come to grips with their world.

19.3 Toys can play an important role in both gross and fine motor development if properly selected and properly introduced into the child's environment.

19.4 Toys can promote cognitive and affective development as well as motor development.

19.5 War toys are of dubious value to the child, particularly the use of realistic toys.

19.6 The Child Protection and Toy Safety Act prohibits the sale of toys that may be harmful to children.

19.7 Care should be taken in the selection and purpose of toys. Guidelines are available from toy manufacturers and child development experts.

19.8 The play environment for children should be designed with care in order to maximize its utilization, developmental potential, and lasting enjoyment.

19.9 Indoor play spaces can be designed that requires a minimum of space and provide for a maximum of vigorous physical activity.

19.10 Outdoor play spaces should be designed for the children they are intended to serve and should follow a set of predetermined guidelines that have been established by individuals knowledgeable in child development, play behavior, and motor development.

TERMS TO REMEMBER

Play   Sociodramatic Play
Egocentric   Small Group Play
Imitative Play   Large Group Play

Exploratory Play
Competency Play
Achievement Play
War Toys

Child Protection & Safety Act
Bureau of Product Safety
Indoor Movement Center
Outdoor Movement Center

CRITICAL READINGS

Aldis, O. (1975). *Play Fighting*. New York: Academic Press.

Bruya, L. (Ed.) (1988). *Play Spaces for Children, Volume II: A New Beginning*. Reston, VA: AAHPERD.

Bruya, L. and Langendorfer, S. (Eds.) (1988). *Where Our Children Play, Volume I: Elementary School Playground Equipment*. Reston, VA: AAHPERD.

Csikszentmihalyi, M. (1975). *Beyond Boredom and Anxiety*. San Francisco: Jossey-Bass, (Chapter 4).

Mason, J. (1982). *The Environment of Play*. West Point, NY: Leisure Press, (Chapters 1-3).

Moore, R. C., Goltsman, S. M., and Iacofano, S. (Eds.) (1988). *Play for All Guidelines: Planning, Design and Management of Outdoor Play Settings for All Children*. Reston, VA: AAHPERD.

Quest, Monograph 26 (1976). "Learning How to Play." Brattleboro, VT: The National Association for Physical Education in Higher Education.

Sutton-Smith, B. (1985). "The Child at Play." *Psychology Today*, October, 64-65.

Yawkey, T. D. and Pellegrini, A. D. (1984). *Child's Play: Developmental and Applied*. Hillsdale, NJ: Erlbaum, (Chapter 1 & 2).

20

Education of Young Children

CHAPTER COMPETENCIES

Upon Completion of This Chapter You Should Be Able To:

- *Discuss the place of movement education and motor development in the lives of children.*

- *List and describe various educational programs for young children.*

- *Distinguish between the concepts of "learning to move" and "moving to learn."*

- *Speculate on the future of developmental movement programs for children.*

Traditionally, the education of young children has been assumed almost entirely by the family. The quantity and quality of learning experiences engaged in by children have been left to the discretion of parents. Until recently, little consideration has been given to preschool education outside the home. Many have scoffed at the Soviet practice of education by the State for children beginning at the age of 2 years instead of our more conservative and "acceptable" practice of beginning formal education at around age 5 or 6. This early education of children was often looked on as something that could not and would not be tolerated in our society. We looked at the education of young children as the sole responsibility of the home, except in extreme cases. In recent years, however, there have been three major developments that have resulted in a dramatic reassessment of this position: (1) the marked change in the social structure of our society, (2) the rapidly changing economic structure of our society, and (3) the increased professional interest in the contribution of early learning to later development. A closer look at each of these factors will help us more fully appreciate their significance.

North American society has experienced tremendous changes in the role of women in society. Many women are no longer satisfied with keeping a home and devoting a good portion of their life to the important but often frustrating task of raising children. Instead, they are returning to school, seeking full- or part-time employment, or searching for other expressions of fulfillment outside the home.

Our rapidly changing economic structure has often made it extremely difficult for many families to survive without two incomes. The inflationary spiral has significantly reduced the amount of spendable income for many. This reduction of spendable income is coupled with the "need" of many families to have the luxuries so skillfully advertised by the media. These factors have played an important role in the tremendous increase in the number of children enrolled in some form of day care or nursery school program.

The dramatic growth of interest in the contribution of early experiences to the later development of young children is the third factor leading to increased interest in early childhood education. Jean Piaget was among the first to stress the importance of early experience for future development. His stress on the importance of perceptual-motor experiences as a facilitator of cognitive development as well as physical development has been a prime factor in stimulating this interest. The late entry by the United States into the Space Age, brought about by the "Sputnik Era" of the 1950s, stimulated many to view the potential of the early years as important determiners of later behavior. The 1970 White House Conference on Children and Youth was a first national look into the education of young children. The conference stressed the need for nursery schools, day-care centers, and kindergartens to be open to all children from all walks of life under the qualified direction of persons trained in early childhood education.

Nursery schools, day-care centers, and other organizations are now concerned with the care and education of a large number of our nation's young children for all or part of their day, and the number increases daily. The preschool program's responsibility for the motor, cognitive, and affective development of children has been a continuing topic of considerable debate. As a result, we have witnessed a rapid increase in the types as well as the number of programs available.

THE MOTOR DEVELOPMENT DILEMMA

Movement is of central importance to young children and their optimal development. Contributions to the motor development of children are certainly a worthy goal of any early childhood educational program.

Enhancing children's ability to move efficiently and effectively, with control and with joy, should be as important to the teacher of young children as are their affective and cognitive development. Realization that the balanced motor development of children also has implications for both these areas should amplify the importance of gross motor development. The fact is, however, that the vast majority of educators are: (1) poorly informed about why motor development is important, (2) poorly informed about what forms of physical activity to include in their programs, and (3) inadequately prepared for going about such a task. As a result, the movement education of children is often taken for granted or dealt with solely through loosely supervised free play. Although free-play activities can and should play a part in the school experience, it is not enough to assume that the purchase of expensive pieces of indoor and outdoor play equipment will aid effectively in the development and refinement of the children's movement abilities. Too often children are turned loose on various forms of equipment and expected to magically develop efficient forms of movement behavior on their own. Only through wise guidance, thoughtful interaction, and careful planning can we assure the proper development of children's movement abilities.

The following is a discussion of five types of programs available for young children. The extent to which movement plays a role in each of these programs depends on individual teachers, their expertise, and their commitment to the total development of children.

PROGRAMS FOR YOUNG CHILDREN

The number and types of programs available for preschool children has increased tremendously. Data from the 1980 census indicate that the number of children under 5 years of age is on the increase, even though the general population under 14 was predicted to drop by 1980. There were more than 55 million children under 14 years of age in the United States according to the 1980 census report. Almost 20 million were under 5. The number of working mothers with children under age 6 has increased significantly from 12.8 to 30.4 percent between 1948 and 1969. Over 56 percent of mothers with children in the home were gainfully employed by 1980 according to statistics released by the U.S. government. By 1990, it is anticipated that over 60 percent of all mothers with children will be employed either full or part time.

The rise in the number of preschool children, coupled with the high percentage of working mothers, makes it abundantly clear that millions of children are cared for by persons other than parents, relatives, or babysitters. The need for quality care, supervision, and education is apparent, and many communities are rising to meet this need.

During the past several years a variety of programs have emerged.

Each of these programs represents a particular philosophical outlook and attempts to provide the particular developmental needs of children. The brief review of the major types of programs in existence throughout North America today is designed to provide the reader with a broader perspective of the nature and scope of programs for young children. Although each program differs in its purposes and content, all have a place in our society and can make a positive contribution to the development of young children. Table 20.1 provides a brief overview of the major types of preschool programs.

Day-Care Centers

The *day-care center* or day nursery, as it was previously termed, has come into wide use in recent years. Day-care centers are established

Table 20.1 Types of Preschool Programs

Program	Ages	Description
Day care center	8 weeks to 6 years	Usually a full-day program between 7 A.M. and 6 P.M. Programs vary greatly in quality and trained leadership.
Head Start Child Development Programs	3 to 6 years	Federally supported compensatory program designed to provide enrichment experiences for culturally deprived children. Half-day and full-day sessions, medical and dental programs, and hot meals. Trained staff, volunteers, and parent help.
Nursery schools	2 to 5 years	Generally privately supported but some publicly supported programs. Half-day session. "Traditional" and "modern" approach. Trained staff, volunteers, and aids.
Parent cooperatives developed	2 to 5 years	Formed, programmed, and staffed by parents. Cost is minimal and quality varies greatly.
Home day care	2 to 6 years	Private facilities often need to be licensed. Babysitting service for groups of three to ten children. Half- or full-day care.
Kindergarten	5 to 6 years	Publicly and privately supported. Certified teachers staff the program. Geared to prepare children for the first grade.

primarily to serve the needs of working mothers. Upon their inception, they were often places where children could be safely "stored" for the day, with general assurance that their basic physical needs would be met. Little was done beyond serving their needs for basic physical care and ensuring that they were returned home in more or less the same condition in which they came. Today, however, day-care centers are broadening their scope and beginning to hire trained professionals who are developing sound programs dealing with the affective and cognitive growth of children.

The typical day-care center is open on weekdays from 7 A.M. until 6 P.M. and beyond. There are no set hours of attendance for the children; they come and go based on their parent's schedule. A great number of children require full-day care. Most of these children are from families with two working parents or only one parent, or from broken homes or low-income families.

The cost of quality day care is high. The cost is high due to the number of hours involved per week, the high demand for the low supply of quality centers, and the limited number of trained professionals. Many communities and county governments, as well as church-affiliated organizations, have aided in the support of the many children in day-care centers from low-income families. Communities far-sighted enough to help share the burdens of the disadvantaged home by making quality day care available are aiding society greatly. Their early concern for good care may help alleviate later delinquency, emotional problems, and frustrations, and may do much to help children develop into happy, healthy, contributing members of society. The day-care center is in a unique position to have a tremendously positive effect on the lives of children and will pay dividends in the future.

The continued upgrading of day-care programs through hiring trained professionals and meeting state certification requirements is an important community matter. Day-care centers need to concern themselves more with the development of children and must cease to view their purpose as simply a storage place for children. The opportunities are great and so are the responsibilities. The early years are too important to be left to chance, and quality day care can go a long way toward ensuring for our society a large segment of the care and nurturing it requires.

Head Start Child Development Programs

Head Start Child Development Programs are a relatively recent phenomenon in American society. They were established as a result of the Economic Opportunity Act of 1964 which authorized the establishment of programs for economically deprived preschool children. Head Start programs were designed to help prepare children for public school as a part of the federal government's war against poverty.

The 1960s became known to many as the decade of the disadvantaged. Head Start programs were one means by which the government made vast attempts at breaking the poverty cycle and alleviating cultural deprivation. The culturally deprived have been defined as "individuals or a group of people who lack social amenities and cultural graces associated with middle-class society" (Leeper et al. 1974, p. 86).

Head Start is an all-inclusive program designed to meet the physical, mental, and emotional needs of young children in an effort to prepare them for success in school. The program involves medical and dental services, social and psychological services, and nutritional care. Parents and local community volunteers are encouraged to take an active role whenever possible, performing many of the nonprofessional duties.

The program itself stresses development of language skills, personal health, self-concept, curiosity, and self-discipline. Head Start programs broaden the range of children's experiences and help them learn how to cope with their environment. They attempt to help children overcome some of the deficiencies of their environment by providing early enrichment experiences in order to help them more effectively meet the demands of school.

Children are selected on the basis of a minimum family income, where the family lives (rural or urban), and the number of children in the family. The vast majority of children come from low-income homes.

In a good Head Start program, classes are small. Children receive individual help, and the school is well staffed. Parents and community volunteers share in the decision making. Home and school are closely correlated in the program in an effort to help the home as well as the individual child better share in the responsibilities and benefits of our society.

The Head Start program has had a tremendous impact on early childhood education: (1) national attention has been focused on preschool education, especially that of culturally disadvantaged children, (2) the philosophy of early education of the young has undergone radical changes, (3) facilities and materials for young children have been vastly expanded, and (4) it has been documented that young children learn faster and earlier than previously thought. Head Start has truly had a lasting impact on our society. It is through the early enrichment of countless young lives that the poverty cycle can be broken and the culturally disadvantaged can become valued, contributing members of society.

Nursery Schools

The nursery school should not be confused with the day-care center. Unlike the day-care center, nursery schools are established primarily to enhance the cognitive and affective development of children. They operate for only a portion of the school day. The children generally attend for 2 to 3 hours daily or every other day for the same period of time. The nursery school is the first in the series of units that make up elementary education. Public nursery schools generally begin at age 4. When operated privately, they often include children 2 to 4 years of age.

The nursery school is an educational experience that has been the primary form of preschool education for over fifty years. At their inception, nursery schools were primarily conducted as laboratory schools by colleges and universities. They were used extensively as training and testing grounds for teachers and materials. The early laboratory schools served a valuable purpose in enhancing our insight into the nature and characteristics of preschool children. Many laboratory schools continue to serve as valuable information-gathering research centers.

Today, nursery schools are conducted on both public and private bases throughout North America, the premise being that early experiences offered in the proper setting by trained professionals will have a positive effect on children's development. Today's nursery school serves the needs of 2- to 5-year-old children by providing them with experiences based on what is known about their development needs. It shares with parents the responsibility for promoting meaningful learning during a period when growth is rapid and significant.

The typical nursery school is an active one in which the open classroom concept is extensively employed. The children generally work in small groups at various interest centers such as the doll corner, carpentry corner, block area, and reading and puzzle corner. The teacher acts as a stimulator or motivator for involvement, encouraging experimentation and exploration of new ideas and ways of doing things.

Nursery school programs vary greatly but may be classified into two general types. The first is sometimes termed the *traditional nursery school*. The traditional nursery school emphasizes the development of affective competencies. The learning of social skills such as sharing, taking turns, working constructively with others, and accepting simple responsibilities is an important aspect of the traditional program. Formal means of instruction are frowned on, and informal play experiences are the primary mode of instruction. The teacher establishes an environment conducive to learning and social interaction. Play experiences are utilized as a means of learning socialization skills. Less emphasis is placed on the formal development of cognitive abilities, although considerable cognitive development often occurs as a byproduct of a good program.

The *modern nursery school*, or *academic nursery school* as it is frequently called, is the second type of nursery school program. Unlike the traditional nursery school, greater emphasis is placed on the development of cognitive abilities. A more complete balance between affective and cognitive development is sought. Sometimes teachers in the academic nursery school view motor development as an integral part of their program. The program in the modern nursery school utilizes a portion of the day for directed activities and the remainder for relatively free activities. The concepts that children learn in the directed aspect of the program are reinforced during play by the teacher's directing the child's attention to factors in the environment that may otherwise be missed or minimized. Concern has been expressed by many that over emphasis on academic readiness and skill development is inappropriate for the developmental level of the young child (NAEYC, 1987).

Parent Cooperatives

Parent cooperatives have become a popular form of preschool education in recent years. The cooperative is formed by parents and is often completely staffed by them. Parents are regularly required to participate in the program and to plan and supervise its activities. The parent cooperative enables children to attend a preschool program at minimum cost. The quality of cooperatives varies greatly, depending on the parents' commitment to the program, their ability to work constructively with groups of children, and the number of people involved.

Some cooperatives are able to hire a qualified professional to provide leadership, guidance, and training. Programs that are fortunate enough to enlist the aid of a trained professional often blossom into excellent programs. On the other hand, a great many parent cooperatives flounder for lack of leadership. Problems often arise in scheduling, planning, staffing, and providing continuity when the duties are rotated between parents.

Home Day Care

The number of *home day care* facilities has increased rapidly during the past few years. Home care programs are those in which a mother cares for from three to ten children in her home. Several states require licensing of home care facilities, but the quality of such programs runs from excellent to terrible. The home care program often is primarily one of babysitting for a group of children for either half or full days.

The licensing requirements of many states for home care are quite rigid. These regulations have been established in order to help, as much as possible, to ensure a safe and hygienic environment for the children.

Kindergarten

Kindergartens have been in existence for over a century. The first public kindergarten was established in St. Louis, Missouri, in 1873. The first private one was established in Watertown, Wisconsin, in 1855. Many kindergartens operate on a private basis. The number of children attending both public and private kindergartens has been increasing steadily for the past twenty years, and many states include kindergarten programs as a portion of the total public school program. In states that do not have public kindergartens, several licensed and privately operated church-related kindergarten programs exist.

Kindergarten enrolls 5-year-old children for a one-year series of generally half-day programs designed to prepare them for the first grade. They are operated by licensed teachers and one or two assistants. Programs are usually individualized to meet each child's needs within a low-pressure, group setting atmosphere in which exploration and investigation experiences are encouraged. The purpose of such programs is to encourage inquiry and wonder, self-direction, self-selection, and the discovery of meaning. The kindergarten program helps children form the basis for lifelong habits of disciplined, joyful learning.

The objectives of the kindergarten include:

1. Recognizing the value and dignity of all people.
2. Emphasizing the importance of self-worth and realization of one's goals.
3. Developing an appreciation of different social, cultural, and ethnic groups.
4. Promoting emotional stability in a world of rapid change, opportunities, and responsibilities.
5. Encouraging independent thinking and fostering creativity within each individual.
6. Providing experiences geared to the needs and ability levels of each child.
7. Fostering positive attitudes toward learning and school.
8. Developing basic readiness skills necessary for success in school.
9. Encouraging the development and refinement of fundamental movement abilities.
10. Enlarging the concept of reliable citizenship, at both individual and group levels.

The kindergarten is for most children an exciting first step into the world of learning. It is an integral part of the elementary school that makes available the type of experience best suited to the immediate needs of children. It provides an atmosphere in which children develop new skills and ideas, increase their fund of information, and gain a better understanding of their neighborhood and community. It is a place where they learn to plan and think through simple tasks. They learn to share and take responsibility for themselves and their work. Kindergarten is a happy place filled with eager faces, bright smiles, and active bodies. It helps prepare children for the challenges forthcoming in the elementary school.

LEARNING TO MOVE, MOVING TO LEARN

The directed play experiences of young children can serve as a primary vehicle by which they learn about themselves and their environment. Play and work are not opposites, as is often thought. For children, play is their way of exploring and experimenting while they gain information about themselves and their world. Through directed play experiences that have been carefully structured and preplanned (but that avoid teacher domination), children learn to come to grips with their world, to cope with life's tasks, to master fundamental movements, and to gain confidence in themselves as individuals, moving effectively and efficiently through space. These early years serve as a time when children are intently involved in the process of *learning to move* and *moving to learn*. Although it is impossible to separate these two processes, it is important that the differences implied by the terms be understood.

Learning to move involves the continuous development of children's fundamental movement abilities. Preschoolers have passed through the period of infancy and are no longer immobilized by the confines of their crib or playpen. They can now move through their environment (locomotion), impart force to objects (manipulation), and maintain their equilibrium in response to the force of gravity (stability). The development of effective patterns of movement permits them to move about freely and in control of their bodies. Children involved in learning to move are constantly exploring, experimenting, practicing, and making a variety of spontaneous decisions based on their perceptions of the moment and of past experiences. They are involved in a continuous process of sorting out their many daily experiences to gain increased knowledge about their body and its potential for movement.

While involved in learning to move, children are simultaneously involved in *moving to learn,* a process that involves utilizing movement as a means to an end rather than as an end in itself. Children involved in moving to learn use their bodies to gain increased knowledge about themselves and their world. Their basic inability to conceptualize at a sophisticated level makes it difficult for them to learn through formal means of education. As a result, movement becomes one of the primary agents by which they grasp fundamental cognitive and affective concepts of direction, space, time, peer relations, and self-assurance. Movement serves as a medium by which they can increase their fund of knowledge in all aspects of their behavior and is not limited to the physical self.

The balanced motor development of children can and must become a concern of the teacher of young children. The important contributions of movement to learning to move and learning through movement should be carefully studied by all. Figure 20.1 presents a schematic representation of the different types of preschool programs and the obligation of these programs to the development of the total child. The extent to which any program incorporates meaningful movement depends on the specific program, its educational goals, and the expertise of the teacher.

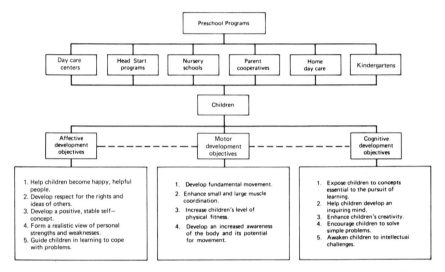

Figure 20.1 Preschool programs are responsible for the development of children in the affective, psychomotor, and cognitive domains of behavior. The extent to which children develop in each of these areas depends on the type of program offered and the expertise of the teacher

SUMMARY

Parents, teachers, psychologists, and pediatricians are becoming increasingly aware of the critical need for children to move about freely in order to grow and develop their potential. The literature on child growth and development is replete with information indicating that the child's experiential background in movement plays an important role in the total developmental process.

Teachers should be concerned with developing a variety of fundamental movement and sport-skill abilities. This may be accomplished by structuring the environment and providing opportunities for the performance of movement activities, with a judicious degree of teacher direction and interaction. For individuals untrained in this area of education, it may be difficult initially to structure movement experiences and provide the proper degree of guidance, but with practice and study, successful experiences will be forthcoming.

Teachers need to develop a keen awareness of the importance of directed movement experiences in the lives of children and to become knowledgeable about how to implement successful programs in this area. It is time that the so-called frivolous play experiences of children be viewed in the light of their potential educational value. Motor development must be put into proper perspective in the education of children, for it truly plays an integral part in their total growth and development.

CHAPTER CONCEPTS

20.1 The changing complexion of North American society has created a situation where over half of all preschoolers are involved in some form of education or care outside the home.

20.2 In most preschool programs a movement education program is absent or takes the form of loosely supervised free play.

20.3 Free play is of value to the developing child, but it cannot take the place of a planned program of developmentally appropriate movement experiences.

20.4 A variety of preschool programs are available to young children. Each type has a different emphasis and all have a place in our society.

20.5 The directed play experiences of preschool and elementary school children can do much to enhance their movement abilities.

20.6 Movement can serve as an effective avenue for moving to learn as well as for learning to move.

TERMS TO REMEMBER

Day-Care Center	Parent Cooperatives
Head Start Child Development Program	Home Day-Care
Traditional Nursery School	Kindergarten
Modern Nursery School	Learning to Move
Academic Nursery School	Moving to Learn

CRITICAL READINGS

Bredekamp, S. (Ed.) (1987). *Developmentally Appropriate Practice in Early Childhood Programs Serving Children from Birth through Age 8.* Washington, D.C.: National Association for the Education of Young Children.

Lewis, B. J. and Cherrington, D. (1984). "Movement Education With Young Children." In Fontana, D. (ed.) *The Education of the Young Child.* New York: Basil Blackwell.

Luke, M., and Warrell, E. (Eds.) (1986). *Looking at Movement: Physical Education in Early Childhood.* Burnaby, British Columbia: Simon Fraser University Publications.

Morgan, G. et. al. (1985). *Quality in Early Childhood Programs: Four Perspectives.* Ypsilanti, MI: High/Scope Educational Research Foundation.

Riggs, M. L. (1980). *Jump to Joy.* Englewood Cliffs, N.J.: Prentice-Hall.

Time-Life Books, Eds. (1987). *Developing Your Child's Potential.* Alexandria, VA: Time-Life Books.

21

Developmental Physical Education: A Curricular Model

CHAPTER COMPETENCIES

Upon Completion of This Chapter You Should Be Able To:

* *Individualize physical education instruction to accommodate developmental levels of each learner.*

* *Plan physical activity programs for all age groups.*

* *Demonstrate awareness of within-age individual differences in planning physical activity programs for any portions of the life span.*

• *Diagram the sequential basis for a developmentally-based physical education program.*

• *Discuss what is meant by the term "developmental physical education" and how it is related to scientific study of motor development.*

Throughout the discussions in the preceding chapters, we have continually focused on the developmental stages that infants, children, and adolescents pass through in their acquisition of motor, cognitive, and affective abilities. The thesis of this entire text has focused on the process of motor development and factors that impinge on its normal sequential progression in the development of movement and physical abilities. If the phases and stages of motor development presented in Chapter 3 and elaborated on throughout this text are to have any real meaning, we should be able to construct a curricular model congruent with these phases. This curricular model should be able to serve as a blueprint for action. In other words, it should make up the basic structure around which the daily lesson is planned and carried out by the teacher or coach in the gymnasium or on the playing field. What has been discussed in the preceding chapters is of little value if we cannot bring order to it and practically apply it to the lives of children. The value of theory and research that fails to foster models for implementation is limited at best. Curricular models not based on sound research and theory are little better. It is, therefore, the purpose of this chapter to propose a developmentally based curricular model for implementing the physical education program during the preschool, elementary and adolescent school years.

CURRICULAR MODELS IN PHYSICAL EDUCATION

Curricular rationales take many forms. Bain (1978) identified six curricular rationales that are in use today by physical education teachers: (1) movement forms, (2) movement analysis, (3) human movement disciplines, (4) developmental stages, (5) motor learning tasks analysis, and (6) student motives and purposes. The movement analysis and developmental stage models are most often found at the elementary school level and are the most common choices for curriculum development. These two approaches were debated by Tanner (1979) and Gallahue (1979) and are summarized in an article by Ward and Werner (1981).

The *developmental approach* to physical education aims to educate children in the use of their bodies so they can move more efficiently and effectively in a wide variety of fundamental movements and be able to apply these basic abilities to a wide variety of movement skills that may or may not be sport-related. At the heart of the developmental model is a focus on developmentally appropriate movement experiences that promote increased proficiency at all levels. Games, sports, dances, and the like serve as vehicles for skill improvement.

The *movement analysis approach* to physical education is defined as that approach to physical education which teaches children to move skillfully, meaningfully, and with knowledge of how they move (Ward and Werner, 1981). The movement analysis model is exemplified by movement education programs that place emphasis on both understanding and application of the movement concepts originally proposed by Laban and Lawrence (1947). These movement concepts are important but, like the content areas of physical education, should serve as a vehicle by which appropriate movement skills are developed and refined.

The developmental model presented here for teaching physical education recognizes the validity of both the developmental stage and movement analysis curriculum rationales. It places the child, not the content areas or movement concepts, at the center of the curricular process. The text *Developmental Physical Education for Today's Elementary School Children* (Gallahue, 1987) represents an attempt to unite both the developmental and movement analysis approaches to teaching children's physical education.

In order to facilitate presentation of the developmental model, we will first review the three categories into which movement may be classified and the appropriate movement skill themes that may be extracted from each category. We will then discuss the three major content areas of physical education and the elements of movement education. Next we will look at the stages in the process of movement skill learning and the implications for emphasizing indirect or direct methods of teaching. A model will be presented for both preschool and primary grades, upper elementary, middle school, and beyond. No attempt will be made to provide scope and sequence charts, lesson plans, or suggestions for developmentally appropriate activities. The reader is instead referred to *Developmental Physical Education For Today's Elementary School Children* (Gallahue, 1987)

CATEGORIES OF MOVEMENT AND MOVEMENT SKILL THEMES

The three *categories of movement* as they relate to motor development have been discussed extensively. Briefly, a category of movement is a classificatory scheme based on common underlying principles of movement. The terms "locomotion," "manipulation," and "stability" are used here to represent these underlying principles. Although others have used the term "nonlocomotor" rather than "stability" for category of movement, I have chosen to give recognition to the term "stability" as a movement category. Doing so is not arbitrary or without support from others. Smith and Smith (1966), Riggs (1980), and Keough and Sugden (1985) have all chosen to classify movement behavior into the categories of locomotion, manipulation, and stability. These three categories serve as the organizing centers of the developmental physical education curriculum and as the basis for the formation of movement skill themes (Figures 21.1 and 21.2).

A *developmental skill theme* is a particular fundamental movement or sport skill around which a specific lesson or series of lessons is organized. In the developmental curriculum a category of movement serves as the organizing center of each unit of the curriculum, while skill themes serve as the organizing centers of the daily lesson plan. Each category of movement is briefly reviewed here, and a few examples of possible skill themes are given.

Fundamental Stability Movements Stressed	Fundamental Locomotor Movements Stressed	Fundamental Manipulative Movements Stressed
Bending	Walking	Throwing
Stretching	Running	Catching
Twisting	Jumping	Kicking
Turning	Hopping	Trapping
Swinging	Skipping	Striking
Inverted supports	Sliding	Volleying
Body rolling	Leaping	Bouncing
Landing	Climbing	Ball rolling
Stopping		Punting
Dodging		
Balancing		

Figure 21.1 Selected fundamental movement skill themes

Stability

Stability refers to the ability to maintain one's balance in relationship to the force of gravity even though the nature of the force's application may be altered or parts of the body may be placed in unusual positions. The classification of stability extends beyond the concept of balance and includes various axial movements and postures in which a premium is placed on controlling one's equilibrium. Stability is the most basic form of human movement. It is basic to all efficient movement and permeates the categories of locomotion and manipulation. Bending, stretching, pivoting, dodging, and walking on a balance beam are examples of skill themes that may be incorported into the daily lesson plan at the fundamental or sport-skill phase of development.

Locomotion

Locomotion refers to changes in the location of the body relative to fixed points on the ground. To walk, run, hop, jump, slide, or leap is to be involved in locomotion. The movement classification of locomotion develops in conjunction with stability, not apart from it. Fundamental aspects of stability must be mastered before efficient forms of locomotion may take place. The vertical jump, rebounding, and high jumping are examples of skill themes that may be incorporated into the daily lesson plan at the fundamental or sport-skill phase of development.

Manipulation

Gross-motor or *object manipulation*, as it is frequently termed, is concerned with giving force to objects and absorbing force from objects by

Sport Skill Themes	Locomotor Skills Stressed		Manipulative Skills Stressed		Stability Skills Stressed
Basketball sport skills	Running Sliding Leaping Jumping		Passing Catching Shooting Dribbling Rebounding	Tipping Blocking	Selected axial movement skills Pivoting Blocking Dodging Cutting Guarding Picking Faking
Combative sport skills	Steping Sliding Hopping(karate)		Dexterity (fencing) Striking (kendo)		All axial movement skills Dodging and feinting Static balance skills Dynamic balance skills
Dance skills	Running Leaping Jumping	Hopping Skipping Sliding Stepping	Tossing Catching		All Axial Movement skills Static balance postures Dynamic balance postures
Disc sport skills	Stepping Running Jumping		Tossing Catching		All axial movement skills Static balance postures Dynamic balance postures
Football sport skills	Running Sliding Leaping	Jumping	Passing Catching Carrying	Kicking Punting Centering	Blocking Pivoting Tackling Dodging
Gymnastic skills	Running Jumping Skipping	Leaping Hopping Landing			Inverted supports Rolling, landing All axial movement skills Static balance tricks Dynamic balance tricks
Implement Striking sport skills (tennis, squash, racketball, hockey, lacrosse, golf)	Running Sliding Leaping Skating Walking		Forehand Backhand Striking Driving Putting Chipping	Lob Smash Drop Throwing Catching Trapping	Dynamic balance skills Turning Twisting Stretching Bending Dodging Pivoting
Skiing sport skills	Stepping Walking Running Sliding		Poling		All axial movement skills Dynamic balance skills Static balance skills
Soccer sport skills	Running Jumping Leaping Sliding		Kicking Trapping Juggling Throwing Blocking	Passing Dribbling Catching Rolling	Tackling Feinting Marking Turning Dodging
Softball/baseball skills	Running Sliding Leaping	Jumping	Throwing Catching	Pitching Batting Bunting	Selected axial movement skills Dynamic balance skills Dodging
Target sport skills			Aiming Shooting		Static balance skills
Track and field skills	Running Hopping Vertical jumping	Horizontal jumping Leaping Starting	Shot put Discus Javelin	Hammer Pole vault Baton passing Throwing	All axial movement skills Dynamic balance skills
Volleyball sport skills	Running Sliding	Jumping Diving Sprawling Rolling	Serving Volleying Bump	Dig Spike Dink Block	Dynamic balance skills Selected axial movements

Figure 21.2 Selected sport skill themes

use of the hands or feet. The tasks of throwing, catching, kicking, trapping, and striking are included in the category of manipulation. Manipulation also refers to the fine motor controls required for tasks such as buttoning, cutting, printing, and writing. The scope of this book, however, has been limited to gross motor aspects of manipulation. Large muscle manipulative abilities tend to develop somewhat later than stability and locomotor abilities. This is due, in part, to the fact that most manipulative movements incorporate elements of both stability and locomotion. Throwing a ball, passing a football, and pitching a baseball are examples of skill themes within the manipulative category of movement.

CONTENT AREAS OF PHYSICAL EDUCATION

Fundamental movements and sport skills within the three categories of movement outlined above may be developed and refined through the three major *content areas* of physical education: "games and sports," "rhythms," and "self-testing activities." The learning of particular games, rhythms, or self-testing activities is a means of developing stability, locomotor, and manipulative abilities appropriate to the developmental level of the child. Teachers must not lose sight of this goal. Every activity used in the program should be selected with an awareness that it can contribute to developing and refining certain movement abilities and to the fitness objectives of physical education. For children, their primary objective may be fun, but for teachers of movement the objectives should involve the children's learning to move and learning through movement. The possibility of fun as the motivation to learn is a by-product of any good educational program, and is an important objective. This point cannot be overemphasized. But when fun becomes, for the teacher, the primary objective of the program, the physical education program becomes a recreation period.

Games and Sports

Games and sports are used as a mean of enhancing movement abilities appropriate to the child's developmental level. They often are classified into subcategories that proceed from the simple to the complex as follows.

1. Low organized games and relays
2. Lead-up games
3. Official sports

Rhythms

Rhythms are an important content area of the movement program. All coordinated movement is rhythmical and involves the temporal sequencing of events and the synchronizing of one's actions. Rhythmic dance activities are generally categorized into the following subcategories:

1. Rhythmic fundamentals
2. Creative rhythms
3. Folk and square dance
4. Social dance

Self-Testing

Self-testing is the third major content area of the program. This area represents a wide variety of activities in which children work on their own and can improve their performance through their own efforts. Self-testing activities may be classified in a variety of ways. The following is a common classification scheme for typical self-testing activities.

1. Fundamental movement activities
2. Sport skill activities
3. Physical fitness activities
4. Stunts
5. Tumbling
6. Small (hand) apparatus
7. Large apparatus

Achieving effectiveness and efficiency in each of the three categories of movement at either the fundamental or the specialized phase is the primary reason for incorporating games, rhythms, and self-testing activities in the program. The degree to which this is achieved depends on the particular developmental level of the children and the teacher's expertise in structuring developmentally appropriate movement experiences. Games, rhythms, and self-testing activities serve only as the vehicle by which these experiences are applied.

MOVEMENT CONCEPTS OF MOVEMENT EDUCATION

Fundamental movements and sport skills within the three categories of movement may be elaborated upon and dealt with in terms of *movement concepts* or *elements*. The development of particular movement concepts, namely, effort, space, and relationships, is the central focus of many movement education programs and is omitted from most traditional physical education programs. In a developmental curriculum, the elements of movement are included and represent an emphasis of the program along with the three content areas discussed in the preceding section. The primary focus of the developmental curriculum is on fundamental movement and sport-skill development through implementation of skill themes. These skill themes are applied to the understanding and application of movement concepts and to the content areas of physical education.

A brief explanation of the three movement concept areas in relationship to movement skill development follows and is also highlighted in Table 21.1.

Effort

The movement concept of *effort* deals with how the body moves. Children need to learn about the concept of effort. Effort may be subdivided into three categories, with the possibility for a wide variety of movement experiences combined with locomotor, manipulative, and stability movements.

1. *Force* refers to the degree of muscular tension required to move the body or its parts from place to place or to maintain its equili-

Table 21.1 The Movement Concepts of Movement Education

Effort (How the body moves with varying amounts of–)	*Space* (Where the body moves at different–)	*Relationships* (Moving with–)
–Force strong light	**–Levels** high/medium/low	**–Objects** (or people) over/under in/out
	–Directions forward/backward diagonally/sideward up/down various pathways (curved, straight, zig-zag, etc.)	between/among in front/behind lead/follow above/below through/around
–Time fast slow medium sustained sudden		
		–People mirroring
–Flow free bound	**–Ranges** body shapes (wide narrow, curved, straight, etc.) body spaces (self-space, and general space) body extensions (near/far, large/small, with & without implements)	shadowing in unison together/apart alternating simultaneously partner/group

brium. Force may be heavy or light or between these two extremes.

2. *Time* refers to the speed at which movement takes place. A movement may be fast or slow, gradual or sudden, erratic or sustained.
3. *Flow* refers to the continuity or coordination of movements. A movement may be smooth or jerky, free or bound.

Space

The movement concept of *space* deals with where the body moves. In addition to understanding how their bodies move, children need to understand where in space their bodies can move. The following movement concepts of space can be directly related to all locomotor, manipulative, and stability movements.

1. *Level* refers to the height at which a movement is performed. A movement may be performed at a high, medium, or low level.
2. *Direction* refers to the path of movement. Movement may occur in a forward, backward, diagonal, up, down, left, or right direction, or it may be in a straight, curved, or zigzag pattern.
3. *Range* refers to the relative location of one's body (self-space/general space) and how various extensions of the body (wide/narrow, far/near, long/short, large/small) are used in movement.

Relationships

The movement concept of *relationships* deals with both how and where the body moves in harmony with objects and other people. It is important that children understand this concept and experience it through the medium of movement.

1. *Objects* are what we station ourselves in relation to. Object relationships may be over/under, near/far, on/off, behind/in front, alongside, front/back, underneath/on top, in/out, between/among, and so on.
2. *People* we move in various forms with. People relationships include solo, partner, group, and mass movement.

LEVELS OF MOVEMENT SKILL LEARNING

The content areas and the movement concepts just discussed may be implemented in a variety of ways. The teacher must, however, be aware that individuals tend to pass through typical learning levels as they develop and refine new movement skills. These levels are based on two developmental concepts: First, that the acquisition of movement abilities progresses from the simple to the complex; Second, that children proceed gradually from general to specific in the development and refinement of their abilities. Based on these two concepts and fortified with the models of Fitts and Posner (1967), Gentile (1972), and Lawther (1977), it is possible to view the learning of a movement skill as a phenomenon that occurs in the following sequence (Figure 21.3):

1. Exploration
2. Discovery
3. Combination
4. Application
5. Performance
6. Individualization.

When involved in developing new stability, locomotor, or manipulative skills to be used in games, sports, rhythm, or self-testing activities, we generally go through the following sequence of learning experiences.

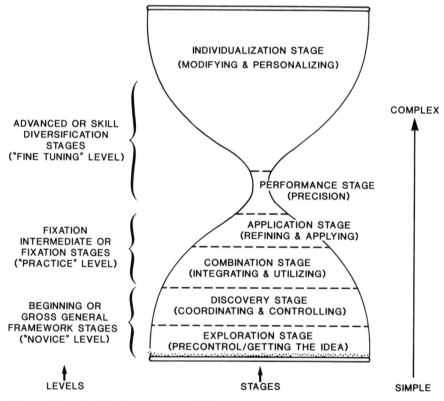

Figure 21.3 Levels of movement skill learning

1. We *explore* the movements involved in the task in relative isolation to one another. The learner does not have control of movement but gets used to the task and forms a gross general framework of the pattern or skill.
2. We *discover* ways and means of better execution of these movements through indirect means such as the observation of pictures, films, books, or of others performing. During this aspect of achieving a gross general framework, the learner begins to gain control and to coordinate the task. It becomes relatively automatic.
3. We *combine* the isolated movements with others and experiment with them in various ways. This is a practice stage in which we integrate, elaborate upon, and begin to utilize separate tasks in varying ways.
4. We *apply* the best ways of combining each of these movements through a variety of lead-up games, informal means of competition, and presentation. This aspect of practice is more specific and detailed than the previous stage, and more attention is given to the entire utilization of several skill-related tasks.
5. We produce a *refined performance* of the selected movements and perform the particular activity through formal or informal means of competition or through leisure-time pursuits. This is often called the "automatic or skill diversification stage" and is a time for refining and smoothing performance.
6. We *individualize* or personalize the movement skill to our particular needs, interests, or desires. Creative application of means to achieve desired ends is possible.

This sequential progression of learning a new movement skill is similar for adolescents and adults as well as for children, although it may not be as apparent. This is because the adolescent and adult are generally at the specialized skill phase and may spend less time with exploration, discovery, and the combination of new skills and more time in the application and refined performance aspects of the sequence. Preschool and primary grade children at the fundamental movement pattern phase of development spend a great deal of time exploring, discovering, and combining new movements and less time with the application of best ways of moving and with the refined performance of activities.

Facilitating Exploration

Exploration represents the first level of the movement skill learning heirarchy. In order to take advantage of this level, the teacher focuses on indirect teaching approaches that encourage exploration. The *movement exploration* technique of teaching movement helps enhance knowledge of the body and its potential for movement in space. Individuals are encouraged to explore and experiment with the movement potentials of their bodies. Accuracy and skill in performance are not stressed. This is accomplished by the leader not establishing a performance model for the movement being explored. Instead, participants are presented with a series of movement questions or challenges posed by the leader and are given an opportunity to solve these problems as they see fit. Any reasonable solution to the problem is regarded as correct. At this time there is not a "best" method of performance to be elicited. The leader is more concerned with creative involvement in the learning process.

Movement exploration experiences stress not so much the product of the movement act as the acceptable execution of fundamental movements. But, the learning process involved is of great importance. In other words, the leader is not particularly concerned with how far David Lee can jump but is interested in his achieving some degree of success within the level of his particular abilities. The leader also places value on David Lee's ability to think and act as an individual.

This is not to imply that success or goal-directed behavior is not important. On the contrary, movement exploration techniques are particularly appropriate for young children and novice learners because they structure the environment for success simply by considering correct all reasonable solutions to the movement problems posed. Success and goal-directed behavior are individual standards that do not require emulation of a performance model or competition with one's peers, but permit success within the limits of one's own abilities. In doing so, the individual is continually encouraged to explore and experiment with endless variations that influence the performance of all locomotor, manipulative, and stability movements in both the content areas (games, rhythms, and self-testing activities) and the movement concepts (effort, space, and relationships).

Facilitating Discovery

Discovery represents the second classification of the movement skill learning hierarchy. Movement experiences that incorporate discovery may be included in the lesson by the leader in an indirect manner similar to the use of movement exploration techniques. The *guided discovery* teaching method is often used when the learner is in the process of discovery. The use of this technique requires that the leader not establish a model for "correct" performance at the outset of the experience. Problems are stated in the form of questions or challenges posed by the leader. These questions result in emphasis being placed on movement pattern development rather than on skill development. Both the movement exploration and the limitation methods utilize *problem-solving* techniques as a common tactic in developing the movement abilities. Gilliom (1970, p. 21), defined problem solving as:

> original thinking, an individual's technique of productive thinking, his techniques of inquiry, which is characterized by (1) a focus on an incomplete situation, (2) the freedom to inquire, and (3) the desire to put together something new to him, on his own, to make the incomplete situation into a complete one.

It is the method employed by the individual in the solution of the problems posed that causes exploration and guided discovery to be considered separately here. Whereas movement exploration considers all solutions correct in the absence of a performance model, the guided discovery technique incorporates an observation phase into the total experience. This phase takes the form of observing the solutions of fellow learners, the leader, or individuals on film in relation to the problem presented. Only after the learners have had an opportunity to solve the problem within the limits of their own understanding and ability is the observation phase utilized.

Instead of problems being entirely open-ended, as in movement exploration, there is a gradual funneling of questions in such a manner that they lead learners to discover for themselves how to perform the particular movement under consideration. The absence of a best way to move at this stage of development allows performance of several "best" ways. After attempting solutions to the problem at hand, the learners have an opportunity to evaluate their interpretations in light of the solutions of others. They are then given an opportunity to reassess their solutions in light of the performance of others (Figure 21.4).

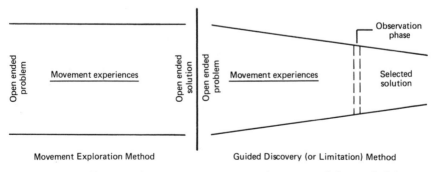

Figure 21.4 Differences between movement exploration and the guided discovery teaching techniques, both of which utilize indirect methods

Facilitating Combination

Combination represents a transitional category in the hierarchical sequence of learning experiences. Movement experiences that use a combination of movement patterns or skills are incorporated into the lesson by the leader through the use of both indirect and direct styles of teaching.

Indirect combination is a logical extension of the movement exploration and guided discovery approaches. These experiences differ only in that activities involving stability, locomotion, and/or manipulation are combined through the problem-solving approaches used at the exploration and discovery stages of learning.

Direct combination experiences follow a more traditional approach to developing and refining combinations of stability, locomotor, and/or manipulative movements. Direct, or traditional, teaching approaches involve establishing a model for correct performance through explanation, and demonstrating the skills to be learned before they are practiced. The learners then duplicate in a short practice session or drill the movement characteristics of the model as nearly as possible within the limits of their abilities. The activity is interrupted and the model is presented again along with general comments concerning problems that the group as a whole may be encountering. The group is then involved in an activity that incorporates these skills. The leader circulates among the learners and aids those individuals who may still be having difficulty executing the skills with a general level of proficiency. Direct combination experiences require establishment of a performance model before the movement experience begins, while indirect experiences do not. The task and the command styles of teaching as proposed by Mooston (1981) are two of the most commonly used teacher-directed methods (Figure 21.5).

Facilitating Application

Application represents the fourth level of the learning hierarchy. To take advantage of this level of experience, the leader aids the students in making conscious decisions concerning the best methods of performing the numerous combinations of stability, locomotor, or manipulative skills rather than merely refining combinations of fundamental movements. Learners begin to select and apply preferred ways of moving in a wide variety of sport, game, and dance activities. Application experiences follow the same direct progression of explanation, demonstration, and practice, followed by general and specific correction and drill that is used with direct combination experiences. Application experiences, however, use more advanced activities than those found in the combination stage. These experiences generally take the form of advanced lead-up activities to dual, team, and individual sports, not low organized games and sport-

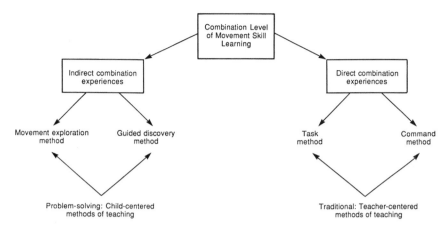

Figure 21.5 At the combination stage of movement skill learning, the leader often utilizes both indirect and direct methods of teaching

skill practice. Lead-up activities combine two or more selected skills into an approximation of the official sport. Advanced lead-up activities used during this period incorporate numerous elements of the official sport. They are modified in terms of the time, equipment, and facilities required and are a close approximation of the final desired combination of specialized movement skills that will be performed in the official sport.

Facilitating Refined Performance

Refined performance is the fifth level in the movement skill learning hierarchy. Individuals at this stage are ready to pit their skills and abilities against those of others. Refined performance here refers to the actual implementation of activities from the application stage in youth sports, interscholastic sports, intramurals, and informal recreational activities. As the performance becomes more refined, greater stress is placed on accuracy, form, and performance of a best way. The job of the teacher is to provide children with a series of experiences that contribute to the fundamental movement skill development that forms the basis for specialized skill development in later years.

Facilitating Individualization

The process of *individualization* is unique to each performer. At this level one is able to make fine adjustments in his or her movement pattern in order to maximize performance. Adjustments are made based on body size, weight, limb length, fitness level, motor abilities and other factors that may influence one's level of performance. The individual nuances in one's golf game, lay-up shot, or swimming are representative of the individualized level of movement skill learning. Occasional breakthroughs in skill performance come about at this level. The individual at this level is able to critically examine his strengths and weaknesses and thoroughly conceptualizes the skill, thus enabling himself to create entirely new ways of moving. The Fosberry method of high jumping pioneered by Bill Fosberry, a previously mediocre high jumper in the 1960s, and the two-handed backhand tennis stroke introduced by Christ Evert in the 1970s are but two examples. Both were able to individualize or personalize skills from their respective sports, and in doing so vastly improved their performance.

In short, the person at the individualized stage is able to use both inductive and deductive thought processes in concert with his or her movement abilities in order to maximize individual performance potentials. To adapt, personalize, and individualize one's movement to the demands of the environment, and to do so successfully, is the zenith of the movement skill learning hierarchy. It is the essence of developing a skillful mover.

THE DEVELOPMENTAL CURRICULAR MODEL

Unfortunately, programs stressing specialized skill development for young children abound throughout North America. Specialized skill development places primary emphasis on refined performance and little emphasis on the other aspects of the learning sequence outlined above. There is nothing inherently wrong with skill specialization, but we must ask ourselves whether skill specialization in the preschool and elementary school is really in the best interest of most children. If it is considered to be in the children's best interest, it should only supplement the regular program in the form of after-school activities. Specialized skill development should never overshadow, replace, or serve as the primary purpose of the regular physical education program. The regular program at the preschool and elementary school levels should stress the development and refinment of fundamental movement skills and the introduction of a wide variety of sport skills instead of specialized skill development through refined performance experiences.

We must involve children in a series of coordinated movement experiences that go beyond the learning of isolated skills and the in-school playing of specific sports they would probably learn on their own through organized activity outside the school.

The developmental model of physical education is based on the proposition that the development of movement abilities occurs in distinct but often overlapping "phases" in each of the "categories of movement." This is achieved through participation in "skill themes" applied to the various "content areas" of physical education and the "movement concepts" of movement education at the appropriate level of "movement skill learning" that is recognized through the implementation of various "indirect techniques" and "direct techniques" of teaching (Figure 21.6).

Preschool and Primary Grades

Developmental teaching recognizes that preschool and primary grade children are involved in developing and refining their fundamental movement abilities in the three categories of movement. These categories serve as the organizing centers of the developmental curriculum and

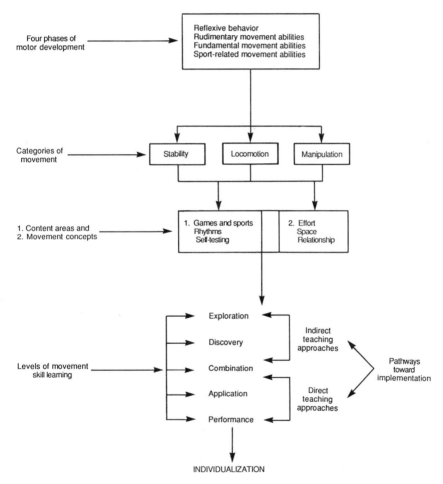

Figure 21.6 Outline of a sequentially based model for the developmental physical education of children and youth

enable formation of skill themes at this level. Each pattern of movement found under these three categories can be dealt with in relative isolation from the others (see Figure 21.1). These fundamental movements are the basis for specialized movements. They are developed and refined at the exploration, discovery, and combination stages of learning primary through indirect styles of teaching that make use of games, rhythms, and self-testing activities and the application of effort, space, and relationship concepts to aid in their development (Figure 21.7).

Upper Elementary, Middle School and Beyond

When the developmental model is applied to the upper elementary and middle school grades and beyond, the focus of the curriculum changes from the fundamental movement phase to the specialized movement phase of development. During this phase of development, children are constantly combining various stability, locomotor, and manipulative patterns of movement in a wide variety of sport skills. Because of this, it becomes impossible to implement movement skill themes that focus on only one category of movement. Instead, skill themes at this level are viewed in the context of the sport area to which they are being applied. The skills inherent within the game of softball, for example, become a "sport skill theme" and involve combinations and elaborations of fundamental manipulative abilities (throwing, catching, and striking), locomotor abilities (base running and sliding) and stability abilities (twisting, turning, and stretching). The teacher at this level gives attention to the development of sport skills related to a particular sport skill theme. This is applied to the various content areas and *knowledge concepts* (rules, strategies, understandings, and appreciation) of physical education. The teacher recognizes that the children's major learning focus at this level is on the combination of skills and application of best ways of performing; therefore, the teacher uses direct teaching methods as his or her primary but not exclusive approach to teaching (Figure 21.8).

SUMMARY

For too many years, both teachers of physical education, and the general population have had only a vague notion of why the balanced motor development and movement education of children are important. The developmental model presented here is based on the Phases of Motor Development. Movement experiences and teaching methodologies are used that recognize the developmental level of the child. The use of games, rhythms, and self-testing activities, as well as the movement concepts of effort, space, and relationships is viewed as a means to achieving increased skill rather than as an end in itself. Learning to move is too

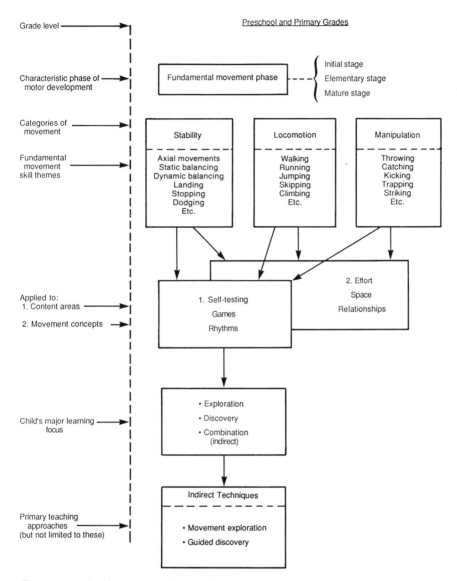

Figure 21.7 Implementing the developmental curricular model at the preschool and primary grade levels

important to be left to chance or to the whims of untrained persons. The individual with knowledge of (1) the Phases of Motor Development, (2) how children learn, and (3) how to implement developmentally appropriate programs for children can serve a vital role in developing one's movement abilities and physical abilities.

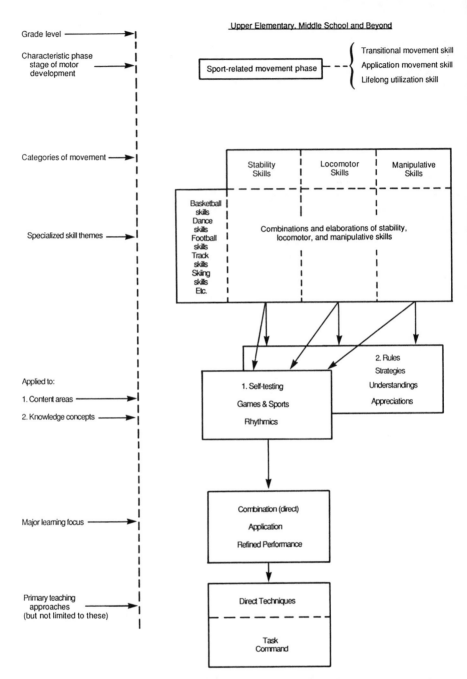

Figure 21.8 Implementing the developmental curricular model in the upper elementary grades and beyond

CHAPTER CONCEPTS

21.1 There are a variety of curricular rationales for organizing the physical education curriculum.

21.2 If research and theory concerning motor development cannot be brought to a practical level, it is of little use.

21.3 If curricular models are not based on sound research and theory, they have little value.

21.4 The developmental stage and movement analysis rationales are among the most popular curricular models at the elementary school level.

21.5 A fundamental movement theme or a sport-skill theme is the focal point of the daily lesson and is composed of one or more movement skills from the locomotor, manipulative, and/or stability categories of movement.

21.6 The content areas of physical education (games and sports, rhythms, and self-testing activities) and the movement concepts of movement education (effort, space, and relationships) are important to the development of skilled movers.

21.7 When learning a new skill, we all pass through a series of levels of movement skill learning that focus on particular aspects of skill development (exploration, discovery, combination, application, refined performance, and individualization).

21.8 Indirect teaching approaches involving problem-solving techniques encourage exploration, discovery, and the indirect combination of movements.

21.9 Direct teaching approaches involving command and task teaching techniques are best suited for combining skills, for selecting best ways to move, and for refining the performance of movement skills.

21.10 A curricular model can be constructed for children at the preschool and primary grade levels to encourage development and refinement of fundamental movement abilities through the incorporation of indirect teaching techniques.

21.11 A curricular model can be constructed for older individuals that encourages development and refinement of a wide variety of sport-related movement abilities through the incorporation of direct teaching techniques.

21.12 The developmental curricular model emphasizes indirect styles of teaching at the preschool and primary grade levels and direct styles of teaching later on. This does not mean, however, that one is limited to the use of these techniques; it simply means that the emphasis switches from indirect to direct techniques.

TERMS TO REMEMBER

Developmental Approach

Movement Analysis Approach

Categories of Movement

Developmental Skill Theme

Stability

Locomotion

Manipulation

Content Areas

Games and Sports

Rhythms

Self-Testing

Movement Concepts (Elements)

Effort

Space

Relationships
Levels of Movement Skill Learning
Individualization
Movement Exploration
Guided-Discovery
Problem-Solving
Combination

Knowledge Concepts
Indirect Combination
Direct Combination
Application
Refined Performance
Individualization

CRITICAL READINGS

Gallahue, D. L. (1987). *Developmental Physical Education for Today's Elementary School Children*. New York: Macmillian. (Chapter 14).

Graham, G., Holt/Hale, S. A. and Parker, M. (1987). *Children Moving A Reflective Approach*. Mountain View, CA: Mayfield, (Chapters 1 & 2).

Holt/Hale, S. A. (1988) *On the Move*. Mountain View, CA: Mayfield, (Parts II and III, C/F/L).

Sage, G. H. (1984). *Motor Learning and Control*. Dubuque, IA: Wm. C. Brown. (Chapter 22).

22

Assessing Motor Behavior

```
┌─────────────────────────────────────────────────────────────────────┐
│                                                                       │
│  CHAPTER COMPETENCIES                                                  │
│                                                                       │
│     Upon Completion of This Chapter You Should Be Able To:            │
│                                                                       │
│  *  Demonstrate understanding of various types of analysis that have  │
│     been used in the study of human development (performance scores,  │
│     motor sequence descriptions, etc.).                               │
│                                                                       │
│  *  View an individual's motor behavior as more or less advanced on   │
│     a developmental continuum rather than as good or bad.             │
│                                                                       │
│  *  Discuss advantages and shortcomings of the major methodologies    │
│     associated with the study of change.                              │
│                                                                       │
│  *  Discuss the use of developmental sequence checklists for          │
│     evaluating motor development.                                     │
│                                                                       │
│  *  Critique current motor development screening tests/scales.        │
│                                                                       │
│  *  Correctly administer at least one motor development test and      │
│     interpret its results.                                            │
│                                                                       │
│  *  Identify resources for referral testing of motor problems.        │
│                                                                       │
└─────────────────────────────────────────────────────────────────────┘
```

There is no lack of tests that purport to measure the motor abilities. Wade (1981) has conservatively estimated that there are at least 250 assessment instruments, 91 of which have been published. The problem lies not in the quantity of instruments available but in their quality. The vast majority of tests have little or no rationale for development and are based on quantitative measures (i.e., how far, how fast, how many), rather than on qualitative measures (how the child moves). Furthermore, the majority of these assessment instruments fail to compare individuals to their own previous performance but instead establish performance criteria based on the performances of their chronological peers. Tests of this nature, although potentially reliable, objective, and relatively easy to administer, reveal little about the motor development of the child. They may be valuable, however, in that they describe the status of the child at that particular time in terms of the criterion measures and in comparison with his or her peers. If, however, we view the term "development" as the process of change over time and are interested in assessing this change, there is little to be gained from administering a battery of tests that merely describe the quantity of an individual's performance at a given point. Tests of this nature have little to do with development and may be more properly labeled "motor performance tests."

There are essentially two types of assessment instruments available to assess motor behavior: product instruments and process instruments. Product, task-oriented, or norm-referenced measures, as they are often termed, are by far the most prevalent. They are probably best exemplified by the devices designed by Apgar (1953), Frankenburg and Dodds (1967), Bayley (1969), Brazelton (1973), Roach and Kephart (1966), and Bruininks (1978). Each of these assessment instruments will be briefly described and critiques will be given in the following sections. The process-oriented or criterion-referenced assessment instruments designed by McClenaghan (1976) Seefeldt and Haubenstricker (1976), Ulrich (1985) and others will also be discussed.

PRODUCT-ORIENTED ASSESSMENT INSTRUMENTS

There is an abundance of descriptive performance tests designed to screen children and to assess their current level of ability as measured by a variety of behavioral events. *Screening tests* are designed to provide a relatively quick and simple means of differentiating normal infants or children from those who may not be developing normally. *Behavioral assessment instruments*, on the other hand, tend to be more varied in intent and design. They may attempt to distinguish between normal and abnormal behavior, predict later abilities, or measure individual differences.

Many product-oriented assessment tools are *norm-referenced*. That is, the quantitative scores obtained on one's performance abilities can be compared against others representing similar backgrounds, ages, and gender. Norm-referenced tests are based on statistical samplings of hundreds or even thousands of individuals. They permit one to compare an individual against a statistical sample that is intended to be representative of the population at large. Caution should be used when interpreting results from norm-referenced tests. Norms are population-specific and serve little specific value. That is, one can not generalize beyond the population on which the norms were generated, and they simply provide a general idea of where one ranks in comparison to others. Scores from norm-referenced assessment tests provide little information into specific needs and programming possibilities. The screening and behavioral assessment instruments that follow are all norm-referenced.

Screening Tests

Three widely used screening devices are the Apgar screening technique used at birth, the Denver Developmental Screening Test used from infancy through early childhood, and the Purdue Perceptual Motor Survey used from early childhood through childhood.

Apgar. Virginia Apgar (1953) developed the Apgar screening technique as a quick and reliable method of assessing the newborn one minute after birth. Supplemental ratings can be made at three, five, and ten minutes after birth. The newborn is evaluated on five items and given a score of 0, 1, or 2 on each for a total of up to 10, depending on its condition. A score of 0 is given if the sign to be observed is absent, a 1 if all of the conditions are not met for a score of 2. Ten is the highest score possible for the five-test total. Infants are rated on (1) heart rate, (2) respiratory effort, (3) irritability, (4) muscle tone, and (5) color. Table 22.1 provides a summary of the five items and how they are scored.

Apgar scores appear to be quite reliable. The test was standardized by Apgar and James (1962) on 27,715 infants. The standardization showed that infants with the lowest Apgar scores had the highest mortality rates and that the device was useful in predicting infant mortality. Self and Horwitz (1979) indicated that Apgar scores are directly related to the type of delivery. Breech deliveries have the lowest average scores, followed by caesarian section deliveries, with spinal anesthesia and natural childbirth deliveries receiving the highest scores. Yang et al. (1976) did note, however, that maternal drug dosage is directly related to Apgar scores. Yang found that the more drugs the mother is given, the lower is the infant's five-minute Apgar score.

The Apgar system has been helpful in screening newborns in need of special attention. It is quick, easy to administer, appears to be highly reliable, and has been used successfully for almost a quarter of a century as a diagnostic tool for the physician.

Denver Developmental Screening Test. The Denver Developmental Screening Test (DDST) developed by Frankenburg and Dodds (1967) is a helpful device used to screen infants and young children. The DDST is one of the most widely recognized and widely used standardized tests for assessing the motor development of young children. It has been success-

Table 22.1 Scoring the Apgar Screening Test

Item tested	Scoring		
	2	1	0
Heart rate	100-140 bpm	Under 100	No heartbeat
Respiratory effort	Regular breathing and lusty crying	Irregular or shallow breathing	No breathing
Reflex irritability (measured by a slap to the soles of the feet)	Lusty crying when soles of feet are slapped	No crying but grimace or movement when soles of of feet are slapped	No reaction when soles of feet are slapped
Muscle tone	Spontaneously flexed arms and legs resist attempts at extension	Spontaneously flexed arms and legs offer little resistance from attempts at extension	Completely flaccid
Color[1]	Entirely pink	Some pink	Other than pink

[1]This is the most controversial item in the test. Few infants receive at 2 at one minute, and the item is, of course, invalid with dark-skinned babies.

fully used to detect evidence of retarded development so effective intervention techniques may be implemented at an early age. Both gross and fine motor skills are evaluated along with language and personal-social skills. The 105 items on the test are scaled according to their normal developmental order of appearance in children. Table 22.2 provides a brief overview of the test and some of the items assessed.

Although the DDST has been roundly criticized for underscreening, it does offer the advantage of indicating the age at which 25, 50, 75, and 90 percent of the population pass each item. Benchmarks of behavior for each of the items assessed are displayed with bar graphs on a screening chart. These graphs illustrate the overlapping but sequentially-based skills of infancy and early childhood. Seldom are more than 20 of the 105 items administered to provide a profile of the child's developmental level.

The DDST has been standardized on a sample of 1,036 children ranging in age from 2 weeks to 6 years. This sample has been criticized as unrepresentative (Buros, 1971). Furthermore, Herkowitz (1978) has stated that:

Table 22.2 Sample Items from the Denver Developmental Screening Test

Area Tested	Sample Items Measured
Gross motor (31 items measured)	Rudimentary stability abilities: control of head, neck, trunk, rolling over, sitting, standing with support, pulling to stand, cruising, standing alone, walking Fundamental manipulative abilities: kicking, throwing, tricycle riding, catching Fundamental locomotor abilities: jumping in place, long-jumping, hopping Fundamental stability abilities: balancing on one foot, heel-toe walk
Fine motor (30 items measured)	Rudimentary manipulative abilities: reaching, grasping, and releasing, cube stacking, scribbling, copying, draw-a-person
Language localization, (21 items measured) language	Vocalizing, laughing, squealing, sound imitation of speech sounds, rudimentary combining words, following directions, recognizing colors, defining words
Personal-social (22 items measured)	Smiling, feeding, drinking from cup, imitating housework, helping in house, removing garment, putting on clothing, washing and drying hands, playing interactive games, separating from mother easily, dressing without supervision

So—although easy to administer, and capable of being used by relatively untrained testers—the DDST is not so reliable or valid as its authors had hoped. Its use for children under 30 months old should be discouraged because of questionable reliability at that age. (p. 168)

The usefulness of the DDST is questionable. It should only be used as a gross screening measure that may provide some clues to the developmentally-delayed child. It should not, at this time, be considered a valid or reliable instrument for research or placement purposes.

The Purdue Perceptual-Motor Survey. The Purdue Perceptual-Motor Survey (PPMS), developed by Roach and Kephart (1966), is not a test. It is a behavioral assessment survey that provides the examiner with an opportunity to observe a broad spectrum of behaviors. In fact, Roach and Kephart note that "at its present level of development, the survey should be regarded merely as an instrument which allows the examiner to observe a series of perceptual-motor behaviors and to isolate areas which may need further study" (pp. 10-11). The survey is based on Kephart's theory that all learning is based on the sensorimotor experiences of childhood.

The PPMS is designed for children from 6 to 10 years of age but is often used with both younger and older children in an effort to gain clues concerning possible perceptual-motor problems. Table 22.3 outlines the various components of the survey and how they are measured.

Table 22.3 Test Items from the Purdue Perceptual-Motor Survey

Items Assessed	Method
Balance and posture walking	Walking forward, backward, sideways on board; performing a series of eight tasks evaluating ability to jump, hop, and skip while maintaining balance.
Body image and differentiation	Identification of body parts, imitation of movement, obstacle course activities, Kraus-Weber Test, angels-in-the-snow.
Perceptual-motor match performing	Making circle, double circle, lateral line, and vertical line on chalkboard; eight rhythmic writing tasks.
Ocular control	Ocular pursuits of both eyes, right eye, left eye, and convergence are tested.
Form perception square,	Seven geometric forms are drawn on sheet of paper: circle, cross, triangle, horizontal, diamond, vertical diamond, and divided rectangle.

The PPMS has been used successfully for several years to discriminate between children who are experiencing problems in their motor development and those who are not. As a survey, however, interpretation and generalization of results are limited. Standardization of the PPMS was conducted on only 200 children from the same school using Kephart's original scale rather than the one published later by Roach and Kephart (Buros, 1971). Reliability scores within subjects and between raters has been reported at .95 (Buros, 1971). The question of validity still has not been answered to the satisfaction of many. Several of the tasks on the PPMS require multiple skills, and some demonstrate the need for more cognitive than motor ability. Also, factor-analytic studies have shown that items are not appropriately grouped. Factors do not remain stable through grades K to 4, nor do they develop at similar or even rates (Dunsing, 1969). Despite its many shortcomings, the PPMS may be of use by the teacher as an observational assessment survey that may offer important clues to the perceptual and motor functioning of the child.

Behavioral Assessment Tests

There are a wide variety of behavioral assessment tests available. Only a few are presented here. They represent, however, a sampling of the most widely used behavioral assessment tests in North America and provide a cross section of tests appropriate for use with neonates, infants, young children, and older children.

Brazelton Neonatal Behavioral Assessment Scale. The Brazelton Neonatal Behavioral Assessment Scale (BNBAS) was developed by Brazelton (1973) with the intention of scoring the infant's responses to his or her environment. The test is designed for use with normal neonates and is divided into 20 elicited neurological items and 27 behavioral items. Table 22.4 provides an overview of the items measured on the BNBAS.

Scoring of the majority of the infant's behavior is done after administration of all the test items. The elicited neurological responses are scored on a four-point scale ranging from 0 to 3 points (0, absent; 1, low; 2, medium; 3 high) for intensity of response. The behavioral items are scored on a scale of 1 to 9 points. This scale represents the state of arousal of the infant. A score of 1, for example, signifies that the infant is sleeping, while a 9 indicates that the infant is actively crying. The ideal state of the infant for assessment lies somewhere between 1 and 9 and varies from item to item. The testing conditions as well as overall impressions of the neonate are also recorded along with general biographical data such as length, weight, and age in days.

Unfortunately, the Brazelton scale has not been standardized beyond the report by Heidelise et al. (1979), in which a homogeneous

Table 22.4 Test Items for the Brazelton Neonatal Behavioral Assessment Scale

	Behavioral Responses	
Elicited Neurological Responses	Specific	General
1. Plantar grasp	1. Response decrement to light (2,3)[a]	1. Degree of alertness (4)
2. Hand grasp	2. Response decrement to rattle (2,3)	2. General tonus (4,5)
3. Anal colonus	3. Response decrement to bell (2,3)	3. Motor maturity (4,5)
4. Babinski reflex	4. Response decrement to pinprick (1,2,3)	4. Cuddliness (4,5)
5. Standing reflex		5. Consolability with intervention (6 to 8)
6. Primary stepping reflex	6. Inanimate visual orientation response (focusing and following an object) (4)	6. Peak to excitement (6)
7. Placing		7. Rapidity of buildup (1,2 to 6)
8. Incurvation	6. Inanimate auditory orientation response (reaction to an auditory stimulus) (4,5)	8. Irritability (3,4,5)
9. Reflex crawling		9. Activity (alert states)
10. Glabulla reflex	7. Animate visual orientation (reaction to persons) (4)	10. Tremulousness (all states)
11. Tonic deviation of head and eyes		11. Amount of startle (3,4,5,6)
12. Nystagmus	8. Animate auditory orientation (reaction to a voice) (4,5)	12. Lability of skin color (all states) (1-6)
13. Tonic neck reflex		13. Liability of states (all states)
14. Moro reflex	9. Animate visual and auditory orientation (reaction to a person's face and voice) (4)	14. Self-quieting activity (6,5 to 4,3,2,1)
15. Rooting reflex intensity		15. Hand-to-mouth facility (all states)
16. Sucking reflex intensity	10. Pull-to-sit (3,5)	
17–20. Passive movements (right arm, left arm, right leg, left leg)	11. Defensive movements (4)	

[a]Numbers in parentheses represent the ideal state for assessment.

group of 54 healthy, full-term white newborns were assessed over a 10-day period. Brazelton himself (Brazelton et al. 1979) has recognized the problem of standardization based on his findings that newborns from different cultures behave differently. The problem, therefore, is to be able to identify a group of newborns that are in fact representative of the population at large. To date, this difficult feat has not been accomplished. Interrated reliability of the BNBAS, however, has been reported to be quite high ranging from .85 to 1.00 (Horowitz and Brazelton, 1973; Heidelise et al. 1979). Its predictive validity is also good, having been reported at 80 percent in a sample of 43 children followed over a 7-year period (Tronick and Brazelton, 1975).

The Brazelton scale appears to be a useful device for identifying high-risk infants and for studying the effects of obstetrical medication, cross-cultural infant behavior, and caregiver intervention. It is a helpful measure for assessing the general, specific, and neurological behavior of the neonate.

Bayley Scale of Infant Development. The Bayley Scales of Infant Development (Bayley, 1969) are a revision of Bayley's (1935) earlier work which attempted, through behavioral assessment, to measure the intellectual development of the child. Very little relationship was found between the infant's score on mental scales and later intelligence or later performance on mental scales. As a result, the current Bayley Scales of Infant Development (BSID) purport to assess only the child's developmental status from 1 month of age to 2+ years.

The BSID is divided into three separate scales. Table 22.5 presents a brief overview of these three scales and the general items measured. Space limitations do not permit a full description of each of the scales. The Mental Scale contains 163 items. The Motor Scale is made up of 81 items measuring progressive change in gross motor abilities such as sitting, standing, walking, stair climbing, and fine motor abilities. Materials for the Motor Scale are expensive and require special equipment.

The BSID has been standardized on 1,262 children from 2 to 3 months of age (Self and Horwitz, 1979). Observer agreement of trained observers (i.e., a minimum of six months training) for the Mental Scale was rated at 89.4 percent and 93.4 percent for the Motor Scale (Werner and Bayley, 1966). Werner and Bayley (1966) also achieved test-retest reliability ratings of .76 for the Mental Scale and .75 for the Motor Scale. Validity data for the BSID have never been published.

The BSID scales are probably the best standardized behavioral assessment techniques available for infants. They have had the most extensive use as a research instrument of any of the infant assessment scales and have proven to be helpful in determining the developmental

Table 22.5 General Description of the Items Measured on the Bayley Scales of Infant Development

Scale	Items Assessed
Mental scale	Sensory-perceptual acuities
	Object discrimination
	Object constancy
	Memory
	Learning
	Problem solving
	Vocalization
	Verbal communication
	Generalizations and classifications
Motor scale	Control of the body
	Gross motor coordination
	Fine motor coordination
Infant behavior record	Administered after the Mental and Motor Scales. Assesses the child's social development, interests, emotions, energy, and tendencies to approach or withdraw from situations.

status of individual infants at a given age. When administered and interpreted by a trained examiner, they can be a valuable research tool.

Bruininks-Oseretsky Test of Motor Proficiency. The Bruininks-Oseretsky Test of Motor Proficiency (BOTMP) was developed by Bruininks (1978, p. 11) as an "individually administered test that assesses the motor functioning of children from 4+ to 14+ years of age." The BOTMP is based, in part, on the adapatation by Doll (1946) of the original Oseretsky Tests of Motor Proficiency and is designed to assess the motor skills of children. The BOTMP is composed of eight subtests designed to measure important aspects of motor development. Table 22.6 provides an overview of the BOTMP. The gross motor skill and fine motor skill sections of the test may be administered separately and will yield separate composite scores. In order to arrive at a composite score for the entire battery of tests, a combination gross and fine motor skills test must be taken along with the separate gross motor items and separate the fine motor items. A short form of the BOTMP is also available.

The BOTMP has been standardized on a sample of 765 children carefully proportioned on the bases of age, sex, race, community size, and geographic location as indicated by 1970 census figures. Norms have been developed and test-retest reliability scores average .87 for the battery composite of the long form and .86 for the short form of the test

Table 22.6 Test Items from the Bruininks-Oseretsky Test of Motor Proficiency

Area Tested	Subtest	Items
Gross motor skills	1. Running—Designed to measure running speed.	Shuttle run.
	2. Balance (8 items)—Designed to measure static and dynamic balance abilities.	Static balance (3 items). Dynamic balance (5 items).
	3. Bilateral coordination (8 items)—Designed to measure simultaneous coordination of upper and lower limbs.	Foot and finger tapping (3 items). Jumping in place (4 items). Drawing lines and crosses simultaneously (1 item).
	4. Strength (3 items)—Designed to measure upper arm and shoulder girdle strength, abdominal strength, and leg strength.	Standing broad jump. Sit-ups. Knee push-ups (boys under 8 and all girls). Full push-ups (boys 8 and older).
Gross and fine motor skills	5. Upper limb coordination (9 items)—Designed to measure gross and fine eye-hand coordination.	Ball bounce and catch (2 items). Catching tossed ball (2 items). Throwing a ball (1 item). Touching swinging ball (1 item). Precise upper limb movements (3 items).
Fine motor skills	6. Response speed (1 item)—Designed to measure response to a moving object.	Yardstick drop (1 item).
	7. Visual-motor control (8 items)—Designed to measure coordition of eye-hand movements.	Cutting (1 item). Drawing and copying (7 items).
	8. Upper limb speed and dexterity (8 items)—Designed to measure hand and finger dexterity, hand speed, and arm speed.	Penny placing (2 items). Card sorting (1 item). Bead stringing (1 item). Peg displacing (1 item). Lines and dots (3 items).

(Bruininks, 1978). The validity of the BOTMP according to Bruininks (1978, p. 28) "is based on its ability to assess the construct of motor development of proficiency." In terms of motor proficiency as measured by the performance of a given child on a given day, the BOTMP is indeed a valid test. It is, however, too much to assume that the BOTMP is a valid test of motor development if the term "development" is viewed as progressive change over time.

The relative merits and drawbacks of the BOTMP were debated at a meeting of the Motor Development Academy of the AAHPERD (Bruininks, 1981; Haubenstricker, et al., 1981; Broadhead, 1981). The test is not without either fault or need for improvement. Despite its limitations, however, it does seem to have good potential for assessing the motor proficiency of children. It should also be of value as a research tool, and as an aid for identifying children with special needs.

PROCESS-ORIENTED ASSESSMENT INSTRUMENTS

Process-oriented, or *criterion-referenced*, assessment instruments as they are frequently termed evaluate the qualitative aspects of one's movement behavior. They differ from norm-referenced instruments in that they compare individuals to themselves over time, not to a standardized population. Criterion-referenced assessment instruments are concerned with the mechanics (quality) of one's movement behavior rather than with his or her performance (quantity) level.

Few formalized tests exist that examine the process of movement. There is, however, a growing body of research oriented toward the quality of children's movement. What is needed now is careful longitudinal study of a variety of movement behaviors to generate developmental continuums. Roberton (1981, p. 3), notes: "Motor development ought to be assessed by observing a child's movement and locating what is seen within a developmental sequence." The three-stage developmental sequence of fundamental movements presented in Chapter 11 offers a means by which the quality of a child's movements can be observed and his or her progress charted over time. It should be stressed, however, that several of the developmental sequences presented in Chapter 11, although based on careful observational assessment, are merely proposed developmental descriptions of fundamental movements. Only through film analysis and longitudinal study can these sequences be validated or refuted. A description of the observational assessment instruments developed by McClenaghan (McClenaghan, 1976; McClenaghan and Gallahue, 1978b), Seefeldt and Haubenstricker (1976), and Ulrich (1985) follows.

Fundamental Movement Pattern Assessment Instrument

The Fundamental Movement Pattern Assessment Instrument (FMPAI) designed by McClenaghan (1976) and later published by McClenaghan and Gallahue (1978b) is a carefully developed observational assessment instrument. It is used to classify individuals at the "initial," "elementary," or "mature" stage of development in five different movements (throwing, catching, kicking, running, and jumping). The developmental sequence for each of these movements is based on an exhaustive review of the biomechanical literature on each fundamental movement.

Validity of the FMPAI was established through the research base on which the developmental progressions of the five movement patterns were formulated and by the opinions of a panel of motor development experts. Interrater reliability for each of the assessed items ranged from a high of 95 percent agreement for throwing to a low of 80 percent agreement for running, with 94 percent, 91 percent, and 90 percent agreement for jumping, catching, and kicking, respectively. Subject performance reliability was rated at 88.6 percent on a retest five days after the original assessment.

The FMPAI is an easy-to-use motor development test designed to measure the present status of children and to assess change over time. It attempts to view the quality of the child's movement and is based on documented developmental sequences for acquiring selected fundamental movement abilities. The FMPAI does not, however, yield a quantitative score, nor can it be used for comparing one child with another. This instrument is intended instead to assess developmental changes over time, using observational assessment as a valid and reliable method of data collection and comparison within individuals.

Developmental Sequence of Fundamental Motor Skills Inventory

The Developmental Sequence of Fundamental Motor Skills Inventory (DSFMSI) assessment instrument was developed by Seefeldt and Haubenstricker (1976) and Haubenstricker et al. (1981). The DSFMSI categorizes each of ten fundamental motor patterns into four or five stages. The fundamental movements of walking, skipping, hopping, running, striking, kicking, catching, throwing, jumping, and punting have been studied. These developmental sequences are based on combinations of longitudinal and cross-sectional data obtained from film analysis. Children are observed and matched to both visual and verbal descriptions of each stage. Individuals are classified along a continuum from stage one (immature) to stage five (mature).

Although reliability scores have not been reported, personal communication with the developers has indicated that, with training using specially designed films and a stop-action projector, interrater reliability is quite high.

Test of Gross Motor Development

The Test of Gross Motor Development (TGMD) was developed by Ulrich (1985) as a means of assessing movement skills in children 3 to 10 years of age. Selected locomotor and manipulative skills comprise the twelve item test. Locomotor skills include: running, galloping, hopping, leaping, horizontal jumping, skipping, and sliding. Manipulative skills include: two-hand striking, stationary ball bouncing, catching, kicking, and overhand throwing.

Administration of the TGMD takes approximately 15 minutes per child. A manual with a clear set of test instructions is available. Mean test-retest reliability coefficients are reported to be .96 for the locomotor items, and .97 for the manipulative items. Interrater rates reliability estimates are similarly high. Content validity was established by having three experts judge the appropriateness and representativeness of the items for preschool and elementary school children. Construct validity was determined through factor analytic techniques.

The TGMD is easy to administer, and can be used with a minimum amount of special training. It provides both norm-referenced and criterion-referenced interpretations, and places emphasis on the sequence and qualitative aspects of gross motor skill acquisition rather than on the product and quantitative aspects of performance.

Other Process-Oriented Assessment Instruments

There are a few other useful process-oriented approaches to motor development assessment. Roberton's (1978c) method represents an expansion of stage theory and analyzes the components of movement within a given pattern. Her longitudinal study of the development of throwing abilities lends support to the concept of developmental stages and offers hope for validation of developmental sequences. The Ohio State University Scale of Intra-Gross Motor Assessment (OSU Sigma) developed by Loovis (1979) and the De Oreo Fundamental Motor Skills Inventory developed by De Oreo (1977) also represent promising efforts at assessing the process of movement.

Ongoing research is providing a great deal of the descriptive data on which future process-oriented motor development tests will be based. The mixed longitudinal data collection process is long and tedious. It requires considerable patience and years of effort before sound, validated developmental progressions can be formulated.

SUMMARY

There is an ever-increasing number of published and unpublished tests purported to be measures of motor development. The vast majority of these assessment instruments are product-oriented and provide information concerning the present status of the child in a variety of areas. These tests are descriptive and generally establish a standard of performance based on certain expectations for each chronological age.

Product-oriented assessment instruments can be of value to the motor development specialist if they are both valid and reliable. Unfortunately, the validity of many tests is suspect because of the lack of a sound rationale, or because of inadequate correlational attempts with other tests purporting to measure the same thing.

Product-oriented tests may be classified as either screening devices or behavioral assessment devices. The Apgar, Denver Developmental Screening Test, and Purdue Perceptual-Motor Survey are easy-to-use tools available for quick but gross classification of children. The Brazelton Neonatal Assessment Scale, Bayley Scales of Infant Development, and Bruininks-Oseretsky Test of Motor Proficiency are among the most widely-used behavioral assessment instruments for neonates, infants, and children, respectively.

There are far fewer process-oriented tests than product-oriented tests, although there is great need to know more about the developmental progression of movement skill acquisition. The Fundamental Movement Pattern Assessment Instrument, the Developmental Sequence of Fundamental Motor Skills Inventory, and the Test of Gross Motor Development represent three attempts at assessing the quality, rather than the quantity, of movement.

CHAPTER CONCEPTS

22.1 Several hundred tests that purport to measure children's motor abilities exist.

22.2 The quality of the vast majority of motor assessment instruments is questionable.

22.3 The validity of many motor assessment instruments is highly questionable.

22.4 Most tests of motor abilities are based on quantitative measures of how far, how fast, or how many.

22.5 Most assessment instruments are scored on chronologically-based criteria.

22.6 Many tests that purport to be motor *development* tests are really measures of motor *performance*.

22.7 Tests of motor behavior in children may be classified as product-oriented or process-oriented.

22.8 Product-oriented tests are sometimes referred to as task-oriented or descriptive measures.

22.9 Product-oriented tests may be classified as either screening or behavioral assessment instruments.

22.10 Screening tests are designed to differentiate normal from abnormal behaviors.

22.11 Behavioral assessment instruments attempt to distinguish, predict, and measure individual differences.

22.12 The Apgar, Denver Developmental Screening Test, and Purdue Perceptual-Motor Survey are three easy-to-administer screening devices designed for newborns, infants, and young children, respectively.

22.13 The Brazelton Neonatal Behavioral Assessment Scale, Bayley Scales of Infant Development, and Bruininks-Oseretsky Test of Motor Proficiency are three behavioral assessment devices designed for neonates, infants, and children, respectively.

22.14 Process-oriented tests of motor development are concerned with the quality of one's movements, are based on developmental references, and are scored in a diagnostic manner.

22.15 The Fundamental Movement Pattern Assessment Instrument, Developmental Sequence of Fundamental Motor Skills Inventory, and Test of Gross Motor Development are process-oriented motor development tests that are reliable, valid, and easy to administer.

22.16 The ongoing research of a variety of investigators is providing a basis for the development of motor development tests that view the quality of the child's movement.

TERMS TO REMEMBER

Product Instruments
Screening Test
Behavioral Assessment Instrument
Norm-Referenced
Apgar
Denver Developmental Screening Test
Purdue Perceptual-Motor Survey
Brazelton Neonatal Behavioral Assessment Scale
Bayley Scale of Infant Development
Bruiniks-Oseretsky Test of Motor Proficiency
Process Instruments
Criterion-Referenced
Fundamental Movement Pattern Assessment Instrument
Developmental Sequence of Fundamental Motor Skills Inventory
Test of Gross Motor Development

CRITICAL READINGS

Adrian, M. J., and Cooper, J. M. *Biomechanics of Human Movement.* Indianapolis: Benchmark Press, (Chapter 8 "Qualitative and Quantitative Assessment).

Gallahue, D. L. (1983). "Assessing Motor Development in Young Children." *Studies in Educational Evaluation*, 8, 247-252.

Haubenstricker, J. (1978). "A Critical Review of Selected Perpetual-Motor Tests and Scales Currently Used in the Assessment of Motor Behavior," In Landers, D. M. and Christina, R. W. (eds.) *Psychology in Motor Behavior and Sport—1977*, Champaign, IL: Human Kinetics.

Herkowitz, J. (1978). "Assessing the Motor Development of Children: Presentation and Critique of Tests," In Ridenour, M. V. (ed.) *Motor Development Issues and Applications*, Princeton, NJ: Princeton.

Paget, K.D. and Bracken, B.A. (1983). *The Psychoeducational Assessment of Preschool Children*. New York: Greene & Stratton (Chapters 11 & 12).

Self, P. A., and F. D. Horwitz. (1979). "The Behavioral Assessment of the Neonate: An Overview," In Osofsky, J. D. (ed.) *The Handbook of Infant Development*. New York: Wiley.

BIBLIOGRAPHY

—A—

AAHPER. (1968). *What Every Parent Should Know About the New Physical Education.* Reston, VA: AAHPERD.

AAHPER. (1973). *Annotated Bibliography of Perceptual-Motor Development.* Reston, VA: AAHPERD.

AAHPERD. (1975). *Testing for Impaired, Disabled and Handicapped Individuals.* Reston, VA: AAHPERD.

AAHPERD. (1976). *Youth Fitness Test Manual: Revised 1976 Edition.* Reston, VA: AAHPERD.

AAHPERD. (1980). *Health Related Physical Fitness Test, Manual.* Reston, VA: AAHPERD.

AAHPERD. (1987). "Summary of Findings from National Children and Youth Fitness Study II." *Journal of Physical Education, Recreation and Dance.* 58-59, 50-96.

Adrian, M. J. and Cooper, J. M. (1989). *Biomechanics of Human Movement.* Indianapolis: Benchmark Press.

Alexander, G. J. et al. (1967). "Injection in Early Pregnancy Produces Abnormalities in Offspring of Rats." *Science,* 157, 459-460.

Aldis, O. (1975). *Play Fighting.* New York: Academic Press.

Alford, C. A. et al. (1975). "Toxoplasmosis: Silent Congenital Infection." In Krogman, S., and Gershon, A. A. (eds.). *Infections of the Fetus and the Newborn Infant.* New York: Alan R. Liss.

Alford, C. A. et al. (1983). "Chronic Cognital Infections Common Environmental Causes for Severe and Subtle Birth Defects." In Finley, S. C. et al. (eds). *Birth Defects: Clinical and Ethical Considerations.* New York: Alan R. Liss.

Amateur Athletic Union. (1988). *The Chrysler Fund—Amateur Athletic Union Physical Fitness Program.* Bloomington, IN: Poplars Building.

American College of Obstetricians and Gynecologists. (1985). "Exercise During Pregnancy and the Postnatal Period." *American College of Obstetricians and Gynecologists Home Exercise Programs.* Washington, D.C. ACOG.

American College of Sports Medicine Position Statement on the Use and Abuse of Anabolic-Androgenic Steroids in Sports. (1977). *Medicine and Science in Sports,* 9, 11-13.

American Academy of Pediatrics Committee on Sports Medicine. (1983). "Weight Training and Weight Lifting: Information for the Pediatrician." *News and Comments,* 33, 7-8.

Ames, II (1937). "The Sequential Patterning of Prone Progression in the Human Infant." *Genetic Psychology Monographs,* 19, 409-460.

Anastasiow, N. J. (1965). "Success in School and Boys' Sex Role Patterns." *Child Development,* 33, 1053-1066.

Anderson, K. L., et al. (1978). "The Rate of Growth in Maximal Aerobic Power of Children in Norway." In Borms, J. and Hebbelinck M. (eds.). *Medicine and Sport Science Series: Pediatric Work Psychology.* Basel, Belgium: S. Karger.

Andrish, J. T. (1984). "Overuse Syndromes of the Lower Extremities in Youth Sports." In Boileau, R. A. (ed.). *Advances in Pediatric Sport Sciences Biological Issues.* Champaign, IL: Human Kinetics.

Apgar, V. (1953). "A Proposal for a New Method of Evaluation of the Newborn Infant." *Current Research in Anesthesia and Analgesia,* 32, 260-267.

Apgar, V., and James L. S. (1962). "Further Observations on the Newborn Scoring System." *American Journal of the Diseases of Children,* 104, 419-428.

Armstrong, D. B. et al. (1951). "Obesity and its Relation to Health and Disease." *Journal of the American Medical Association,* 147, 1007.

Armussen, E. (1973). "Growth in Muscular Strength and Power." In Rarick, G. L. (ed.). *Physical Activity: Human Growth and Development.* New York: Academic Press.

Aslin, R. N. (1977). "Development of Binocular Fixation in Human Infants." *Journal of Experimental Child Psychology,* 23, 133-150.

Aslin, R. N. (1981). "Developmental of Smooth Pursuit in Human Infants." In Fisher, D. F. et al. (eds.). *Eye Movements: Cognition and Visual Perception.* Hillsdale, NJ: Erlbaum.

Aslin, R. N. (1984). "Motor Aspects of Visual Development in Infancy." In Salapatek, P., and Cohen, L. B. (eds.). *Handbook of Infant Perception.* New York: Academic Press.

Aslin, R. N. et al. (1983). "Auditory Development and Speech Perception in Infancy." In Mussan, P. H. (ed.). *Handbook of Child Psychology.* New York: Wiley.

Aslin, R. N., and Dumais, S.T. (1980). "Binocular Vision in Infants: A Review and a Theoretical Position." *Advances in Child Development and Behavior,* 15, 53-94.

Aslin, R. N. and Salapatek, P. (1975). "Saccadic Localization of Peripheral Targets by the Very Young Human Infant." *Perception and Psychophysics.* 17, 292-302.

Astrand, P. O. (1952). *Experimental Studies of Working Capacity in Relation to Sex and Age.* Copenhagen, Denmark: Munksgaard.

Astrand, P. O. and Rodahl, K. (1970). *Textbook of Work Physiology.* New York: McGraw-Hill.

Athletic Institute: (1975) *National Youth Sports Directors' Conference.* November 19-21, Proceedings Report. Chicago: Athletic Institute.

Atkinson, J. and Braddick, O. (1982). "Sensory and Perception Capacities of the Neonate." In Stratton, P. (ed.). *Psychobiology of the Human Newborn.* New York: Wiley.

—B—

Bailey, D. A. et al. (1978). "Size Dissociation of Maximal Aerobic Power During Growth in Boys." In Borms, J. and Hebbelinck, M. (eds.). *Medicine and Sport Science Series, Pediatric Work Psysiology.* Basel, Belgium: S. Karger.

Bailey, D. A. and Burton, E. C. (1982). *The Dynamic Self: Activities to Enhance Infant Development.* St. Louis: Mosby.

Bain, L. (1978). "Status of Curriculum Theory in Physical Education." *Journal of Physical Education and Recreation,* 49, 25.

Bandura, A. (1982). "Self Efficacy: Toward a Unifying Theory of Behavioral Change." In Rosenberg, M., and Kaplan, H. B. (eds.). *Social Psychology of the Self-Concept.* Arlington Heights, IL: Harlan Davidson.

Banks, M. (1980). "The Development of Visual Accommodation During Early Infancy." *Child Development.*

Barness, L. W. (1975). "Nutrition for the Low Birth Weight Infant." *Clinical Perinatology,* 2, 345-352.

Bar-Or, O. (1983). *Pediatric Sports Medicine for the Practitioner.* New York: Springer-Verlag.

Bar-Or, O. (1987). " A Commentary to Children and Fitness: A Public Health Perspective." *Research Quarterly for Exercise and Sport,* 58, 4, 304-307.

Bar-Or, O. (Ed.) (1989). *Advances in Pediatric Sport Sciences (Volume 3: Biological Issues).* Champaign, IL: Human Kinetics.

Barrow, H. M. and McGee, R. (1979). *A Practical Approach to Measurement in Physical Education.* Philadelphia: Lea and Febiger.

Barsch, R. (1965). *Achieving Perceptual-motor Efficiency.* Seattle: Special Child Publications.

Bayley, N. (1935). "The Development of Motor Abilities During the First Three Years." *Monograph of the Society for Research on Child Development,* 1, 1-26.

Bayley, N. (1954). "Some Increasing Parent-Child Similarities During the Growth of Children." *Journal of Educational Psychology,* 45, 1-21.

Bayley, N. (1969). *Manual for the Bayley Scales of Infant Development.* New York: Psychological Corporation.

Bee, H. (1985). *The Developing Child.* New York: Harper & Row.

Behar, M. (1968). "Prevalence of Malnutrition Among Preschool Children." In Scrimshaw, N.S. and Gordon, J. E. (eds.). *Malnutrition, Learning and Behavior.* Cambridge, MA: MIT Press.

Bench, J. et al. (1972). "A Comparison Between the Neonatal Sound-Evoking Startle Response and the Head-Drop (Moro) Reflex." *Developmental Medicine and Child Neurology.* 14, 308-314.

Bergel, R. (1978). "Motor Performance and Physical Growth Components of Headstart and Non-Headstart Pre-School Children." In *Symposium Papers,* 1, 53-56. AAHPERD Research Consortium: Reston, VA.

Bernard, J. and Sontag, L. W. (1947). "Fetal Reactivity to Tonal Stimulation: A Preliminary Report." *Journal of Genetic Psychology,* 70, 205-210.

Bernuth, G. A. et al. (1985). "Age, Exercise, and the Endocrine System." In Fotherby, K. and Pal, S. B. (eds.), *Exercise Endocrinology.* New York: Walter de Gruyter.

Beumen, G. et al. (1980). "Learning Effects of Repeated Measure Designs." In Berg, K. and Erickson, B. (eds.), *Children and Exercise IX.* Baltimore: University Park Press.

Birch, H. G. and Gussow, J. D. (1970). *Disadvantaged Children.* New York: Harcourt, Brace & World.

Blatt, G. T., and Cunningham, J. (1981). *It's Your Move: Expressive Movement Activities for the Language Arts Class.* New York: Teachers College Press.

Bloom, B. S. (1985). *Developing Talent in Young People.* New York: Ballentine Books.

Bloom, B. S. et al (1956). *Taxonomy of Educational Objectives: Handbook I: Cognitive Domain.* New York: David McKay.

Bolby, J. (1958). "The Nature of the Child's Tie to His Mother." *International Journal of Psychoanalysis,* 39, 350-373.

Bonds, D. R. and Delivoria-Papadopoulos, M. (1985). "Exercise During Pregnancy-Potential Fetal and Placental Metabolic Effects." *Annals of Clinical and Laboratory Science,* 15, 29-99.

Bonica, J. J. (1967). *Principles and Practices of Obstetric Analgesia and Anesthesia.* Philadelphia: F. A. Davis.

Bornstein, M. H. et al. (1976). "The Categories of Hue in Infancy." *Science,* 191, 201-202.

Bornstein, M. H. (1976). "Infants are Trichomats." *Journal of Experimental Child Psychology,* 21, 421-445.

Bouchard, C. (1985). "Reproducibility of Body-Composition and Adipose-Tissue Measurements in Humans." In *Body-Composition Assessment in Youths and Adults.* Report of the Sixth Ross Conference on Medical Research. Columbus, OH: Ross Laboratories.

Bower, T. G. R. (1966). "The Visual World of Infants," *Scientific American,* 215, 80-97.

Bower, T. G. R. (1976). *Development in Infancy.* San Francisco: W. H. Freeman.

Bower, T. G. R. (1976). "Repetitive Processes in Child Developmnt." *Scientific American*, 225, 38-47.

Bower, T. G. R. (1977). *The Perceptual World of the Child*. Cambridge, MA: Harvard University Press.

Bower, T. G. R. et al. (1970). "Demonstration of Intention in the Reaching Behavior of Neonate Humans." *Nature*, 228-234.

Brackbill, Y. (1970). "Continuous Stimulation and Arousal Level in Infants: Additive Effects." *Proceedings, 78th Annual Convention, American Psychological Association*, 5, 271-272.

Brackbill, Y. (1979). "Obstetrical Medication and Infant Behavior." In Osofsky, J. D. (ed.), *The Handbook of Infant Development*. New York: Wiley.

Brain, D. J. and Moslay, I. (1968). "Controlled Study of Mothers and Children in Hospital." *British Medical Journal*, 278-280.

Branta, C. et al. (1987). "Gender Differences in Play Patterns and Sport Participation of North American Youth." In Gould, D. and Weiss M. R. *Advances in Pediatric Sport Sciences* (Volume 2, Behavioral Issues). Champaign, IL: Human Kinetics.

Brazelton, T. B. (1973). *Neonatal Behavior Assessment Scale, Clinics in Developmental Medicine, No. 50* Philadelphia: Lippincott.

Brazelton, T. B. et al. (1979). "Specific Neonatal Measures: The Brazelton Neonatal Behavior Assessment Scale." In Osofsky, J. D. (ed.), *The Handbook of Infant Development*. New York: Wiley.

Bredekamp, S. Ed. (1987). *Developmentally Appropriate Practice In Early Childhood Programs Serving Children From Birth Through Age 8*. Washington, D.C.: National Association for the Education of Young Children.

Bredemeier, B. J. and Shields, D. L. (1987). "Moral Growth Through Physical Activity: A structural/Developmental Approach." In Gould, D. and Weiss, (eds.), M. R. *Advances in Pediatric Sport Sciences* (Volume 2, Behavioral issues). Champaign, IL: Human Kinetics.

Bril, B. (1985). "Motor Development and Cultural Attitudes." In Whiting, H. T. A. and Wade, M. G. (eds.) *Themes in Motor Development*. Dordrecht: The Netherlands: Martinus Nyhoff Publishers.

Broadhead, G. D. (1981). "Motor Performance Assessment in a Special Education Context." Paper presented in the Motor Development Academy at the AAHPERD Convention. Boston, April 13.

Broer, M. (1973). *Efficiency in Human Movement*. Philadelphia: W. B. Saunders.

Broer, M. R. and Zernicke, R. F. (1979). *Efficiency of Human Movement*. Philadelphia: W. B. Saunders.

Brookover, W. B. et al. (1967). *Self Concept of Ability and School Achievement*. U.S. Office of Education, Cooperative Research Project, No. 2831. East Lansing: Michigan State University.

Brown, C. H. et al. (1972). "The Effects of Cross-Country Running on Pre-Adolescent Girls. *Medicine and Science in Sports*, 4, 1-5.

Brown, E. W., and Branta, C. F. (1988). *Competitive Sports For Children and Youth: An Overview of Research and Issues*. Champaign, IL: Human Kinetics.

Brown, N. A. et al. (1979). "Ethanol Embryotoxicity: Direct Effects on Mammalian Embryos in Vitro," *Science*, 206, 573-575.

Bruch, H. (1940). "Energy Expenditure of Obese Children." *American Journal of Diseases of Children*, 60, 5.

Bruch, H. (1979). *The Golden Cage—The Enigma of Anorexia Nervosa*. New York: Vintage Books.

Bruch, H. (1986). "Anorexia Nervosa: The Therapeutic Task." In Brownell, K. D., and Foreyt, J. P. (Eds.) *Handbook of Eating Disorders*. New York: Basic Books

Bruininks, R. H. (1978). *Bruininks-Oseretsky Test of Motor Proficiency*. Cricle Pines, MN: American Guidance Service.

Bruininks, R. H. (1981). "Asssssing the Motor Performance of Children: An Overview of the Bruininks-Oseretsky Test of Motor Proficiency." Paper presented in the Motor Development Academy at the AAHPERD Convention, Boston, MA, April 13.

Bruner, J. S. (1961). "The Act of Discovery." *Harvard Educational Review*, 31, 1.

Bruner, J. S. (1965). *The Process of Education*. Cambridge, MA: Harvard University Press.

Bruner, J.S. (1969). "Processes of Growth in Infancy." In Ambrose, A. (ed.), *Stimulation in Early Infancy*, New York: Academic Press.

Bruya, L. (Ed.) (1988). *Play Spaces for Children, Volume II: A New Beginning*. Reston, VA: AAHPERD.

Bruya, L., and Langendorfer, S. (Eds.) (1988). *Where Our Children Play; Volume I: Elementary School Playground Equipment*. Reston, VA: AAHPERD.

Burd, B. (1986). "Infant Swimming Classes: Immersed in Controversy." *The Physician and Sports Medicine*, 14, 3, 239-244.

Burnett, C. N. and Johnson, E. W. (1971). "Development of Gait in Childhood, Part II." *Developmental Medicine and Child Neurology*, 13, 207-212.

Buros, O. K. (ed.) (1971). *The Seventh Mental Measurement Yearbook*, Highland Park, NJ: Gryphon Press.

Butler, R. N. et al. (1972). "Cigarette Smoking in Pregnancy: Its Influence on Birth Weight and Prenatal Mortality." *British Medical Journal*, 2, 127-130.

—C—

Cabrera, R. (1980). "The Influence of Maternal Age Birth Order, and Socioeconomic Status on Infant Mortality." *American Journal of Public Health*, 70, 174-177.

CAHPER (1980). *Canadian Association for Health, Physical Education, and Recreation: Manitoba Physical Fitness Performance Test Manual and Fitness Objectives*, Ottawa, Canada, CAHPER.

Cain, D. J. and Broekhoff, J. (1987). "Maturity Assessment: A Viable Preventive Measure Against Physical and Psychological Insult to the Young Athlete?" *The Physician and Sportsmedicine*, 15, 3, 67-79.

Caine, D. J. and Lindner, K. (1984). "Growth Plate Injury: A Threat to Young Distance Runners?" *The Physician and Sportsmedicine*, 12, 4, 118-124.

Campbell, R. M. (1984). *The New Science: Self-Esteem Psychology*. San Diego: University Press of America.

Campos, J. J. et al. (1982). "The Emergence of Self-Produced Locomotion." In Brecker, D. D. (Ed.) *Intervention With At-Risk and Handicapped Infants*. Baltimore: University Park Press.

Caplan, F. (1981). *The First Twelve Months of Life*. New York: Bantam.

Caputo, A. J. et al. (1978). "Primitive Reflex Profile: A Pilot Study." *Physical Therapy*, 58, 1061-1065.

Caputo, D. V. and Mandell, W. (1970). "Consequences of Low Birth Weight." *Developmental Psychology*, 3, 363-383.

Carmichael, L. (1925). "Heredity and Environment: Are They Antithetical?" *Journal of Abnormal and Social Psychology*, 20, 245-260.

Carnegie Report (1987), "Preparing for Life: The Critical Transition of Adolescence." Carnegie Corporation of New York.

Carpenter, G. (1975). "Mother's Face and the Newborn." In Lewin, R. (ed.), *Child Alive*. New York: Doubleday.

Chausow, S. A. et al. (1984). "Metabolic and Cardiovascular Responses of Children During Prolonged Physical Activity." *Research Quarterly for Exercise and Sport*, 55, 1, 1-7.

Chess, S. and Thomas, A. (1973). "Temperament in the Normal Neonate." In Westman, J. C. (ed.), *Individual Difference in the Child*, New York: Wiley.

Chez, R. A. (1977). "Clinical Application of Nutrition in Perinatal Practice." In Moghiss, K. S. and Evans, T. N. (eds.). *Nutritional Impacts on Women Throughout Life With Emphasis on Reproduction*. New York: Harper & Row.

Clapp, J. F. and Dickstein, S. (1984). "Endurance Exercise and Pregnancy Outcome." *Medicine and Science in Sports and Exercise*, 16, 556-562.

Clark, J. E. and Phillips, S. J. (1985). "A Developmental Sequence of the Standing Long Jump." In Clark, J. E. and Humphrey, J. H. (eds.). *Motor Development: Current Selected Research*. Princeton, NJ: Princeton Book Co.

Clarke, D. (1974). "Predicting Certified Weight of Young Wrestlers" *Medicine and Science in Sports*, 6, 52-57.

Clark, H. H. (1971). *Physical Motor Tests in the Medbord Boys Growth Study*. Englewood Cliffs, N. J.: Prentice-Hall.

Clifford, E. and Clifford, M. (1967). "Self Concepts Before and After Survival Training." *British Journal of Social and Clinical Psychology*, 6, 241-248.

Coakley, J. (1983). "Play, Games, and Sports: Developmental Implications for Young People." In Harris, J. C. and Park, R. J., (eds.), *Play, Games, and Sports in Cultural Contexts*. Champaign, IL: Human Kinetics.

Coakley, J. J. (1987). "Children and The Sport Socialization Process." In Gould, D. and Weiss, M. R. (eds.) *Advances in Pediatric Sport Sueno*. (Volume 2, Behavioral Issues). Champaign, IL: Human Kinetics.

Cocherty, D. and Bell, R. D. (1985). "The Relationship Between Flexibility and Limb Measures in Boys and Girls 6-15 Years of Age." *Journal of Human Movement Studies*, 11, 279-288.

Cohen, G. C. et al. (1989). "Intense Exercise During the First Two Trimesters of Unapparent Pregnancy." *The Physician and Sports Medicine*, 17, 1, 87-94.

Cohen, L. B. et al. (1979). "Infant Visual Perception." In Osofsky, J. D. (ed.). *Handbook of Infant Development*. New York: Wiley.

Collings, C. A. et al. (1983). "Maternal and Fetal Responses to a Maternal Aerobic Exercise Program." *American Journal of Obstetrics and Gynecology*. 145, 6, 702-707.

Collingswood, T. B. and Willett, L. (1971). "The Effects of Physical Training Upon Self-Concept and Body Attitude." *Journal of Consulting Psychology*, 2, 411-412.

Comalli, P. E. et al. (1959). "Perception of Verticality in Middle and Old Age," *Journal of Psychology*, 47, 259-266.

Combs, A. W. and Snygg, D. (1959). *Individual Behavior*. New York: Harper & Row.

Conger, J. J. and Peterson, A. C. (1984). *Adolescence and Youth*. New York: Harper and Row.

Congressional Report (1978). "Alcohol Labeling and Fetal Alcohol Syndrome." Hearing Before the Subcommittee on Alcohol and Drug Abuse, 95-102.

Conway, E. and Brackbill, Y. (1970). "Delivery Medication and Infant Outcomes." *Monographs of the Society for Research in Child Development*, 35, 24-34.

Cooley, C. H. (1902). *Human Nature and the Social Order*. New York: Scribner.

Cooper, J. M. and Andrews, W. (1975). "Rhythm as a Linguistic Art." *Quest*, 65, 61-67.

Cooper, J. M. et al. (1982) *Kinesiology*. St. Louis: Mosby.

Cooper, K. H. (1968). *Aerobics*. New York: Bantam.

Cooper, S. (1987). "The Fetal Alcohol Syndrome." *Journal of Child Psychology and Psychiatry*, 49, 1, 223-227.

Coopersmith, S. (1967). *The Antecedents of Self-Esteem*. San Francisco: W. H. Freeman.

Coopersmith, S. (1977). "A Method of Determining Types of Self Esteem." *Journal of Abnormal and Social Psychology*, 59, 87-94.

Corbin, C. B. (ed.) (1980). *A Textbook of Motor Development*. Dubuque, IA: W. C. Brown.

Cratty, B. J. (1967). *Social Dimensions of Physical Activity*. Englewood Cliffs, NJ: Prentice-Hall.

Cratty, B. J. (1968). *Psychology and Physical Activity*. Englewood Cliffs, NJ: Prentice-Hall.

Cratty, B. J. (1972). *Physical Expressions of Intelligence*. Englewood Cliffs, NJ: Prentice-Hall.

Cratty, B. J. (1973). *Intelligence in Actions*. Englewood Cliffs, NJ: Prentice-Hall.

Cratty, B. J. (1986). *Perceptual and Motor Development in Infants and Children*. Englewood Cliffs, NJ: Prentice-Hall.

Cratty, B. J. and Martin, M. (1969). *Perceptual-Motor Efficiency in Children*. Philadelphia: Lea and Febiger.

Crawford, J. W. (1982). "Motor-Infant Interaction in Premature and Full-Term Infants." *Child Development*, 53, 957-962.

Cruishank, R. M. (1941). "The Development of Visual Size Consistence in Early Infancy." *Journal of Genetic Psychology*, 58, 327-351.

Cumming, G. R. et al. (1967). "Repeated Measurements of Aerobic Capacity During a Week of Intensive Training at a Youth's Track Camp." *Canadian Journal of Physiology and Pharmacology*, 45, 805-811.

Cumming, G. R. et al. (1969). "Failure of School Physical Education to Improve Cardiorespiratory Fitness." *Canadian Medical Association Journal*, 101, 69-73.

Cumming, G. R. and Friesen, W. (1967). Bicycle Ergometer Measurement of Maximal Oxygen Uptake in Children." *Canadian Journal of Physiology and Pharmacology*, 45, 937-946.

Cumming, G. R. and Hnatiuk, A. (1980). "Establishing of Normal Values for Exercise Capacity in a Hospital Clinic." In Berg, K. and Erickson, B. (eds.), *Children and Exercise IX*, Baltimore: Academic Press.

Cunningham, D. A. et al. (1976). "The Cardiopulmonary Capacities of Young Hockey Players—Age 10." *Medicine and Science in Sports*, 8, 23-25.

Cunningham, D. A. et al. (1977). "Reliability and Reproducibility of Maximal Oxygen Uptake Measures in Children." *Medicine and Science in Sports*, 9, 104-105.

Curry, N. (1974). "Self Concept and the Educational Experience in Physical Education." *The Physical Educator*, 31, 116-119.

Czikszentmihalyi, M. (1975). *Beyond Boredom and Anxiety*. San Francisco: Jossey-Bass.

—D—

Daniels, J. and Oldridge, N. (1971). "Changes in Oxygen Consumption of Young Boys During Growth and Training." *Medicine and Science in Sports*, 3, 161-165.

Davids, A. et al. (1961). "Anxiety, Pregnancy and Childbirth Abnormalities." *Journal of Consulting Psychology*, 25, 74-77.

Davidson, H. P. (1934). "A Study of Reversals in Children." *Journal of Genetic Psychology*, 44, 452-465.

Davies, P. and Stewart, A. L. (1975). "Low Birth-Weight Infants: Neurological Sequelae and Later Intelligence." *British Medical Bulletin*. 31, 85-91.

Daw, S. F. (1974). "Age of Boy's Puberty in Leipzig, 1727-49, as indicated by Voice Breaking in J. S. Bach's Choir Members," *Human Biology*, 46, 381-384.

Dayton, G. O. and Jones, M. H. (1964). "Analysis of Characteristics of Fixation Reflexes in Infants by Use of Direct Current Electroculography." *Neurology*, 14, 1152-1157.

Deach, D. F. (1951). "Genetic Development of Motor Skills in Children Two Through Six Years of Age." Unpublished doctoral dissertation. University of Michigan.

Dean, R. F. (1965). "Effects of Malnutrition, Especially of Slight Degree, on the Growth of Young Children. *Curier* 15, 78-83.

Delacato, C. (1959). *Treatment and Prevention of Reading Problems*. Springfield, IL: Charles C. Thomas.

Delacato, C. (1966). *Neurological Organization and Reading*. Springfield, IL: Charles C. Thomas.

Delozier, M. G., et al. (1988) "Conducting Treadmill Tests on Preschool Children." *Journal of Physical Education, Recreation and Dance*, 59, 9, 83-87.

De Myer, W. (1974). "Congenital Anomalies of the Central Nervous System." In Tower, D. B. (ed.), *The Nervous System*. New York: Raven.

Denhoff, E. (1981). "Current Status of Infant Stimulation of Enrichment Programs for Children With Developmental Disabilities," *Pediatrics*, 67, 32-36.

Dennis, W. (1935). "The Effect of Restricted Practice Upon the Reaching, Sitting, and Standing of Two Infants." *Journal of Genetic Psychology*, 47, 17-32.

Dennis, W. (1940). "Does Culture Appreciably Affect Patterns of Infant Behavior?" *Journal of Social Psychology*, 12, 307-317.

Dennis, W. (1960). "Causes of Retardation Among Institutional Children: Iran." *Journal of Genetic Psychology*, 96, 47-59.

Dennis, W. and Najarian, P. (1957). "Infant Development Under Environmental Handicap." *Psychology Monographs*, 71, 7.

De Oreo, K. L. (1971). "Dynamic and Static Balance in Preschool Children." Unpublished doctoral dissertation, University of Illinois.

De Oreo, K. L. (1977). "De Oreo Fundamental Motor Skills Inventory." Unpublished paper, Kent State University.

De Oreo, K. L. (1980). Performance of Fundamental Motor Tasks." In Corbin C. B. (ed.). *A Textbook of Motor Development*. Dubuque, IA: William C. Brown.

DeVires, J. I. P. et al. (1982). "The Emergence of Fetal Behavior In Qualitative Aspects." *Early Human Development*, 7, 301-322.

Dickstein, E. (1977). "Self and Self-Esteem: Theoretical Foundations and Their Implications for Research." *Human Development*, 20, 129-140.

Dietz, W. H. (1983). "Do We Fatten Our Children at the Television Set? Obesity and Television Viewing in Children and Adolescents." *Pediatrics*, 75:807-812.

DiNucci, J. M. (1976). "Gross Motor Performance: A Comprehensive Analysis of Age and Sex Differences Between Boys and Girls Ages Six to Nine Years." In Browkhoff, J. (ed.), *Physical Education, Sports and the Sciences*. Eugene, OR: Micorform Publications.

Documenta, G. (1970). "Scientific Tables." In Dierm, K. and Lentner, C. (eds.), *Scientific Tables*. Barie, Switzerland: Ciba-Geigy.

Doll, E. A. (1946). *The Oseretsky Tests of Motor Proficiency*. Circle Pines, MN: American Guidance Service.

Dorfan, P. W. (1977). "Timing and Anticipation: A Developmental Perspective." *Journal of Motor Behavior*, 9, 67-79.

Drillien, C. M. (1964). *Growth and Development of the Prematurely Born Infant*. Edinburgh, Scotland: Livingstone.

Drillien, C. M. (1970). "The Small-for-Dates Infant-Etiology and Prognosis." *Pediatric Clinics of North America*, 17, 9-23.

Drillien, C. M. et al. (1980). "Low Birth Weight Children at Early School Age." *Developmental Medicine and Child Neurology*, 22, 26-47.

Duda, M. (1986). "Prepubescent Strength Training Gains Support." *The Physician and Sportsmedicine*, 14, 2, 157-161.

Duke, R. M. et al. (1980). "Adolescence' Self-Assessment of Sexual Maturation." *Pediatrics*, 66, 918-920.

Dunsing, J. D. (1969). "Perceptual-Motor Factors in the Defleopment of School Measures: An Analysis of the Purdue Perceptual-Motor Survey." *American Journal of Optometry*. 46, 760-765.

—E—

Easton, T. A. (1972). "On the Normal Use of Reflexes." *American Scientist*, 60, 591-599.

Eckert, H. (1987). *Motor Development*. Indianapolis: Benchmark Press.

Eckert, H. (1973). "Age Changes in Motor Skills." In Rarick, G. L. (ed.), *Physical Activity: Human Growth and Development*. New York: Academic Press.

Eckert, H. M. and Rarick, G. L. (1975). "Stabliometer Performance of Educable Mentally Retarded and Normal Children." *Research Quarterly*, 47, 619-621.

Egan, D. F. et al. (1969). *Developmental Screening 0-5 Years*. London: Spastic International Medical Publications.

Eichenwald, H. P. and Fryer, P. C. (1969). "Nutrition and Learning." *Science*, 163, 644-648.

Eichorn, D. H. (1968). "Biology of Gestation and Infancy." *Merrill-Palmer Quarterly*, 14, 47-81.

Eichorn, D. H. (1970). "Physiological Development." In Mussen, P. H. (ed.). *Carmichael's Manual of Child Psychology*. New York: Wiley.

Eichorn, D. H. (1979). "Physical Development: Current Foci of Research." In Osofsky, J. (ed.), *The Handbook of Infant Development*. New York: Wiley.

Eisenberg, R. B. et al. (1966). "Habituation to an Acoustic Pattern as an Idea of Differences Among Neonates." *Journal of Auditory Research*, 6, 239-248.

Ekbolm, O. (1969). "Effect of Physical Training on Adolescent Boys." *Journal of Applied Physiology*, 27, 350-355.

Ellis, M. J. (1973). *Why People Play*. Englewood Cliffs, N. J.: Prentice-Hall.

Engen, T. et al. (1963). "Olfactory Responses and Adaptation in the Human Neonates." *Journal of Comparative Physiological Psychology*, 56, 73-77.

Egen, T. and Lipsett, L. P. (1965). "Decrement and Recovery of Responses of Olfactory Stimuli in the Human Neonate." *Journal of Comparative and Physiological Psychology*, 59, 312-316.

Enos, W. F. et al. (1955). "Pathogenesis of Coronary Disease of American Soldiers Killed in Korea." *Journal of the American Medical Association*, 158, 912-914.

Erdelyi, G. J. (1962). "Gynecological Survey of Female Athletes." *Journal of Sports Medicine and Physical Fitness*, 2, 174-179.

Erhartic, M. (1977). "Stability of Global Self-Concepts of Children from Three Different Elementary Schools During Their First Year in a Regionalized Junior High School." Unpublished doctoral dissertation, Boston University.

Erikson, E. (1963). *Childhood and Society*. New York: Norton.

Erikson, E. (1980). *Identity and the Life Cycle*. New York: Norton.

Eriksson, B. D. and Gunter K. (1973). "Effect of Physical Training on Hemodynamic Response During Submaximal and Maximal Exercise in 11-13 Year Old Boys." *Acta Physiologica Scandinavica*, 87, 27-39.

Erkkola, R. (1976). "The Physical Work Capacity of Expectant Mothers and Effect on Pregnancy, Labor and the Newborn." *International Journal of Gynecology and Obstetrics*, 14, 153-159.

Errecart, M. T. et al. (1987). "The National Children and Youth Fitness Study II: Sample Design." *Journal of Physical Education, Recreation and Dance*, 58-59, 63-65.

Errecart, M. T. (1985). "The National Children and Youth Fitness Study: Sampling Procedures. *Journal of Physical Education, Recreation and Dance*, 56, 1, 54-56.

Espenschade, A. S. and Eckert, H. M. (1980) *Motor Development*. Columbus, OH: Merill.

Eveleth, P. B. and Tanner, J. M. (1976). *Worldwide Variation in Human Growth*. Cambridge, MA: Cambridge University Press.

—F—

Falls, H. B. (1980). "Modern Concepts of Physical Fitness." *Journal of Health, Physical Education and Recreation*, 51, 25.

Fantz, R. L. (1963). "Pattern Vision in Newborn Infnts." *Science*, 140, 296-297.

Fantz, R. L. et al. (1975). "Early Visual Selectivity." In Cohen, L. B., and Salapatek, P. (eds.). *Infant Perception From Sensation to Cognition*. New York: Academic Press.

Felker, D. W. (1974). *Building Positive Self-Concepts*. Minneapolis, MN Burgess.

Field, J. (1976). "The Adjustment of Reaching Behavior to Object Distance in Early Infancy." *Child Development*, 47, 304-308.

Fiorentino, M. R. (1963). *Reflex Testing Methods for Evaluating C.N.S. Development*. Springfield, IL: Charles C. Thomas.

Fisch, R. O. et al. (1975). "Obesity and Leanness at Birth and Their Relation to Body Habitus in Later Childhood." *Pediatrics*, 56, 421-428.

Fishbein, H. D. (1976). *Evolution, Development, and Children's Learning*. Pacific Palisader: Goodyear.

Fitts, P. M. (1962). "Factors in Complex Skill Learning." In Glasser R. (ed.). *Training Research and Education*. Pittsburgh: University of Pittsburgh Press.

Fitts, P. M. and Posner M. I. (1967). *Human Performance*. Belmont, CA: Brooks/Cole.

Fleishman, E. A. "Toward a Taxonomy of Human Performance." *American Psychologist*, 30, 1127-1149.

Ford, E. H. T. (1973). *Human Chromosomes*. New York: Academic Press.

Fox et al. (1980). Stereopsis in Human Infants." *Science*, 207, 323-324.

Frank, L. K. (1968). "Play is Valid." *Childhood Education*, 3, 433-440.

Frankenburg, W. K. and Dodds J. B. (1967). "The Denver Developmental Screening Test." *Journal of Pediatrics*, 71, 181-191.

Frederick, S. D. (1977). "Performance of Selected Motor Tasks By Three, Four and Five Year Old Children." Unpublished doctoral dissertation, Indiana University.

Freeman, R. K. and Pescar, S. C. (1982). *Safe Delivery: Protecting Your Baby During High Risk Pregnancy*. New York: McGraw Hill.

Freud, A. (1965). *Normality and Pathology in Childhood: Assessment of Development*. New York: International Universities Press.

Freud, S. (1927). *The Ego and the Id*. New York: Norton.

Frost, R. B. (1972). "Physical Education and Self-Concept." *Journal of Physical Education*, 36.

Frostig, M. (1969). *Move Grow and Learn*. Chicago: Follett.

Frostig, M. et al. (1966). *Administration and Scoring Manual: Frostig Developmental Test of Visual Perception*. Palo Alto, CA: Consulting Psychologists Press.

—G—

Gad-Elmawla, E. K. G. (1980). "Kinematic and Kinetic Analysis of Gain in Children at Different Age Levels in Comparison with Adults." Unpublished doctoral dissertation, Indiana University.

Galambos, J. W. (1970). *Organizing Free Play*. Office of Child Development. Department of HEW.

Gallahue, D. L. (1968). "The Relationship Between Perceptual and Motor Abilities." *Research Quarterly*, 39, 948-952.

Gallahue, D. L. (1974). *Yes I Can! Movement and the Developing Self* (film strip). Bloomington, IN: Phi Delta Kappa.

Gallahue, D. L. (1979). "Movement Education: Its Place in the Elementary School Physical Education Program." *In Proceedings of the Contemporary Elementary School Physical Education Conference*. Georgia State University, Atlanta, GA.

Gallahue, D. L. (1982). *Developmental Movement Experiences for Children*. New York: Wiley.

Gallahue, D. L. (1982). "Effects of Movement and Vision on Visual-Motor Adjustment to Optical Rearrangement." *Perceptual Motor Skills*, 54, 935-942.

Gallahue, D. L. (1983). "Assessing Motor Development in Young Children." *Studies in Educational Evaluation*, 8, 247-252.

Gallahue, D. L. (1987). *Developmental Physical Education for Today's Elementary School Children*. New York: Macmillian.

Gallahue D. L. (1989). Motor Developmentalistic All? *Motor Development Academy Newsletter*, 10, 1.

Gangirly, P. (1977). "The Problem of Human Adaptation: An Overview." *Man in India*, 57, 1-22.

Gentile, A. (1972). "A Working Model of Skill Acquisition with Application to Teaching." *Quest*, 17, 3-23.

Gentile, A. M. (1981). "Developmental Aspects of Motor Learning." Paper presented at the Motor Development Academy at the AAHPERD Convention, Boston, MA.

Gerber, M., and Dean R. F. A. (1957). "Gessell Tests of African Children." *Pediatrics*, 20, 1055-1065.

Gessell, A. (1928). *Infancy and Human Growth*. New York: Macmillan.

Gessell, A. (1945). *The Embryology of Behavior*. New York: Harper.

Gesell A. et al. (1949). *The First Five Years of Life: A Study of the Preschool Child*. New York: Harper.

Gesell A. and Thompson H. (1929). "Learning and Growth in Identical Twins." *Genetic Psychology Monographs*, 6, 1-124.

Gesell A. and Thompson H. (1934). *Infant Behavior, Its Genesis and Growth*. New York: McGraw-Hill.

Getman, G. N. (1952). *How to Develop Your Child's Intelligence (a research publication)*. Lucerne, Minn: G. N. Getman.

Gibson, E. J. and Walk R. B. (1960). "The Visual Cliff." *Scientific American*, 4, 67-71.

Gilliam, T. B. (1981). "What Volunteer Coaches and Youth Sport Administrators Should Know About Training, Conditioning, and Injury Prevention." Paper presented at the Second Annual Youth Sports Forum, Youth Sports Institute, Michigan State University, April 27.

Gilliam, T. B. et al. (1981). "Physical Activity Patterns Determined by Heart Rate Monitoring in 6-7 Year-Old Children." *Medicine and Science in Sports and Exercise*, 131, 65-67.

Gilliam, T. B. and Macconnie, S. E. (1984). "Coronary Heart Disease Risk in Children and Their Physical Activity Patterns." In Boileau, R. A. (ed.) *Advances in Pediatric Sport Sciences: Volume One, Biological Issues*. Champaign, IL: Human Kinetics.

Gillion, B. C. (1970). *Basic Movement Education for Children: Rationale and Teaching Units*. Reading, MA: Addison-Wesley.

Glassow, R. L. and Kruse, P. (1960). "Motor Performance of Girls Age 6-14 Years." *Research Quarterly*, 31, 426-431.

Goetzinger, C. P. (1961). "Re-evaluation of Heath Rail Walking 1951 to 1967." *Journal of Education Research*, 54, 187-191.

Goldstein, K. M. et al. (1976). "The Effects of Prenatal and Perinatal Complications on Development at One Year of Age." *Child Development*, 47, 613-621.

Gordon, R. L. (1981). "A Neurological Paradigm: An Analysis of Swimming and Walking Acquisition." Unpublished paper, School of HPER, Ohio State University.

Gortmaker, S. L. et al. (1987). Increasing Pediatric Obesity in the U.S." *American Journal of Diseases in Children*, 14, 1, 535-540.

Gortmarker, S. L. et al. (1987). "Increasing Pediatric Obesity in the U.S. *American Journal of Diseases of Children*, 14, 1, 535-540.

Gould, D. (1987). "Understanding Attrition in Children's Sports." In Gould, D., and Weiss, M. R. (eds.) *Advances in Pediatric Sport Sciences*: (Volume II, Behavioral Issues). Champaign, IL: Human Kinetics.

Graham, G. et al. (1987). *Children Moving: A Reflective Approach*. Mountain View, CA: Mayfield.

Greendorfer, S. L. (1987). "Psycho-Social Correlates of Organized Physical Activity." *Journal of Physical Education, Recreation and Dance*, 58, 69-64.

Greendorfer, S. L. (1977). "Role of Socializing Agents in Female Sport Involvement." *Research Quarterly*, 48, 304-310.

Greendorfer, S. L. and Lewko, J. H. (1978). "Role of Family Members in Sport Socialization of Children." *Research Quarterly*, 49, 149-152.

Greenspan, E. (1983). *Little Winners: Inside the World of the Childs Sports Star*. Boston: Little Brown.

Greulich, W. W. and Pyle, S. I. (1959). *Radiographic Atlas of Skeletal Development of the Hand and Wrist*. Stanford, CA: Stanford University Press.

Grieve, D. W. and Gaer, R. J. (1966). "The Relationship Between the Length of Stride, Step, Frequency, Time of Swing and Speed of Walking for Children and Adults." *Ergonomics*, 9, 379-399.

Groves, D. (1988). "Is Childhood Obesity Related to TV Addiction?" *The Physician and Sports Medicine*, 16, 11, 117-122.

Gumbs, V. L. et al. (1982). "Bilateral Distal Radius and Ulnar Fractures in Adolescent Weight Lifters." *The American Journal of Sports Medicine*, 10, 375-379.

Gustafson, J. (1978). "Teaching for Self-Esteem." The Physical Educator, 35, 67-70.

Guttridge, M. (1939). "A Study of Motor Achievements of Young Children." *Archives of Psychology*, 244, 1-178.

—H—

Haase, R. (1968). *Designing the Child Development Center.* U. S. Office of Education, Project Head Start, Washington, D.C.: U.S. Government Printing Office.

Hagberg, B. M. (1975). "Pre-, Peri-, and Postnatal Prevention of Major Neuropediatric Handicaps." *Neuropaediatrics,* 6, 331-338.

Hagstrom, J. and Morrill, J. (1979). *Games Babies Play.* New York: A & W Visual Library.

Haith, M. M. (1966). "The Response of the Human Newborn to Visual Movement." *Journal of Experiemental Child Psychology,* 3, 235-243.

Haith, M. M. (1980). *Rules That Babies Look By.* Hillsdale, NJ: Erlbaum.

Halverson, H. M. (1937). "Studies of the Grasping Responses in Early Infancy." *Journal of Genetic Psychology,* 51, 437-449.

Halverson, H. M. et al. (1931). "An Environmental Study of Prehension in Infants by Means of Systematic Cinema Records." *Genetic Psychology Monographs,* 10, 107-186.

Halverson, L. (1980). "The Motor Development Academy." *Journal of Physical Education and Recreation,* 51, 38.

Halverson, L. (1966). "Development of Motor Patterns in Young Children." *Quest,* 6, 44-53.

Halverson, L. E. and Robertson, M. A. (1966). "A Study of Motor Pattern Development in Young Children." Paper presented at the AAHPER Conference, Chicago.

Halverson, L. E. and Roberton, M. A. (1979). *Motor Development Laboratory Manual.* Madison, WI: American Printing and Publishing.

Halverson, L. E., and Williams, K. (1985). "Developmental Sequences For Hopping Over Distance: A Prelongitudinal Study." *Research Quarterly for Exercise and Sport,* 56, 37-44.

Harbison, R. D., and Mantilla-Plata, B. (1972). "Prenatal Toxicity, Maternal Distribution and Placental Transfer of Telralydrocan-Malinol." *Journal of Pharmacology Experimental Therapeutics,* 180, 446-453.

Harrow, A. J. (1971). *A Taxonomy of the Psychomotor Domain.* New York: David McKay.

Harter, S. (1978). "Effectance Motivation Reconsidered: Toward a Developmental Model." *Human Development,* 21, 34-64.

Harter, S. (1981). The Development of Competence Motivation in the Mastry of Cognitive and Physical Skills: Is There Still a Place for Joy?" In Roberts, G. C. and Landers, D. M. (eds.), *Psychology of Motor Behavior and Sport.* Champaign, IL: Human Kinetics.

Harter, S. (1982). "Development Perspectives on Self-Esteem." In Hetherinton, E. M. (ed.), *Handbook of Child Psychology, Volume IV: Socialization, Personality, and Social Developments.* New York: Wiley.

Harter, S. (1982). "The Perceived Competence Scale for Children." *Child Development,* 53, 87-97.

Harter, S., and Connell, J. P. (1984). "A Model of the Relationship Among Children's Academic Achievement and Children's Perceptions of Competence, Control, and Motivational Orientation." In Nicholls, J. (ed.), *The Development of Achievement-Related Cognitions and Behaviors.* Greenwich, CT: J. A. I. Press.

Harter, S. and Pike, R. (1984). "The Pictoral Scale of Perceived Competence and Social Acceptance for Young Children." *Child Development,* 55, 1967-1982.

Hasselmeyer, E. G. (1964). "The Premature Neonates' Response to Handling." *American Nurses Association,* 11, 15-24.

Haubenstricker, J. (1978). "A Critical Review of Selected Perceptual-Motor Tests and Scales Currently Used in the Assessment of Motor Behavior." In Landers, D. M. and Christina, R. W. (eds.), *Psychology in Motor Behavior and Sport — 1977.* Champaign, IL: Human Kinetics.

Haubenstricker, J. Inter-Rater Reliability of the Developmental Sequences of Fundamental Motor Skills, Personal Communication, October, 1980.

Haubenstricker, J. et al. (1981). "The Efficiency of the Bruininks-Oseretsky Test of Motor Proficiency in Discriminating Between Normal Children and Those with Gross Motor Dysfunction." Paper presented at the Motor Development Academy at the AAPERD Convention, Boston, MA, April 13.

Haubenstricker, J. et al. (1983). "Preliminary Validation of Developmental Sequences of Throwing and Catching." Paper presented at the annual meeting of the North American Society for the Psychology of Sport and Physical Activity, May, East Lansing, MI.

Haubenstricker, J. and Seefeldt, V. (1986). "Acquisition of Motor Skills During Childhood." In Seefeldt, V. (ed.) *Physical Activity and Well-Being.* Reston, VA: AAHPERD.

Havighurst, R. (1952). *Developmental Tasks and Education.* New York: David McKay.

Havighurst, R. (1953). *Human Development and Education.* New York: Longmans Green.

Havighurst, R. (1972). *Developmental Tasks and Education.* New York: David McKay.

Havighurst, R., and Levine, R. (1979). *Society and Education.* Reading, MA: Allyn and Bacon.

Hayes, H. et al. (1965). "Visual Accommodation in Human Infants." *Science,* 148, 525-530.

Heald, F. P. and Hung, W. (eds.). (1970). *Adolescent Endocrinology.* Englewood Cliffs, NJ: Appleton-Century-Crofts.

Heath, S. R. (1949). "The Railwalking Test: Preliminary Motivational Norm for Boys and Girls." *Motor Skills Research Exchange,* 1, 34.

Hebb, D. O. (1949). *The Organization of Behavior*. New York: Wiley.

Heidelise, A. et al. (1979). "Specific Neonatal Measures: The Brazelton Neonatal Behavior Assessment Scale." In Osofsky, J. D. (ed.), *The Handbook of Infant Development*. New York: Wiley.

Hejna, W. F. (1982). "Prevention of Sport Injuries in High School Students Through Strength Training." *NSCA Journal*, 4, 1, 28-31.

Held, R. (1965). "Plasticity of Sensory-Motor Systems." *Scientific American*, 213, 84-94.

Held, R. and Blossom, J. (1961). "Neonatal Deprivation and Adult Rearrangement: Complementary Techniques for Analyzing Plastic Sensory-Motor Coordinations." *Journal of Comparative Physiological Psychology*, 54, 33-37.

Held, R. and Hein, A. (1963). "Movement-Produced Stimulation in the Development of Visually Guided Behavior." *Journal of Comparative Physiological Psychology*, 56, 872-876.

Held, R., and Mikaelian, H. (1964). "Motor Sensory Feedback Versus Need in Adaptation to Rearrangement." *Perceptual Motor Skills*, 18, 685-688.

Hellebrandt, F. et al. (1961). "Physiological Analysis of Basic Motor Skills." *American Journal of Physical Medicine*, 40, 14-25.

Henderson, A. (1982). "Problems in the Assessment of Change in Abnormal Reflex Behavior." In Brecker, D. D. (ed.) *Intervention With At-Risk and Handicapped Infants*. Baltimore: University Park Press.

Henry, F. M. (1960). "Influence of Motor and Sensory Sets: Reaction Latency, and Speed of Discrete Movement." *Research Quarterly*, 31, 459-468.

Henry, F. M. and Rogers, D. (1960). "Increased Response Latency for Complicated Movements and a Memory Drum Theory of Neuromotor Reaction." *Research Quarterly*, 31, 448-468.

Hepner, R. (1958). "Maternal Malnutrition and the Fetus." *Journal of the American Medical Association*, 169, 1774-1777.

Herkowitz, J. (1978). "Assessing the Motor Development of Children: Presentation and Critique of Tests." In Ridenour, M. V. (ed.) *Motor Development: Issues and Applications*. Princeton, NJ: Princeton Book Company.

Herkowitz, J. (1978). "Instruments Which Assess the Efficiency/Maturity of Children's Motor Pattern Performance." In Landers, D. L. and Christina, R. W. (eds.), *Psychology in Motor Behavior and Sport — 1977*. Champaign, IL: Human Kinetics.

Hershenson, M. (1964). "Visual Discrimination in the Human Newborn." *Journal of Comparative Physiological Psychology*, 158, 270-276.

Hess, E. H. (1959). "Imprinting." *Science*, 130, 133-141.

Hicks-Hughes, D. and Langendorfer, S. (1986). "Aquatics for the Young Child: A Survey of Selected programs." *National Aquatics Journal*, 2, 2, 12-17.

Hilgard, J. R. (1932). "Learning and Maturation in Preschool Children." *Journal of Genetic Psychology*, 41, 36-56.

Hockey, R. V. (1981). *Physical Fitness*. St. Louis: Mosby.

Hoepner, B. J. (1967). "Comparison of Motor Ability, New Motor Skill Learning and Adjustment to a Rearranged Visual Field." *Research Quarterly*, 38, 605-614.

Holle, B. (1977). *Motor Development in Children: Normal and Retarded*. St. Louis: Blackwell Scientific Publications.

Holt, J. (1970). *What Do I Do Monday?* New York: Dutton.

Holt/Hale, S. A. (1988). *On the Move*. Mountain View, CA: Mayfield.

Hooker, D. (1952). *The Prenatal Origin of Behavior*. Lawrence, KA: University of Kansas Press.

Horowitz, F. D. (1968). "Infant Learning and Development: Retrospect and Prospect." *Merrill-Palmer Quarterly*, 14, 101-120.

Horowitz, F. D., and Brazelton, T. B. (1973). "Research with the Brazelton Neonatal Scale." In Brazelton, T. (ed.), *Neonatal Behavioral Assessment Scale*. Philadelphia, Lippincott.

Houston, K. B. (1969). "Review of the Evidence and Qualifications Regarding the Effects of Hallucinogenic Drugs on Chromosomes and Embryos." *American Journal of Psychiatry*, 126, 251-254.

Hoyt, L. (1981). "Effects of Marijuana on Fetal Development." *Journal of Drug Education*, 12, 113-123.

Humphrey, J. (1974). *Child Learning*. Dubuque, Iowa: W. C. Brown.

Hunsicker, P. and Reiff, G. (1977). "Youth Fitness Report, 1958—1965—1975." *Journal of Physical Education and Recreation*, 48, 32.

Hupperich, F. L. and Sigerseth, P. (1950). "The Specificity of Flexibility in Girls." *Research Quarterly*, 21, 25-33.

—I/J—

Isaacs, L. D. (1980). "Effects of Ball Size, Ball Color, and Preferred Color on Catching By Young Children." *Perceptual and Motor Skills*, 51, 583-586.

James, W. (1880/1963). *Psychology*. New York: Fawcett.

Jeannerod, M. (1986). "The Formation of the Finger Grip During Prehension A Cortually-Mediated

Visuo-Motor Pattern." In Whiting, H. T. A. and Wade, M. G. (eds). *Themes in Motor Development.* Dordrecht, The Netherlands: Martinus Nijhoff.

Jeffrey, W. E. (1966). "Discrimination of Oblique Lines by Children." *Journal of Comparative Physiological Psychology*, 62, 154-156.

Johnson, L. (1969). "Effects of 5-Day-A-Week Vs. 2- and 3-Day-A-Week Physical Education Classes on Fitness, Skill, Adipose Tissue, and Growth." *Research Quarterly*, 40, 93.

Johnson, M. L. et al. (1956). "Relative Importance of Inactivity and Overeating in the Energy Balance of Obese High School Girls." *American Journal of Clinical Nutrition*, 4, 37.

Johnson, R. (1962). "Measurement of Achievement in Fundamental Skills of Elementary School Children." *Research Quarterly*, 33, 94-103.

Johnson, W. R. et al. (1968). "Changes in Self Concept During a Physical Education Program." *Research Quarterly*, 39, 560-565.

Jones, H. E. (1949). *Motor Performance and Growth.* Berkeley: University of California Press.

Jones, O. H. (1976). "Caesarean Section in Present-Day Obstetrics." *American Journal of Obstetrics and Gynecology*, 126, 521-530.

Joslin, E. P. et al. (1952). *Treatment of Diabetes Mellitus.* Philadelphia: Lea and Febiger.

—K—

Kallen, D. J. (ed.) (1973). "Nutrition, Development, and ocial Behavior." *HEW Publication No. (NIH) 73-242*, Washington, DC: U. S. Government Printing Office.

Kallen, W. B. and Sorlie, P. (1979). "Some Health Benefits of Physical Activity: The Framingham Study." *Archives of Internal Medicine*, 139, 857-861.

Karpovitch, P. V. (1937). "Textbook Fallacies Regarding the Development of the Child's Heart." *Research Quarterly*, 8, 33-37.

Katch, F. I. (1985). "Assessment of Lean Body Tissues by Radiography and by Bioelectrical Impedance." In *Body-Composition Assessments in Youth and Adults.* Report of the Sixth Ross Conference on Medical Research. Columbus, OH: Ross Laboratories.

Katchadourian, H. (1977). *The Biology of Adolescence.* San Francisco: W. H. Freeman.

Kaufman, D. A. (1975). "Fundamentals of Fat." *The Physical Educator*, 32, 77-79.

Kavale, K. and Mattson, P. D. (1983). One Jumped Off the Balance Beam: Meta-Analysis of Perceptual-Motor Training. *Journal of Learning Disabilities*, 16, 165-73.

Kellman, H. C. (1958). Compliance, Identification, and Internalization: Three Processes of Attitude Change." *Journal of Conflict Resolution*, 2, 51-60.

Kemper, H. C. G., et al. (1978). "Investigation into the Effects of Two Extra Physical Education Lessons per Week During One School Year Upon Physical Development of 12- and 13-Year-Old Boys." In Borms, J. and Habbelinck, M. (eds.), *Medicine and Sport Science Series. Vol. II, Pediatric Work Physiology,* Basel, Belgium: S. Karger.

Kennell, J. H. et al. (1974). "Maternal Behavior One Year After Early and Extended Post-Partum Contact." *Developmental Medicine and Child Neurology*, 16, 172-179.

Kennell, J. H. et al. (1979). "Parent-Infant Bonding." In Osofsky, J. D. (ed.), *The Handbook of Infant Development.* New York: Wiley.

Kenyon, G. S. (1968). "Six Scales for Assessing Attitude Toward Physical Activity." *Research Quarterly*, 39, 566-574.

Keogh, J. F. (1965). *Motor Performance of Elementary School Children.* Los Angeles: University of California, Physical Education Department.

Keough, J. and Sugden, D. (1985). *Movement Skill Development.* New York: Macmillian.

Kephart, N. C. (1971). *The Slow Learner in the Classroom.* Columbus, OH: Merrill.

Kessen, W. et al. (1970). "Human Infancy: A Bibliography and Guide." In Mussen, P. H. (ed.), *Manual of Child Psychology.* New York: Wiley.

Kessen, W. et al. (1972). "The Visual Response of the Human Newborn to Linear Contour." *Journal of Experimental Child Psychology*, 13, 9-20.

Klopper, P. et al. (1964). "Maternal Imprinting in Goats." *Proceedings of the National Academy of Science*, 52, 911.

Knuttgen, H. G. (1967). "Aerobic Capacity of Adolescents." *Journal of Applied Physiology*, 22, 655-658.

Kohlberg, L. (1981). *The Philosophy of Moral Development: Moral Stages and the Idea of Justice.* San Francisco: Harper & Row.

Kohlberg, L. (1984). *Essays of Moral Development: Vol. 2. The Psychology of Moral Development.* San Francisco: Harper & Row.

Kopp, C. B. (1982). "The Role of Theoretical Frameworks in the Study of At-Risk and Handicapped Young Children." In Bricker, D. D. (ed.) *Intervention with At-Risk and Handicapped Infants.* Baltimore: University Park Press.

Kopp, C. B. and Parmelee, A. H. (1979). "Prenatal and Perinatal Influence on Infant Behavior." In Osofsky, J. D. (ed.), *The Handbook of Infant Development.* New York: Wiley.

Korner, A. F. (1981). "What We Don't Know About Waterbeds and Apnesis Preterm Infants." *Pediatrics,* 68-306.

Korner, A. F. et al. (1975). "Effects of Waterbed Flotation on Premature Infants: A Pilot Study." *Pediatrics,* 56, 361-367.

Korner, A. F. et al. (1982). "Effects of Waterbeds on the Sleep and Motility of the Theophyeline Treated Preterm Infants." *Pediatrics,* 70, 864-869.

Kraft, R. E. (1978). "Can the Movement Specialist Really Influence Self-Concept?" *The Physical Educator,* 35, 20-21.

Krahenbuhl, G. S., et al. (1977). "Field Estimate of VO2 Max in Children Eight Years of Age." *Medicine and Science in Sports,* 9, 37-40.

Krahenbuhl, G. S. et al. (1985). "Developmental Aspects of Maximal Aerobic Power in Children." In Terjung, R. L. (ed.) *Exercise Science and Sport Research.* New York: Macmillian.

Krathwohl, D. R., Bloom, B. and Masia, B. (1964). *Taxonomy of Educational Objectives, Handbook II: Affective Domain.* New York: David McKay.

Kraus, H., and Hirschlan, R. P. (1954). "Minimum Muscular Fitness Tests in Children." *Research Quarterly,* 25, 178.

Kreig, K. (1978). "Tonic Covergence and Facial Growth in Early Infancy." Unpublished Senior Honors Thesis, Indiana University.

Kreipe, R. E. and Gewanter, H. L. (1983). "Physical Maturity Screening For Participation in Sports." *Pediatrics,* 75, 1076-1080.

Krogman, W. M. (1980). *Child Growth,* Ann Arbor: University of Michigan Press.

Kuoppasalmi, K., and Aldecrevtz, H. (1985). "Interaction Between Catabolic and Anabolic Steroid Hormones in Muscular Exercise." In Fotherby, K., and Pas, S. B. (eds.), *Exercise Endocrinology.* New York: Walter de Gruyter.

—L—

Laban, R. and Lawrence, F. (1947). *Effort.* London: Unwin Brothers.

Lamaze, F. (1970). *Painless Childbirth - The Lamaze Method.* Chicago: Regency.

Lamb, M. E. et al. (1985). *Infant - Mother Attachment.* Hillsdale, NJ: Lawrence Erilbaum Associates.

Landreth, C. (1958). *The Psychology of Early Childhood.* New York: Knoph.

Langendorfer, S. (1987). "Separating Fact From Fiction in Preschool Aquatics." *National Aquatics Journal,* 3, 1, 2-4.

Langendorfer, S. (1988). "Goal of a Motor Task as a Constraint on Developmental Status." In Clark, J., and Humphrey, J. (eds.). *Advances in Motor Development Research.* New York: AMS Press.

Langer, J. (1970). "Werners' Comparative Organismic Theory." In Mussem, P. H. (ed.), *Manual of Child Psychology.* New York: Wiley.

Larson, R. L. (1973). "Physical Activity and the Growth and Development of Bone Structure." In Rarick, G. L. (ed.), *Physical Activity: Human Growth and Development.* New York: Academic Press.

Lawther, J. D. (1977). *The Learning and Performance of Physical Skills.* Englewood Cliffs, NJ.: Prentice-Hall.

Le Boyer, R. (1975). *Birth Without Violence.* New York: Knopf.

Lecky, P. (1945). *Self Consistency: A Theory of Personality.* New York: Island.

Leeper, S. et al. (1974). *Good Schools for Young Children.* New York: Macmillan.

Legwold, G. (1982). "Does Lifting Weights Harm a Prepubescent Athlete?" *The Physician and Sportsmedicine,* 10, 7, 141-144.

Legwold, G. (1983). "Preadolescents Show Dramatic Strength Gains." *The Physician and Sportsmedicine,* 11, 10, 25.

Leifer, A. et al. (1972). "Effects of Mother-Infant Separation on Maternal Attachment Behavior." *Child Development,* 43, 1203-1218.

Leighton, J. R. (1956). "Flexibility Characteristics of Males Ten to Eighteen Years of Age." *Archives of Physical Medicine and Rehabilitation,* 37, 494-499, 1956.

Leonard, E. et al. (1980). "Nutritive Sucking in High Risk Neonates After Perioral Stimulation." *Physical Therapy,* 60, 299-302.

Lerner, P. M. (1986). *Concepts and Theories of Human Development.* Reading, MA: Addison-Wesley.

Leuko, J. H. and Greendorfer, S. L. (1978). "Famiy Influence and Sex Differences in Children's Socialization into Sport: A Review." In Landers, D. M. and Christina, R. W. (eds.), *Psychology of Motor Behavior and Sport—1977.* Champaign, IL. Human Kinetics.

Levanthal, A. and Lipsett, L. P. (1964). "Adaption, Pitch Discrimination and Sound Vocalization in the Neonate." *Child Development,* 37, 331-346.

Lewis, B. J. and Cherrington, D. (1984). "Movement Education With Young Children." In Fontana, D. (Ed.) *The Education of the Young Child.* New York: Basil Blackwell.

Lewis, M. J. et al. (1966). "Pattern of Fixation in the Young Infant." *Child Development*, 37, 331-346.

Lipsett, L. P. et al. (1963). "Developmental Changes in the Olfactory Threshold of the Neonate." *Child Development*, 34, 371-376.

Lipton, E. L. et al. (1961). "Autonomic Function in the Neonate." *Psychosomatic Medicine*, 23, 472-484.

Litch, S. (1978). *Towards Prevention of Mental Retardation in the Next Generation.* Fort Wayne, IN: Fort Wayne Printing.

Lockhart, A. (1964). "What's in a Name?" *Quest*, 2, 9-13.

Logsdon, B. J. et al. (1984). *Physical Education for Children, A Focus on the Teaching Process.* Philadelphia: Lea and Febiger.

Lohman, T. G. (1986). "Applicability of Body Composition Techniques and Constants for Children and Youth." *Exercise and Sports Sciences Review*, 14, 325-357.

Lohman, T. G. (1987). "The Use of Skinfold To Estimate Body Fatness on Children and Youth." *Journal of Physical Education, Recreation and Dance*, 59, 9, 98-102.

Loovis, E. M. and Ersing, W. F. (1979). *Assessing and Programming Gross Motor Development for Children.* Lexington, KY: Wallace's.

Lorenz, K. (1952). King Solomon's Ring. New York: Crowell.

Lotgering, F. K. et al. (1984). "The Interactions of Exercise and Pregnancy: A Review." *American Journal of Obstetrics and Gynecology*, 149, 5: 560-568.

Lotgering, F. et al. (1985). "Maternal and Fetal Responses To Exercise During Pregnancy." *Physiological Reviews*, 65, 1:1-36.

Lubchenco, L. O. et al. (1963). "Sequalae of Premature Birth." *American Journal of Disease of Children*, 106, 101-115.

Luedke, G. C. (1980). "Range of Motion as the Focus of Teaching the Overhand Throwing Pattern to Children." Unpublished doctoral dissertation, Indiana University.

Lugo, J. O. and Hershey, G. L. (1974). *Human Development, a Multi-Disciplinary Approach to the Psychology of Individual Growth.* New York: Macmillan.

Luke, M., and Warrell, E. (Eds.) (1986). *Looking at Movement: Physical Education in Early Childhood.* Burnaby, British Columbia: Simon Fraser University Publications.

Lustick, M. J. (1985). "Bulimia in Adolescents: A Review." Pediatrics, 75, 685-690.

—M—

Macek, M., and Vavra, J. (1971). "Cardiopulmonary and Metabolic Changes During Exercise in Children." *Journal of Applied Physiology*, 30, 200-204.

Magill, R. A. (1982). "Critical Periods: Relation to Youth Sport." In Magill, R. A., et al. (eds.). *Children in Sport.* Champaign, IL: Human Kinetics.

Magill, R. A. (1989). *Motor Learning—Concepts and Applications.* Dubuque, IA: Wm. C. Brown.

Maier, H. W. (1978). *Three Theories of Child Development.* New York: Harper.

Malina, R. M. (1975). *Growth and Development: The First Twenty Years.* Minneapolis, MN: Burgess.

Malina, R. M. (1978). "Secular Changes in Growth and Performance." In Hutton, R. S. (ed.). *Exercise and Sport Science Reviews*, 6, 206-255.

Malina, R. M. (1980). "Environmentally Related Correlates of Motor Development and Performance During Infancy and Childhood." In Corbin, C. (ed.). *A Textbook of Motor Development.* Dubuque, IA: W. C. Brown.

Malina, R. M. (1984). "Human Growth, Maturation and Regular Physical Activity." In Boileau, R. A. (ed.). *Advances in Pediatric Sport Sciences.* Champaign, IL: Human Kinetics.

Malina, R. M. (1986). "Physical Growth and Maturation." In Seefeldt, V. *Physical Activity and Well-Being.* Reston, VA: ASHPERD.

March of Dimes Birth Defects Foundation. (1984). "Public Health Education Information Sheet." 1275 Mamaroneck Avenue: White Plains, NY.

March of Dimes Birth Defects Foundation. (1985). "Drugs, Alcohol, Tobacco Abuse During Pregnancy." 1275 Mamaroneck Avenue: White Plains, NY.

March of Dimes Birth Defects Foundation. (1986). "Sexually Transmitting Disease." 1275 Mamaroneck Avenue: White Plains, NY.

Maresh, M. M. (1948). "Growth of the Heart Related to Bodily Growth During Childhood and Adolescence." *Pediatrics*, 2, 382-404.

Martens, R. (1986). "Youth Sport in the USA." In Weiss, M. R., and Gould, D. (eds.). *Sport for Children and Youth.* Champaign, IL: Human Kinetics.

Martens, R. et al. (1981). *Coaching Young Athletes.* Champaign, IL: Human Kinetics.

Martin, T. P. and Stull, G. A. (1969). "Effects of Various Knee Angle and Foot Spacing Combinations on Performance in the Vertical Jump." *Research Quarterly*, 40, 324.

Martinek, T. and Zaichkowsky, L. D. (1977). *The Martinek-Zaichkowsky Self-Concept Scale for Children.* Jacksonville, IL: Psychologists and Educators.

Marx, J. L. (1975). "Cytomegalovirus: A Major Cause of Birth Defects." *Science*, 190, 1184-1186.

Mason, J. (1982). *The Environment of Play*. West Point, NY: Leisure Press.

Massicotte, L. R. and MacNab, B. J. (1974). "Cardiorespiratory Adaptations to Training at Specific Intensities in Children." *Medicine and Science in Sports*, 6, 242-246.

Masters, W. H. and Johnson, V. E. (1970). *Human Sexual Inadequacy*. Boston: Little Brown.

Mayer, J. (1960). "Exercise and Weight Control." In *Exercise and Fitness*. Chicago: Athletic Institute.

Mayer, J. (1968). *Overweight: Causes, Cost and Control*. Englewood Cliffs, NJ: Prentice-Hall.

Maynard, R. (1973). *Guiding Your Child to a More Creative Life*. New York: Doubleday.

McCandless, B. R. (1976). *Children—Behavior and Development*. New York: Holt, Rinhart and Winston.

McCaskill, C. L. and Wellman, B. L. (1938). "A Study of Common Motor Achievements at the Preschool Ages." *Child Development*, 9. 141.

McClenaghan, B. A. (1976). "Development of an Observational Instrument to Assess Selected Fundamental Movement Patterns of Low Motor Functioning Children." Unpublished doctoral dissertation, Indiana University.

McClenaghan, B. A. and Gallahue, D. L. (1978). *Fundamental Movement: A Developmental and Remedial Approach*. Philadelphia: W. B. Saunders.

McClenaghan, B. A. and Gallahue, D. L. (1978) *Fundamental Movement: Observation and Assessment*. Philadelphia: W. B. Saunders.

McFarlane, A. (1975). "Olfaction in the Development of Social Preference in the Human Neonate." In *Parent-Infant Interaction*. Amsterdam: CIBA Foundation Symposium 33.

McGarrity, W. J. et al. (1958). "Effect on Reproductive Cycle of Nutritional Status and Requirements." *Journal of the American Medical Association*, 168, 2138-2145.

McGillicuddy - Delisi and Sigel, E. (1982). "Effects of the Atypical Child on the Family." In Bond, L. A. and Joffe, J. M. (eds.) *Facilitating Infant and Early Childhood Development*. Hanover, NH: University Press of New England.

McGraw, M. B. (1934). *The Neuromuscular Maturation of the Human Infant*. New York: Hafner.

McGraw, M. B. (1935). Growth: A Study of Johnny and Jimmy. New York: Appleton-Century.

McGraw, M. B. (1939). "Later Development of Children Specially Trained During Infancy." *Child Development*, 10, 1.

McGraw, M. B. (1939). "Swimming Behavior of the Human Infant." *Journal of Pediatrics*, 15, 485-490.

McGraw, M. B. (1954). "Maturation of Behavior." In Carmichael L. (ed.), *Manual of Child Psychology*. New York: Wiley.

McNamera, J. J. et al. (1971). "Coronary Artery Disease in Combat Casualties in Vietnam." *Journal of the American Medical Association*, 216, 1186-1187.

Mehlman, J. (1940). "The Tonic Neck Reflex in Newborn Infants." *Journal of Pediatrics*, 16, 767-769.

Mercer, J. (1973). *Labeling the Mentally Retarded*. Berkeley: University of California Press.

Meredith, H. V. (1952). "North American Negro Infants: Size at Birth and Growth During the First Postnatal Year." *Human Biology*, 24, 290.

Meredith, H. V. (1975). "Somatic Changes During Human Prenatal Life," *Child Development*, 46, 603-610.

Micheli, L. J. (1983). "Overuse Injuries in Children's Sports: The Growth Factor." *Orthopedis Clinics of North America*, 14, 2, April.

Micheli, L. J. and Melhonian, N. (1987). "The Child in Sport." In *Preceedings of the Pan American Sports Medicine Congress XII*. Indiana University, Bloomington, IN.

Micheli, L. J. and Micheli, E. R. (1985). "Children's Running: Special Risks?" *Annals of Sports Medicine*, 2, 61-63.

Milinarie, C. (1974). *Birth*, New York: Harmony.

Miller, S. (1978). "The Facilitation of Fundamental Motor Skill Learning in Young Children." Unpublished doctoral dissertation, Michigan State University.

Mills, C. A. (1942). "Climate Effects on Growth and Development, with Particular Reference to the Effects of Tropical Residence." *American Anthropology*, 41, 1-13.

Minuchin, D. et al. (1978). *Psychosomatic Families—Anorexia Nervosa in Context*. Cambridge, MA: Harvard University Press.

Mitchell, J. and Blomquis, G. (1971). "Maximal Oxygen Uptake." *New England Journal of Medicine*, 284, 1018-1022.

Montague, M. F. A. (1962). *Prenatal Influences*. Springfield, IL: Charles C. Thomas.

Montoye, H. (1970). *Introductin to Measurement in Physical Education*. Indianapolis, IN: Phi Epsilon Kappa Fraternity.

Moore, R. C., et al. (Eds.) (1988) *Play for All Guidelines: Design and Management of Outdoor Play Settings for All Children*. Reston, VA: AAHPERD.

Moore, S. and Kilmer, S. (1973). *Contemporary Preschool Education*. New York: Wiley.

Mooston, M. (1981). *Teaching Physical Education*, Columbus, OH: Merrill.

Morgan, G. et al. (1985). *Quality in Early Childhood Programs. Four Perspectives*. Ypsilanti, MI: High/Scope Educational Research Foundation.

Morison, R. (1969). *A Movement Approach to Educational Gymnastics*. London: J. M. Dent and Sons.

Morley, D. and Woodland, M. (1979). *See How They Grow-Monitoring Child Growth For Appropriate Health Care in Developing Countries*. New York: Oxford University Press.

Morris, G. S. (1977). *Elementary Physical Education: Toward Inclusion*. Salt Lake City: Brighton.

Morris, G. S. (1977). "Dynamic Visual Acuity: Implications for the Physical Educator and Coach." *Motor Skills: Theory into Practice*, 2, 5-10.

Mrzena, B., and Macuek, M. (1978). "Uses of Treadmill and Working Capacity Assessment, in Preschool Children," In Borma, J. and Hebbelinck, M. (eds.), *Medicine and Sports Series, Volume II Pediatric Work Physiology*. Basel, Belgium: S. Karger.

Muller, P. F. et al. (1971). "Prenatal Factors and Their Relationship to Mental Retardation and Other Parameters of Development." *American Journal of Obstetrics and Gynecology*, 109, 1205-1210.

Murray, J. L. (1980). *Infaquatics.-Teaching Kids To Swim*. West Point, NY: Leisure Press.

Myers, C. B. et al. (1977). "Vertical Jumping Movement Patterns of Early Chidhood." Unpublished paper, Indiana University, Physical Education Department.

Myers, P. I., and Hammill, D. D. (1982). *Learning Disabilities: Basic Concepts, Assessment Practices and Instructional Strategies*. Austin, TX: Pro-Ed.

—N—

Naeye, R. L. et al. (1969). "Urban Poverty: Effects of Prenatal Nutrition." *Science*, 166, 1026.

Nagel, C. and Moore, F. (1966). *Skill Development Through Games and Rhythmic Activities*. Palo Alto, CA: National Press.

National Association for the Education of Young Children. (1987). *Developmentally Appropriate Practice in Early Childhood Programs Serving Children From Birth Through Age 8*. Bredenekamp, S. (Ed.) Washington, D.C.: NAEYC.

National Center for Health Statistics (1976). Washington, D. C.: U. S. Department of Health, Education and Welfare (ARA), 25, 76-1120, June 22.

National Children and Youth Fitness Study I. (1985). *Journal of Physical Education, Recreation and Dance*, 56, 1, 43-90.

National Children and Youth Fitness Study II. (1987). *Journal of Physical Education, Recreation and Dance*, 58, 9, 49-96.

National Foundation/March of Dimes (1977). *Birth Defects. Tragedy and Hope*.

National Strength and Conditioning Association (1985). "Position Paper on Prepubescent Strength Training." *National Strength and Conditioning Association Journal*, 7, 4, 27-31.

Nora, J. J. and Fraser, F. C. (1974). *Medical Genetics: Principles and Practices*. Philadelphia: Lee and Febiger.

—O—

Oppenheimer, S. B. (1980). *Introduction to Embryonic Development*. Boston: Allyn and Bacon.

Oscai, L. B. (1973). "The Role of Exercise in Weight Control." In Wilmore, J. H. (ed.) *Exercise and Sport Science Reviews, Volume I*. New York: Academic Press.

Oscai, L. B. (1974). "Exercise and Weight Control." Symposium on Overweight and Obesity, AAHPER Conference, Anaheim, CA., March 30.

Oscai, L. B. et al. (1974). "Effects of Exercise and of Food Restriction in Early Life on Adipose Tissue Cellularity." Abstract of the 21st Annual Meetings of the American College of Sports Medicine. Spring.

Osofsky, J. D. (ed.): (1979). *The Handbook of Infant Development*. New York: Wiley.

Osofsky, J. D. and Conners, K. (1979). "Mother Infant Interaction: An Intergrative View of a Complex System." In Osofsky, J. D. (ed.). *The Handbook of Infant Development*. New York: Wiley.

Oster, H. S. (1975). "Color Perception in Ten-Week Old Infants." Paper presented at the annual meeting of the Society for Research in Child Development, Denver.

Ottenbacker, K. (1983). "Developmental Implications of Clinically Applied Vestibular Stimulation." *Physical Therapy*, 63, 338-341.

Ounsted, M. and Ounsted, C. (1973). "On Fetal Growth Rate." In, Clinics in *Developmental Medicine*. London: William Heinemann Medical Books.

Owen, G. M. et al. (1974). "A Study of the Nutritional Status of Preschool Children in the United States." USDHEW, 53 Part II, Supplement.

—P—

Paffenbarger, R. S. et al. (1986). "Physical Activity, All-Cause Mortality, and Longevity, and Longevity of College Alumni." *New England Journal of Medicine*, 314, 605-613.

Paget, K. D. and Bracken, B. A. (1983). *The Psychoeducational Assessment of Preschool Children*. New York: Grune and Stratton.

Parizkova, J. (1972). "Somatic Development and Body Composition Changes in Adolescent Boys Differing in Physical Activity and Fitness: A Longitudinal Study." *Anthropologie*, 10, 3-36.

Parizkova, J. (1973). "Body Composition and Exercise During Growth and Development." In Rarick, G. L. (ed.), *Physical Activity: Human Development*. New York: Academic Press.

Parizkova, J. (1977). *Body Fat and Physical Fitness*. The Hague, Netherlands: Martinus Nijkoff B. V. Medical Division.

Parizkova, J. (1982). "Physical Training in Weight Reduction of Obese Adolescents." *Annals of Clinical Research*, 34, 69-73.

Parker, D. E. (1980). "The Vestibular Apparatus." *Scientific American*, 243, 118-135.

Parron, D. and Eisenberg, L. (1982). *Infants at Risk for Developmental Dysfunction*. Washington, D. C.: National Academy Press.

Pasamanuck, B., and Knoblach, N. (1966). "Retrospective Studies on the Epidemiology of Reproductive Causality: Old and New." *Merrill-Palmer Quarterly*, 12, 7-26.

Pate, R. R. and Blair, S. N. (1978). "Exercise and the Prevention of Atheroscherosis: Pediatric Implications." In Strong, W. (ed.). *Pediatric Aspects of Atheroscherous*. New York: Greene and Stratton.

Pate, R. R. et al. (1985). "The New Norms: A Comparison with the 1980 AAHPERD Norms." *Journal of Physical Education, Recreation and Dance*, 56, 1, 28-30.

Pate, R. R. et al. (1987). "The National Children and Youth Fitness Study II: The Modified Pull-Up Test." *Journal of Physical Education, Recreation and Dance*, 58, 9, 71-73.

Pawlak-Frazier, P. and Pawlak-Frazier, D. (1978). *Cause and Defect: Fetal Alcohol Syndrome: A Special Report*. Institute for Chemical Survival: Phoenix, AZ.

Payne, V. G., and Isaacs, L. D. (1987). *Human Motor Development: A Lifespan Approach*. Mountain View, CA: Mayfield.

Payne, V. G. (1981). "Effects of Object Size and Experimental Design on Object Reception By Children in the First Grade." *Journal of Human Movement Studies*, 11, 1-9.

Payne, G. (1985). "The Effects of Object Size, Experimental Design and Distance of Projection of Object Reception by Children in the First Grade." Unpublished doctoral dissertation, Indiana University.

Payne, G. (1985). "Infant Reflexes in Human Motor Development." Lauren Productions: Box 666. Mendocino, CA 95460 (video tape).

Payne, G. et al. (1979). *Head Start: A Tragicomedy with Epilogue*. New York: Behavioral Publications.

Peck, E. B., and Ullrich, H. D. (1988). "Children and Weight: A Changing Perspective." 1116 Miller Ave., Berkley, CA: Nutrition Communications Associates.

Pederson, E. J. (1973). "A Study of Ball Catching Abilities of First-, Third-, and Fifth-Grade Children on Twelve Selected Ball Catching Tasks." Unpublished doctoral dissertation, Indiana University.

Peeples, D. R., and Teller, D. Y. (1975). "Color Vision and Brightness Discrimination in Two-Month-Old Human Infants." *Science*, 189, 1102-1103.

Peterson, G. (1967). *Atlas for Somatotyping Children*. The Netherlands: Royal Vagorcum Ltd.

Peterson, K. L. et al. (1974). "Factor Analyses of Motor Performance for Kindergarten, First and Second Grade Children: A Tentative Solution." Paper presented at the Annual Convention of the AAHPER, Anaheim, CA., March 31.

Piaget, J. (1932). *The Moral Judgement of the Child*. New York: Harcourt and Brace.

Piaget, J. (1952). *The Origins of Intelligence in Children*. New York: International Universities Press.

Piaget, J. (1954). *The Construction of Reality and the Child*. New York: Basic Books.

Piaget, J. (1957). *Plays, Dreams and Imitation in Childhood*. London: William Heinemann Medical Books.

Piaget, J. (1962). *Plays, Dreams, and Imitation in Childhood*. New York: W. W. Norton.

Piaget, J. (1969). "The Psychology of the Child." New York: Basic Books.

Piaget, J. (1974). "Development and Learning." In Riple, R. E. and Rockcastle, V. N. (eds.). *Piaget Rediscovered*. Ithaca, NY: Cornell University Press.

Piers, E. V. (1969). *Manual for the Piers-Harris Children's Self-Concept Scale*. Nashville, TN: Counselor Recordings and Tests.

Piers, M. W. (ed) (1972). *Play and Development*. New York: Norton.

Pijpers, J. W. et al. (1984). Effect of Short-Term Maternal Exercise on Maternal and Fetal Cardiovascular Dynamics." *British Journal of Obstetrics and Gynocology*, 91, 1081-1086.

Plummer, G. W. (1952). "Anomalies Occurring in Children Exposed in Utero to Atomic Bomb in Hiroshima." *Pediatrics*, 10, 687-692.

Poe, A. (1976). "Description of the Movement Characteristics of Two-Year-Old Children Performing the Jump and Reach." *Research Quarterly*, 47, 200.

Pontius, A. A. (1973). "Neuro-Ethics of Walking in the Newborn." *Perceptual and Motor Skills*, 37, 235-245.

Poulton, E. C. (1957). "On Prediction in Skilled Movements." *Psychological Bulletin*, 57, 467-478.

Pratt, K. C. (1954). "The Neonate." In Carmichael, L. (ed.), *Manual of Child Psychology*. New York: Wiley.

Prechtl, H. F. R. (1965) "Problem of Behavioral Studies in the New Born Infant." In Leckarman, D. S. et al. (eds)., *Advances in the Study of Behavior, Volume 1*. New York: Academic Press.

Prechtl, H. F. R. (1986). "Prenatal Motor Development." In Wade, M. G. and Whiting, H. T. A. (eds). *Motor Development in Children: Aspects of Coordination and Control*. Dordrecht: The Netherlands: Martinus Nijohoff Publishers.

Prechtl, H. F. R., and Beintema, D. J. (1964). *The Neurological Examination of the Full Term Newborn Infant*. London: William Heinimann Medical Books.

Profiles on Children, 1970. (1970). White House Conference on Children, Washington, D. C., Superintendent of Documents, U. S. Government Printing Office.

—R—

Rarick, G. L. (1973). *Physical Activity, Human Growth and Development*. New York: Academic Press.

Rarick, G. L. (1980). "Motor Development, Its Growing Knowledge Base," *Journal of Physical Education and Recreation*, 51, 20.

Rarick, G. L. (1981). "The Emergence of the Study of Human Motor Development." In Brooks, G. A. (ed.). *Perspectives of the Academic Disciplines of Physical Education*. Champaign, IL: Human Kinetics.

Rarick, G. L. and Dobbins, A. (1975). "Basic Components in the Motor Performance of Children Six to Nine Years of Age." *Medicine and Science in Sports*, 17, 105-110.

Read, D. G. (1968). "The Influence of Competitive—Non-Competitive Programs of Physical Education on Body Image and Self Concept." Unpublished doctoral dissertation, Boston University.

Reilly, M. (ed.). (1974). *Play as Exploratory Behavior*. Beverly Hills, CA: Sage.

Reuschlein, P. and Haubenstricker, J. (eds.). (1985). "1984-85 Physical Education Interpretive Report: Grades 4, 7 and 10." Michigan Educational Assessment Program. State Board of Education, Michigan Department of Education, Lansing.

Richman, L. C. (1980). "General Intellectual and Specific Language Development of Low-Birth Weight Children." Paper presented at the meeting of the APA, Montreal.

Ridenour, M. V. (1974). "Influence of Object Size, Speed, and Direction on the Perception of a Moving Object." *Research Quarterly*, 45, 293-301.

Ridenour, M. V. (ed.). (1978). *Motor Development: Issues and Applications*. Princeton, N.J.: Princeton.

Rissen, A. H., and Aarons, L. (1959). "Visual Movement and Intensity Discrimination of Pattern Vision." *Journal of Comparative Physiological Psychology*, 52, 142-149.

Riggs, M. L. (1980). *Jump to Joy*. Englewood Cliffs, NJ.: Prentice-Hall.

Roach, E. G. and Kephart, N. C. (1966). *The Purdue Perceptual Motor Survey*. Columbus, OH: Merrill.

Roberton, M. A. (1977). "Stability of Stage Categorization Across Trials: Implications for the Stage Theory of Overarm Throw Development." *Journal of Human Movement Studies*, 3, 49-59.

Roberton, M. A. (1978). "Longitudinal Evidence for Developmental Stages in the Forceful Overarm Throw." *Journal of Human Movement Studies*, 4, 167-175.

Roberton, M. A. (1978). "Stability of Stage Categorization in Motor Development." In Landers, D. M. and Christine R. W. (eds.), *Psychology in Motor Behavior and Sport—1977* Champaign, IL: Human Kinetics.

Roberton, M. A. (1978). "Stages in Motor Development." In Ridenour, M. (ed.), *Motor Development: Issues and Applications* Princeton, N.J.: Princeton.

Roberton, M. A. (1981). "Movement Quality Not Quantity." *Motor Development Academy Newsletter*, 2, 2-3.

Roberton, M. A. (1982). "Describing Stages Within and Across Motor Tasks." In Kelson J. A. S. and Clark, J. (eds)., *The Development of Movement Control and Coordination*. New York: Wiley.

Roberton, M. A. (1987). "Developmental Level as a Function of the Immediate Environment." In Clark, J. E. and Humphrey, J. H. *Advances in Motor Development Research*. New York: AMS Press.

Roberton, M. A. (1985). "Changing Motor Patterns During Childhood." In Thomas, J. K. (ed.). *Motor Development During Childhood and Adolescence*. Minneapolis: Burgess.

Roberton, M. A. and Halverson, L. E. (1984). *Developing Children-Their Changing Movement*. Philadelphia: Lea and Febiger.

Roberts, J. A. and Morgan, W. P. (1971). "Effect of Type and Frequency of Participation in Physical Activity Upon Physical Working Capacity." *American Corrective Therapy Journal*, 25, 99-104.

Robson, K. (1967). "The Role of Eye-to-Eye Contact in Maternal-Infant Attachment." *Journal of Child Psychology and Psychiatry and Allied Disciplines*, 8, 13-25.

Rogers, D. R. (1977). *Child Psychology*. Monterey, CA: Brooks/Cole.

Rosenberg, M. (1982). "Psychological Selectivity in Self-Esteem Formation." In Rosenberg, M. and Kaplan, H. B. (eds.) *Social Psychology of the Self-Concept*. Arlington Heights, IL: Harlan Davidson.

Rosenberg, M. (1979). *Conceiving the Self*. New York: Basic Books.

Rosenblith, J. F. and Sims-Knight, J. E. (1985). *In the Beginning: Development in the First Two Years*. Monterey, CA: Brooks/Cole.

Ross, J. G. and Gilbert, G. G. (1985). The National Children and Youth Fitness Study: A Summary of Findings." *Journal of Physical Education Recreation and Dance*, 56, 1, 45-50.

Ross, J. G., et al. (1987). "Changes in the Body Composition of Children." *Journal of Physical Education, Recreation and Dance*, 58, 9, 74-77.

Ross, J. G. and Pate, R. R. (1987) The National Children and Youth Fitness Study II: A Summary of Findings." *Journal of Physical Education, Recreation and Dance*, 58, 9, 51-56.

Ross, J. G. et al. (1987). "Home and Community in Children's Exercise Habits," *Journal of Physical Education, Recreation and Dance*, 58, 9, 85-92.

Ross, J. G. and Gilbert, G. G. (1985). "The National Children and Youth Fitness Study." *Journal of Physical Education, Recreation and Dance*, 56, 1, 45-50.

Rossett, H. L., and Sander, L. W. (1979). "Effects of Maternal Drinking on Neonatal Morphology and State," In Osofsky, J. (ed.). *The Handbook of Infant Development*. New York: Wiley.

Rothenberg, A. (1976). "Understanding the Anorectic Student." *Today's Education*, 65, 48-49.

Rubin, R. A. et al. (1973). "Psychological and Educational Sequel of Prematurity." *Pediatrics*, 52, 352-363.

Rudel, R. G. and Teuber, H. L. (1963). "Discrimination of Direction of Line in Children." *Journal of Comparative Physiological Psychology*, 56, 892-899.

—S—

Sage, G. H. (1984). *Motor Learning and Control A Neurophyschological Approach*. Dubuque, IA: Wm. C. Brown.

Sage, G. H. (1986). "Social Development." In Seefeldt, V. (ed.), *Physical Activity and Well-Being*. Reston, VA: AAHPERD.

Salapatek, P. (1975). "Pattern Vision in Early Infancy." In Cohen, L. B. and Salapatek, P. *Infant Perception*. New York: Academic Press.

Sameroff, A. (1973). "Reflexive and Operant Aspects of Sucking Behavior in Early Infancy." In Bosma, J. F. (eds.) *Oral Sensation and Perception Development in the Fetus and Infant*. Springfield, MO: Charles C. Thomas.

Samuel, M. D., and Samuels, N. (1979). *The Well Baby Book*. New York: Cummit Books.

Santrock, J. W. and Yussen, S. R. *Child Development an Introduction*. Dubuque, IA: Wm. C. Brown.

Sapp, M. (1980). "Developmental Sequence of Galloping." Unpublished materials, Michigan State University.

Saunders, J. E. et al. (1953). "The Major Determinants in Normal and Pathological Gait." *Journal of Bone and Joint Surgery*, 35, 543-558.

Savage, M. P. et al. (1985). "Exercise Training Effects on Serum Lipids of Prepubescent Boys and Adult Men." *Medicine and Science in Sports Exercise*, 8, 97-204.

Schaie, K. W. and Baltes, P. B. (1975). "On Sequential Strategies in Developmental Research: Description or Explanation." *Human Development*, 18, 384-390.

Schaller, M. J. (1975). "Chromatic Vision in Human Infants: Conditioned Fixation to Hues of Varying Intensity." Paper presented at the meeting of the Society for Research in Child Development, Denver.,

Schempp, P. G. et al. (1983). "Influence of Decision-Making on Attitudes, Creativity, Motor Skills and Self-Concept in Elementary Children." *Research Quarterly*, 540, 2, 183-189.

Schmidt, R. A. (1977). "Schema Theory: Implications for Movement Education." *Motor Skills Theory into Practice*, 2, 36-48.

Schneider, B. A. et al. (1980). "High-Frequency Sensitivity in Infants." *Science*, 207, 1003-1004.

Scrimshaw, N. S. (1967). "Malnutrition, Learning and Behavior." *American Journal of Clinical Nutrition*, 20, 493-502.

Seashore, H. G. (1949). "The Development of a Beam Walking Test and Its Use in Measuring Development of Balance in Children." *Research Quarterly*, 18, 246-259.

Seefeldt, V. (1972). "Discussion of Walking and Running." Unpublished research, Michigan State University

Seefeldt, V. (1975). "Critical Learning Periods and Programs of Intervention." Paper presented at the AAHPERD Conference, Atlantic City.

Seefeldt, V. (1980). "Physical Fitness Guidelines for Preschool Children," In *Proceedings of the National Conference on Physical Fitness and Sports for All*, Washington, D. C.: President's Council on Physical Fitness and Sports, 5-19.

Seefeldt, V. (1989). "This is Motor Development." *Motor Development Academy Newsletter*, 10, 1.

Seefeldt, V. (ed.) (1987). "Selling the Potential Rather Than the Record." *Journal of Physical Education, Recreation and Dance*, 158, 42-43.

Seefeldt, V. et al. (1972). "Sequencing Motor Skills Within the Physical Education Curriculum." Paper presented at the AAHPER Conference, Houston, TX.

Seefeldt, V. and Gould, D. (1980). Physical and Psychological Effects of Athletic Competition on Children and Youth, Washington, D. C. ERIC Clearinghouse on Teacher Education.

Seefeldt, V. and Haubenstricker, J. (1976). "Developmental Sequences of Fundamental Motor Skills." Unpublished research, Michigan State University.

Seefeldt, V. and Haubenstricker, J. (1981). "Developmental Sequences of Kicking: Second Revision." Paper presented at the Midwest AAHPERD Conference, Chicago, March 19.

Seefeldt, V. Ed. (1987). *Handbook for Youth Sport Coaches*. Reston, VA: AAHPERD.

Seifert, K. L. and Hoffnung, R. J. (1987). *Child and Adolescent Development*. Boston: Houghton: Houghton-Mifflin.

Self, P. A., and Horwitz, F. D. (1979). "The Behavioral Assessment of the Neonate: An Overview." In Osofsky, J. D. (ed.), *The Handbook of Infant Development*. New York: Wiley.

Sewell, L., and Micheli, L. (1984). "Strength Development in Children." Paper presented to the American College of Sports Medicine, San Diego.

Sheldon, W. H. et al. (1940). *The Varieties of Human Physique*, New York: Harper.

Sheldon, W. H. et al. (1954). *Atlas of Man*. New York: Harper.

Shepard, R. J. (1984). "Physical Activity and 'Wellness' of the Child." In Boileau, R. A. (ed.), *Advances in Pediatric Sport Sciences, Volume I*. Champaign, IL: Human Kinetics.

Shirley, M. (1931). *The First Two Years: A Study of Twenty-Five Babies, 1. Postural and Locomotor Development*. Minneapolis: University of Minnesota Press.

Simmons-Morton, B. G. et al. (1987). "Children and Fitness: A Public Health Perspective." *Research Quarterly for Exercise and Sport*, 58, 4, 295-303.

Sinclair, C. (1973). *Movement of the Young Child*. Columbus, OH: Merrill.

Singer, R. N. (1980). *Motor Learning and Human Performance*. New York: Macmillan.

Siqueland, E. R. and Delucia, C. A. (1969). "Visual Reinforcement of Non-Nutritive Sucking in Human Infants." *Science*, 165, 1144-1146.

Sloan, W. (1954). *Manual for the Lincoln-Oseretsky Motor Development Scale*. Chicago: C. H. Stolting.

Smart, M. S. and Smart, R. C. (1973). *Preschool Children: Development and Relationships*. New York: Macmillan.

Smart, M. S. and Smart, R. C. (1973). *School Age Children: Development and Relationships*. New York: Macmillan.

Smith, D. W. and Witson, A. A. (1973). *The Child with Down's Syndrome (Monogolism)*. Philadelphia: W. B. Saunders.

Smith, H. (1970). "Implications for Movement Education Experience Drawn from Perceptual Motor Research." *Journal of Health, Physical Education and Recreation*, 4, 30-33.

Smith, K. V. and Smith, W. M. (1972). *Perception and Motion: An Analysis of Space-Structured Behavior*. Philadelphia: W. B. Saunders.

Smith, O. W. (1965). "Spatial Perceptions and Play Activities of Nursery School Children." *Perceptual Motor Skills*, 21, 160.

Smith, O. W. and Smith, P. C. (1966). "Developmental Studies of Spatial Judgements by Children and Adults." *Perceptual Motor Skills* (Monograph Supplement), 22, 3-73.

Snyder, E. E. and Spretizer, E. (1973). "Family Influences and Involvement in Sports." *Research Quarterly*, 44, 249-255.

Snyder, E. E. and Spretizer, E. (1979). "Orientation Toward Sport: Intrinsic, Normative and Extrinsic." *Journal of Sport Psychology*, 1, 170-175.

Solkoff, N. et al. (1969). "Effects of Handling on the Subsequent Development of Premature Infants." *Developmental Psychology*, 1, 765-768.

Spears, W. C. (1964). "Assessment of Visual Preference and Discrimination in the 4-Month Old Infant." *Journal of Comparative Physiological Psychology*, 57, 381-386.

Spitz, R. (1945). "Hospitalism: An Inquiry into the Genesis of Psychiatric Conditions in Early Childhood." *Psychoanalytic Study of the Child*, 1, 53-74.

Stallones, R. A. (1980). "The Rise and Fall of Ischemic Heart Disease." *Scientific American*, 243, 53-59.

Standley, K., et al. (1974). "Local-Regional Anesthesia, During Childbirth and Newborn Behavior." *Science*, 18, 634-635.

Stanley, S. (1977). *Physical Education: A Movement Orientation*. Toronto: McGraw-Hill.

Stein, E. A., et al. (1981). "Coronary Risk Factors in the Young." *Annual Reviews of Medicine*, 52, 601-613.

Stevenson, R. (1977). *The Fetus and Newly Born Infant*. St. Louis: C. V. Mosby.

Stewart, K. J., and Gutin, B. (1976). "Effects of Physical Training on Cardiorespiratory Fitness in Children." *Research Quarterly*, 47, 110-120.

Strauss, M. E. et al. (1975). "Behavior of Nicotine-Addicted Newborns." *Child Development*, 46, 887-893.

Streissguth, A., et al. (1985). "Natural History of the Fetal Alcohol Syndrome: A 10-Year Followup of Eleven Patients." *Lancet*, 2, 85-91.

Sundberg, A. L. and Wirsen, C. (1977). *A Child Is Born. The Drama of Life Before Birth*. New York: Delacorts.

Susser, M. et al. (1972). "Birth Weight, Fetal Age and Perinatal Mortality." *American Journal of Epidemiology*, 96, 197-204.

Sutton-Smith, B. (1985). "The Child at Play." *Psychology Today*, October, 64-65.

Svejda, M. and Schmidt, D. (1979). "The Role of Self Produced Locomotion on the Onset of Fear of Heights on the Visual Cliff." Paper presented at the Society for Research in Child Development. San Francisco.

Swartz, D., and Allen, M. (1975). "Residual Reflex Patterns as a Basis for Diagnosing Stroke Faults." In Clarys, J. P. and Levillie, L. (eds.), *Swimming II*. Baltimore: University Park Press.

—T—

Tanner, J. M. A. (1979). "Physical Growth." In Mussen, P. H. (ed.). *Carmichaels' Manual of Child Psychology*. New York: Wiley.

Tanner, J. M. (1962). *Growth at Adolescence*. Oxford, England: Blackwell Scientific Publications

Tanner, J. M. (1978). *Fetus into Man*. Cambridge, MA: Harvard University Press.

Tanner, J. M. et al. (1975). *Assessment of Skeletal Maturity and Prediction of Adult Height*. New York: Academic Press.

Tanner, P. (1979). "Movement Education: A Total Program of Elementary School Physical Education." *Proceedings of the Contemporary Elementary School Physical Education Conference*. Georgia State University, Atlanta, GA.

Taylor, B. J. (1980). "Pathways To a Healthy Self-Concept." In Yaroke, T. D. (ed.), *The Self Concept of the Young Child*. Salt Lake City, Brigham Young Press.

Taylor, W. N. (1987). "Synthetic Anabolic-Androgenic Steroids: A Plea for Controlled Substance Status." *Physician and Sports Medicine*, 15, 5, 140-147.

Thelen, E. (1979). "Rhythmical Stereotypies in Normal Human Infants." *Animal Behavior*, 27, 699-715.

Thelen, E. (1980). "Determinants of Amount of Stereotyped Behavior in Normal Human Infants." *Ethology and Sociobiology*, 1, 141-150.

Thelen, E. (1981). Kicking, Rocking, and Waving: Contextual Analysis of Rhythmical Stereotypies in Normal Human Infants." *Animal Behavior*, 29.

Thelen, E. (1985). Developmental Origins of Motor Coordination: Leg Movements in Human Infants." *Developmental Psychobiology*, 18, 1-22.

Thelen, E. (1985). "Rhythmical Behavior in Infancy: An Ethological Perspective." *Developmental Psychology*, 17, 237-257.

Thelen, E. (1986). "Development of Coordinated Movement. Implications for Early Motor Development." In Wade, M. G. and Whiting, H. T. A. (eds.) *Motor Development in Children: Aspects of Coordination and Control*. Dordrecht, The Netherlands: Martinus Nyhoff.

Thelen, E., Kelso, J. A. S. and Fogel, A. (1987). "Self-Organizing Systems and Infant Motor Development." *Developmental Review*, 7, 39-65.

Thissen, P. et al. (1976). "Individual Growth in Stature: A Comparison of Four Growth Studies in the U. S. A." *Annals of Human Biology*, 3, 529-542.

Thomas, J. H. (1984). *Motor Development During Childhood and Adolescence*, Minneapolis: Burgess.

Thompson, H. and Gesell, A. (1929). "Learning and Growth in Identical Twins: An Experimental Study by the Method of Co-Twin Control." *Journal of Genetic Psychology Monographs*, 6, 1-24.

Thompson, J. D. and Thompson, M. W. (1973). *Genetics in Medicine*. Philadelphia: W. B. Saunders.

Time-Life Books, Eds. (1987). *Developing Your Child's Potential*. Alexandria, VA: Time-Life Books.

Tipton, C. and Tcheng, T. K. (1970). "Iowa Wrestling Study." *Journal of the American Medical Association*, 214, 1269-1274.

Titchner, E. B. (1909). *A Textbook of Psychology*. New York: Macmillan.

Travers, J. F. (1977). *The Growing Child*. New York: Wiley.

Trehub, S. E. et al. (1980). "Infants' Perception of Melodies: The Role of Melodic Contour." *Child Development*, 55, 821-830.

Tronick, E. (1972). "Stimulus Control and The Growth of the Infants' Effective Visual Field." *Perception and Psychophysics*, 11, 373-375.

Tronick, E., and Brazelton, T. B. (1975). "Clinical Uses of the Brazelton Neonatal Behavioral Assessment." In Friedlander B. Z. and Rosenbluml (eds.), *Exceptional Infant* (Vol. III). New York: Brunner/Mazel.

Tuddenham, R. S. (1951). "Studies in Reputation III, Correlates of Popularity Among Elementary School Children." *The Journal of Educational Psychology*, 42, May.

Twitchell, T. E. (1965). "Attitudinal Reflexes." *Physical Therapy*, 45, 411-418.

—U—

Ulrich, B. D. (1984). "The Effects of Stimulation Programs on the Development of High Risk Infants: A Review of Research." *Adapted Physical Activity Quarterly*, 1, 68-80.

Ulrich, B. (1987). Perceptions of Physical Competence, Motor Competence and Participation in Organized Sports: Their Interrelations in Young Children." *Research Quarterly for Exercise and Sport*, 58, 57-67.

Ulrich, D. A. (1985). *Test of Gross Motor Development*. Austin TX: Pro-ED.

U.S. Bureau of the Census (1988). *Statistical Abstract of the United States*. Washington, D. C.: U. S. Department of Commerce.

U. S. Department of Commerce, Bureau of the Census (1987). *Statistical Abstract of the United States*. Washington, D. C.: U. S. Government Printing Office.

—V—

Van Slooten, P. H. (1973). "Performance of Selected Motor-Coordination Tasks by Young Boys and Girls in Six Socioeconomic Groups." Unpublished doctoral dissertation, Indiana University.

Vogel, P. G. (1986). "Effects of Physical Education Programs on Children." In Seefeldt, V. (ed.) *Physical Activity and Well-Being*. Reston, VA AAHERD.

von Bernuth, H. G. L. and Prechtl, H. R. R. (1969). "Reflexes and Their Relationship to Behavioral State in the Newborn." *Acta Pediatric Scandanavia*, 57, 177-185.

von Hofsten, C. (1977). "Binocular Convergence as a Determinant of Reaching Behavior." *Perception*, 6, 139-144.

von Hofsten, C. (1979). "Development of Visually Guided Reaching: The Approach Phase." *Journal of Human Movement Studies*, 5, 160-178.

von Hofsten, C. (1982). "Eye-Hand Coordination in Newborns." *Developmental Psychology*, 18, 450-461.

von Hofsten, C. (1986). "The Emergence of Manual Skills." In Wade, M. G. and Whiting, H. T. A. (eds.). *Motor Development in Children: Aspects of Coordination and Control*. Dorbrecht, The Netherlands: Martinus, Nijhoff.

Vrijens, J. (1969). "The Influence of Interval Circuit Exercise in Physical Fitness in Adolescents." *Research Quarterly*, 40, 595-599.

Vrijens, J. (1978). "Muscle Strength Development in Pre- and Postpubescent Age." In Borms, J. and Hebbelinck, M. (eds.), *Pediatric Work Physiology*. New York: Karjer.

—W—

Wade, M. (1981). "A Plea for Process Oriented Tests." *Motor Development Academy Newsletter*, 2, 1, 1-2.

Wade, M. G. and Whitinig, H. T. A. (1986). *Motor Development in Children: Aspects of Coordination and Control*. Dordrecht, The Netherlands: Martinus Nijhoff Publishers.

Wallace, R. N. and Stuff, J. (1973). "A Perceptual Program for Classroom Teachers, Some Results." *Genetic Psychology Monographs*, 87, 253-288.

Walk, R. D. (1966). "The Development of Depth Perception in Animal and Human Infants." *Monograph of the Society for Research in Child Development*, 31, 5.

Walk, R. D. (1978). "Depth Perception and Experience." In Walk, R. D. and Pick, A. (eds.). *Perception and Experiences*. New York: Plenum Press.

Wapner, S. and Werner, H. (1957). *Perceptual Development: An Investigation Within the Sensory Tonic Field Theory*. Worchester, MA: Clark University Press.

Ward, D. and Werner, P. (1981). "Analysis of Two Curricular Approaches in Physical Education." *Journal of Physical Education and Recreation*, 52, 60-63.

Ward, D. S. et al. (1987). "Effects of a Multicomponent Intervention Program and Reducing Health Risk in Obese Children." *The Physical Educator*, 45, 44-49.

Ward, D. S. and Bar-Or, O. (1986). "Role of the Physician and the Physical Education Teacher in the Treatment of Obesity." *Pediatrician*, 13, 44-51.

Warkany, J. et al. (1961). "Intrauterine Growth Retardation." American Journal of Diseases of Children, 102, 462-476.

Warren, K. and Rosett, H. (1978). "Fetal Alcohol Syndrome." *Alcohol Health and Research World*, HEW, 2, 2-12.

Watson, E. H. and Lowrey, G. H. (1967). *Growth and Development of Children*, Chicago: Year Book.

Watson, R. I. and Lindgreen, H. C. (1979). *Psychology of the Child and the Adolescent*. New York: Macmillan.

Wattenberg, W. and Clifford, C. (1962). *Relationship of Self-Concept to Beginning Achievement in Reading*. U. S. Office of Education, No. 377, Detroit: Wayne State University.

Weiss, M. R. (1987). "Self Esteem and Achievement in Children's Sport and Physical Activity." In Gould, D. and Weiss, M. R. (eds.). *Advances in Pediatric Sport Sciences*, (Volume 2, Behavioral Issues). Champaign, IL: Human Kinetics.

Weiss, M. R. and Bredemeier, B. J. (1986). "Moral Development." In Seefeldt, V. (ed.), *Physical Activity and Well-Being*. Reston, Va: AAHPERD.

Weissbourd, B. (1987). "A Sense of Confidence." *Parents Magazine*, 62, 204.

Wellman, B. (1937). "Motor Achievements of Preschool." *Childhood Education*, 13, 311-316.

Werner, E. E. and Bayley, N. (1966). "The Reliability of Bayley's Revised Scale of Mental and Motor Development During the First Year of Life." *Child Development*, 37, 39-50.

Werner, P. H., and Burton, E. (1979). *Learning Through Movement*. St. Louis: C. V. Mosby.

Wertheimer, M. (1961). "Psychomotor Coordination of Auditory-Visual Space at Birth." *Science*, 134, 1692.

Westman, J. C. (ed.) (1973). *Individual Differences in Children*. New York: Wiley.

Wetzel, N. C. (1948). *The Wetzel Grid for Evaluating Physical Fitness*. Cleveland: NEA Services.

Whitall, J. (1988). "A Dynamical Systems Approach to Motor Development: Applying New Theory to Practice." Paper presented at the International Early Childhood Physical Education Conference, Washington, D.C.

White, B. (1975). *The First Three Years of Life*. Englewood Cliffs, NJ: Prentice-Hall.

White, B., and Held, R. (1966). "Plasticity of Sensorimotor Development in the Human Infant," In Rosenblith, J. P. and Allinsmith, W. (eds.), The Causes of Behavior: *Readings in Child Development and Educational Psychology*. Boston: Allyn and Bacon.

White, R. W. (1959). "Motivation Reconsidered: The Concept of competence." *Psychological Review*, 66, 297-333.

White House Conference on Children and Youth (1970). *Conference Proceedings*. Washington, D. C.: Superintendent of Documents, U. S. Government Printing Office.

Whithurst, G. J. and Varta, R. (1977). *Child Behavior*. Boston: Roughton Mifflin.

Whiting, H. T. A. (1969). *Acquiring Ball Skill*. London: G. Bell and Sons.

Whiting, H. T. A. (1974). "Dynamic Visual Acuity and Performance of a Catching Task." *Journal of Motor Behavior*, 6, 87-94.

Whiting, H. T. A. (1975). *Concepts in Skill Learning*. London: Lepus Books.

Wickstrom, R. (1983). *Fundamental Motor Patterns*. Philadelphia: Lea and Febiger.

Wickstrom, R. L. (1980). "Acquisition of a Ball-Handling Skill." Paper presented at the Annual meeting of the AAHPERD, Detroit.

Wieczorek, R. R. and Natapoff, J. N. (1981). *A Conceptual Approach to the Nursing of Children*. Philadelphia: J. B. Lippincott.

Wierman, M. E. and Crowley, W. F., Jr. (1986). "Neutroendoirine Control of the Onset of Puberty." In Falkner, F. and Tanner, J. M. (eds.) *Human Growth, Volume 2: Postnatal Growth*, revised edition. New York: Plenum.

Wild, M. (1938). "The Behavioral Pattern of Throwing and Some Observations Concerning Its Course of Development in Children." *Research Quarterly*, 3, 20.

Wilkerson, J. A. (1982). "Strength and Endurance Training for the Youthful Performer." In Gallahue, D. L. (ed.), *Directions in Health, Physical Education and Recreation, Monograph*, 2. Bloomington, IN: Indiana University, School of HPER.

Williams, H. (1970). "A Study of Perceptual-Motor Characteristics of Children in Kindergarten Through Sixth Grade." Unpublished paper, University of Toledo.

Williams, H. (1973). "Perceptual-Motor Development in Children." In Corbin, C. (ed.), *A Textbook of Motor Development*. Dubuque, IA: Wm. C. Brown.

Williams, H. G. (1983). *Perceptual and Motor Development*. Englewood Cliffs, NJ: Prentice-Hall.

Williams, K. (1980). "Developmental Characteristics of a Forward Roll." *Research Quarterly for Exercise and Sport*, 51, 4, 703.

Wilmore, J. H. (1974). "The Roll of the Health and Physical Education." Symposium on Overweight and Obesity. AAHPERD Conference. Anaheim, CA: March 30.

Winchester, A. M. (1979). *Human Genetics*. Columbus, OH: Merill.

Winters, A. M. (1973). "The Relationship of Time of Initial Feeding to Success of Breastfeeding." Unpublished paper, University of Washington.

Witti, F. P. (1978). "Alcohol and Birth Defects." *FDA Consumer*, 22, 20-23.

Wyke, B. (1975). "The Neurological Basis of Movement: A Developmental Review." In, Holt, K. S. (ed.), *Movement and Child Development*. London: Williams Heinemann Medical Books.

Wylie, R. (1974). *The Self Concept*. Lincoln: University of Nebraska Press.

Wylie, R. (1974). *The Self Concept, A Critical Survey of Pertinent Research Literature*. Lincoln: University of Nebraska Press.

Wylie, R. (1979). *The Self Concept*. Lincoln: University of Nebraska Press.

—X/Y—

Yakacs, R. F. (1971). "Heart Rate Response of Children to Four Separate Bouts of Training." Unpublished doctoral dissertation, Texas A & M University.

Yamamoto, K. (1972). *The Child and His Image*. Boston: Houghton Mifflin.

Yang, R. K. (1979). "Early Infant Assessment: An Overview." In Osofsky, J. D. (ed.), *The Handbook of Infant Development*. New York: Wiley.

Yang, R. K. et al. (1976). "Successive Relationships Between Maternal Attitudes During Pregnancy, Analgesic Medication During Labor and Delivery, and Newborn Behavior." *Developmental Psychology*, 12, 6-15.

Yarber, W. L. (1985). *STD: A Guide for Today's Young Adult*. Reston, VA: AAHPERD.

Yarber, W. L. (1987). *AIDS: What Young Adults Should Know*. Indianapolis, IN: Indiana State Board of Health.

Yarber, W. L. (1987). *AIDS Education: Curriculum and Health Policy*. Bloomington, IN: Phi Delta Kappa.

Yawkey, T. D. (ed.) (1980). *The Self Concept of the Young Child*. Salt Lake City, UT: Brigham Young Press.

—Z—

Zaichkowsky, L. B. et al. (1975). "Self-Concept and Attitudinal Differences in Elementary Age Children After Participating in a Physical Activity Program." *Movement*, 243-245. October.

Zaichkowsky, L. D. et al. (1980). *Growth and Development: The Child and Physical Activity*. St. Louis, MO: C. V. Mosby.

Zelazo, P. (1976). "From Reflexive to Instrumental Behavior." In Lipsitt, L. P. (ed.). *Developmental Psychobiology: Significance of Infancy*. Hillsdale, NJ: Lawrence Erlbaum.

Zelazo, P. et al. (1972). "Walking in the Newborn." *Science*, 176, 314-315.

Zubek, J. P. and Solberg, P. (1954). *Human Development*. New York: McGraw-Hill.

Appendix A

Equivalent Measures

English-Metric

1 inch = 2.54 centimeter
1 foot = 0.3048 meter
1 yard = 0.9144 meter
1 mile = 1.6093 kilometers

1 ounce = 28.349 grams
1 pound = 0.53 kilograms
1 short ton = 0.907 metric ton

1 fluid ounce = 29.573 millileters
1 pint = 0.473 liter
1 quart = 0.946 liter
1 gallon = 3.785 liters

Metric-English

1 centimeter = 0.3937 inch
1 meter = 3.281 feet
1 meter = 1.0936 yards
1 kilometer = 0.6214 mile

1 gram = 0.35 ounce
1 kilogram = 2.2046 pounds
1 metric ton = 1.1 short ton

1 milliliter = .06 cubic inch
1 liter = 61.02 cubic inch
1 liter = 0.908 dry quart
1 liter = 1.057 liquid quart

Appendix B

Inches-Centimeters: Conversion Table

IN	CM	IN	CM	IN	CM
1/32	.08	24	61.0	52	132.1
1/16	.16	25	63.5	53	134.6
1.8	.32	26	66.0	54	137.2
1/4	.64	27	68.6	55	139.7
1/2	1.27	28	71.1	56	142.2
1	2.5	29	73.7	57	144.8
2	5.1	30	76.2	58	147.3
3	7.6	31	78.7	59	149.9
4	10.2	32	81.3	60	152.4
5	12.7	33	83.8	61	154.9
6	15.2	34	86.4	62	157.5
7	17.8	35	88.9	63	160.0
8	20.3	36	91.4	64	162.6
9	22.9	37	93.8	65	165.1
10	25.4	38	96.5	66	167.6
11	28.0	39	99.1	67	170.2
12	30.5	40	101.6	68	172.7
13	33.0	41	104.1	69	175.3
14	25.5	42	106.7	70	177.8
15	38.1	43	109.2	71	180.3
16	40.6	44	111.8	72	182.9
17	43.2	45	114.3	73	185.4
18	45.1	46	116.8	74	188.0
19	48.2	47	119.4	75	190.5
20	50.8	48	121.9		
21	53.3	49	124.5		
22	55.9	50	127.0		
23	58.4	51	129.5		

Appendix C

Pounds-Kilograms: Conversion Table

LB	Kg	LB	Kg	LB	Kg	LB	Kg
1	0.54	26	11.77	51	23.10	80	36.24
2	0.90	27	12.23	52	23.55	81	36.69
3	1.35	28	12.68	53	24.00	82	37.14
4	1.81	29	13.13	54	24.46	83	37.59
5	2.26	30	13.59	55	24.91	84	38.05
6	2.71	31	14.04	56	25.36	85	38.50
7	3.17	32	14.49	57	25.82	86	38.95
8	3.62	33	14.94	58	26.27	87	39.41
9	4.07	34	15.40	59	26.72	88	39.86
10	4.50	35	15.85	60	27.18	89	40.31
11	4.98	36	16.30	61	27.63	90	40.77
12	5.43	37	16.76	62	28.08	91	41.22
13	5.88	38	17.21	63	28.53	92	41.67
14	6.34	39	17.66	64	28.99	93	42.12
15	6.79	40	18.12	65	29.44	94	42.58
16	7.24	41	18.57	66	29.89	95	43.03
17	7.70	42	19.02	67	30.35	96	43.48
18	8.15	43	19.47	68	30.80	97	43.94
19	8.60	44	19.93	69	31.25	98	44.39
20	9.06	45	20.38	70	31.71	99	44.84
21	9.51	46	20.83	71	32.16	100	45.30
22	9.96	47	21.29	72	32.61		
23	10.41	48	21.74	73	33.06		
24	10.87	49	22.19	74	33.52		
25	11.32	50	22.65	75	33.97		

Index

Hemispherical dominance approach to developmental theory, 30
Hemoglobin electrophoresis, 111
Hereditary factors, 107-112
Hereditary filter, 56-57
High-risk pregnancy, 98
Home day care, 486
Honadotropic hormones, 388
Horizontal jumping, 236-240
Hormonal imbalances, 115
Human Development, theoretical models, 26-28
Hydrostatic weighing, 299, 429-430
Hypertrophy, 218
Hyponatremia, 180
Hypothalamus, 388

Illness, effects on growth and development, 220
Imprinting, 70-72
Inches-Centimeters Conversion Table, 556
Indoor play spaces, 471-473
Inductive method of theory formulation, 45-46
Infant aquatic programs, 179-180
Infant growth, 135-141
Infant perception, methods of study, 184-186
Infant stimulation program, 178-179
Infants, programs for, 177-188
Information decoding, 144
Information encoding, 144
Injuries, growth palate, 219
Insulin, 102-103
Integration as biological factor, 66-67
Internally paced sport skills, 409
Interrater reliability, 11, 418
Intraskill sequences, 227
Inverted supports, 275
Isokinetic strength, 296
Isometric strength, 295, 426-427
Isotonic strength, 295-296, 423-424

James, William, 350-351
Joint flexibility, 298, 428
Jumping, for distance, 434-435; from a height, 242; horizontal, 236-240; vertical, 240-242

Kicking, 260-261
Kindergarten, 486-488
Koop, Dr. C. Everett, 58, 178

Labyrinthine righting reflex, 47, 154
Later childhood, development, 211-216; growth, 210-211
Law of acceleration, 90
Law of action and reaction, 90-91
Law of inertia, 90
Lifestyle filter, 57-58
Line of gravity, 88
Locomotion, 16, 172-175, 234-235, 494
Locomotor movement, 45-46, 234-249
Longitudinal study, 8-9
Lungs, 382-385

Male genitalia, 391
Manipulation, 16, 175-177, 249, 494-496
Manipulative movement, 45-46, 249-264

March of Dimes Birth Defects Foundation, 107
Maternal, drugs, 101-103; emotional stress, 117; infections, 114-115; nutrition, 98-100; separation, long-term effects, 71; syphilis, 114
Maturation, 15
Maturational theory of growth and development, 26
Maturity assessment, 392-394
Maximal oxygen consumption, 291-293
Medford Boys Growth Study, 8
Medical problems, 113-118
Menarche, 385-386
Mesomorphic physique, 218
Metatarsus varus, 109-110
Mixed-longitudinal method of study, 9-10
Monocular depth cues, 327-328
Moral development, 450-452
Moro primitive reflex, 149
Morphological age, 12
Motor behavior, 4, 18; product-oriented assessment instruments, 514-524
Motor control, 4, 18
Motor development, 6, 16; dilemma, 480-481; programs for young children, 481-488; study, terminology, 14-21; as specialized, 4; defined, 17-18; history of study, 7-8; infant studies, 167-168; life span process, 53-58; methods of study, 8-11; neuromaturational theory, 146; phases of, 45-53

Motor fitness, 310-320; as physical factor, 86-88
Motor interpretation, 332
Movement abilities, 16; health-related, 310
Movement activation, 332
Movement competence, 354
Movement conditions, 231-233
Movement control factors, 312
Movement education, concepts, 497-499
Movement hypothesis, 324-325
Movement skill learning, 499-506
Movement skill themes, 493-496
Movement techniques for enhancing self-esteem, 361-368
Movement, axial, 45-46, 271-285; categories of, 16, 493-496; defined, 18-19; developmental differences, 233-234; fundamental, 49-53, 226; learning, 488-489; locomotor, 45-46, 234-239; manipulative, 45-46, 249-264; nonlocomotor, 45; observable, 45; precontrol stage, 49; reflex inhibition stage, 48-49; reflexive, 46-47; rhythmic, 335; rudimentary, 48; specialized, developmental sequence, 398-400; sport related, 51; stability, 45-46, 264-271; studies of, 227-231
Muscular efficiency testing, 290
Muscular endurance, 296-297
Muscular strength, 294-296
Myelination, 202-204
Myelinization, 166

National Center for Health Statistics (NCHS), 302, 430-432
National Children and Youth Fitness Study, 290, 417-440